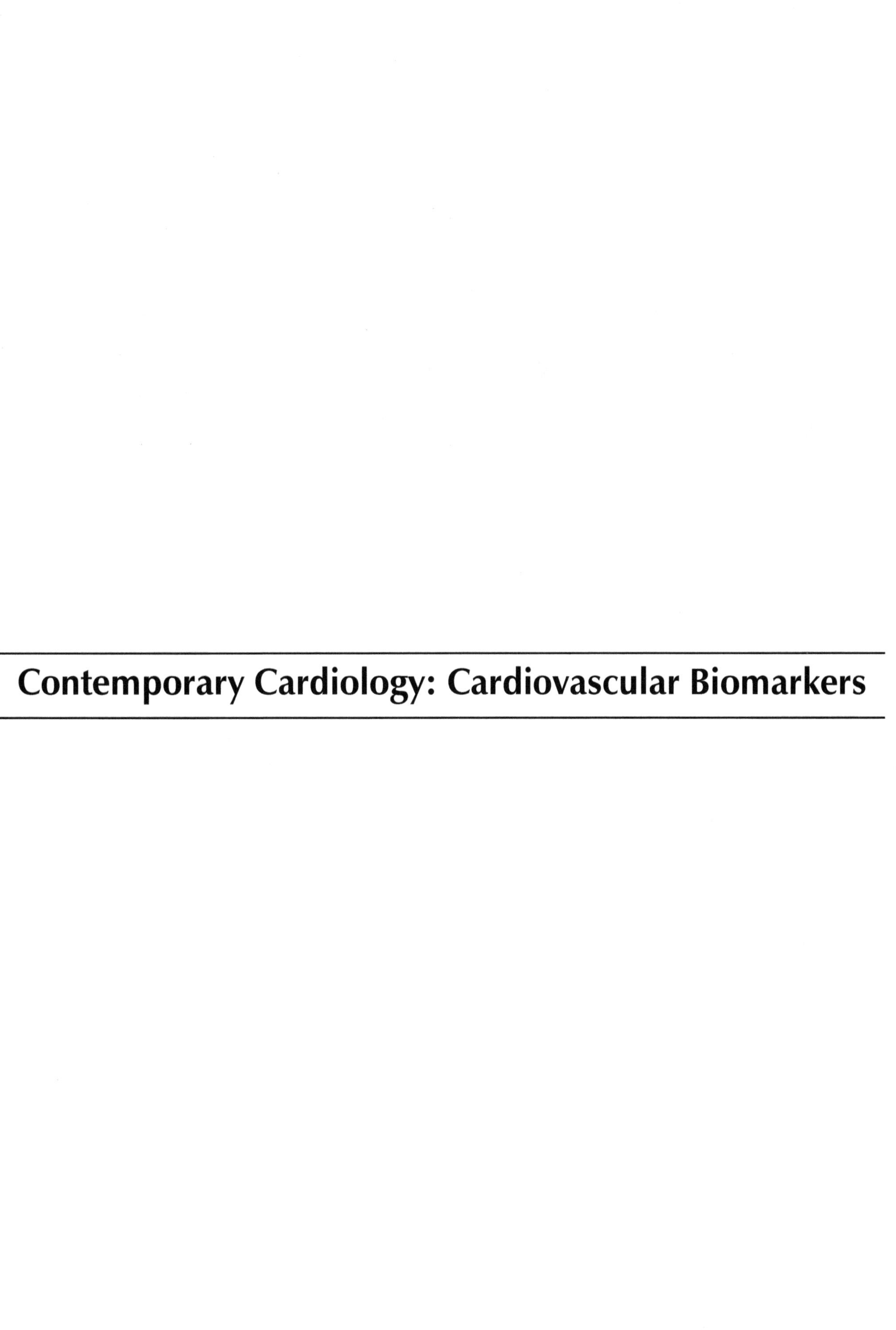

Contemporary Cardiology: Cardiovascular Biomarkers

Contemporary Cardiology: Cardiovascular Biomarkers

Editor: Emily Woods

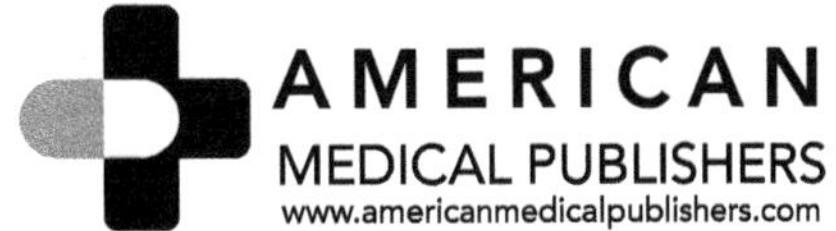

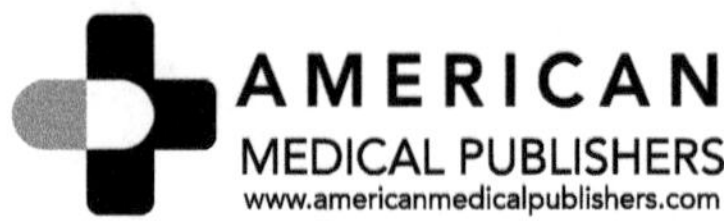

Cataloging-in-Publication Data

Contemporary cardiology : cardiovascular biomarkers / edited by Emily Woods.
p. cm.
Includes bibliographical references and index.
ISBN 978-1-63927-640-0
1. Cardiovascular system--Diseases. 2. Biochemical markers. 3. Cardiology. I. Woods, Emily.
RC669 .C66 2023
616.1--dc23

American Medical Publishers,
41 Flatbush Avenue,
1st Floor, New York,
NY 11217, USA

ISBN 978-1-63927-640-0 (Hardback)

Contents

Preface

Cardiovascular biomarkers are necessary diagnostic tools used in the clinical practices of cardiology. They are useful for the purpose of diagnosis, prognosis, and guiding the course of therapy and medication. Various biomarkers are linked to different cardiovascular conditions. Biomarkers such as natriuretic peptides and troponins are associated with heart failure and acute coronary syndrome respectively. Furthermore, galectin 3 and soluble suppression of tumorigenesis-2 are new biomarkers of cardiovascular diseases. These two biomarkers are also associated with the biomarkers of inflammation, metabolism, and fibrosis. One of the major roles of biomarkers is to identify patients who are at a high risk of developing cardiovascular diseases. They help in the identification of patients who can receive disease-modifying therapies including aggressive blood pressure control, lipid-lowering therapy, and novel agents like sodium-glucose co-transport 2 inhibitors for decreasing the risk of cardiovascular diseases. This book aims to understand the clinical significance of biomarkers in cardiovascular diseases. It is a valuable compilation of topics, ranging from the basic to the most complex advancements in this area of study. This book is appropriate for students seeking detailed information in this area as well as for experts.

The information contained in this book is the result of intensive hard work done by researchers in this field. All due efforts have been made to make this book serve as a complete guiding source for students and researchers. The topics in this book have been comprehensively explained to help readers understand the growing trends in the field.

I would like to thank the entire group of writers who made sincere efforts in this book and my family who supported me in my efforts of working on this book. I take this opportunity to thank all those who have been a guiding force throughout my life.

Editor

1

Possible Use of Blood Tryptophan Metabolites as Biomarkers for Coronary Heart Disease in Sudden Unexpected Death

Kobchai Santisukwongchote [1], Yutti Amornlertwatana [1,*], Thanapat Sastraruji [2] and Churdsak Jaikang [1,*]

1 Department of Forensic Medicine, Faculty of Medicine, Chiang Mai University, Chiang Mai 50200, Thailand; kobchai.san@gmail.com

2 Center of Excellence in Oral and Maxillofacial Biology, Faculty of Dentistry, Chiang Mai University, Chiang Mai 50200, Thailand; s_thanapat@hotmail.com

* Correspondence: yutti.amornlert@cmu.ac.th (Y.A.); Churdsak.j@cmu.ac.th (C.J.)

Abstract: Coronary heart disease (CHD) is the major cause of death in sudden unexpected death (SUD) cases. Tryptophan (TRP) and its metabolites are correlated with the CHD patient but less studies in the SUD. The aim of this study was to evaluate the relationship of TRP and its metabolites with the CHD in the SUD cases. Blood samples and heart tissues were collected from CHD subjects ($n = 31$) and the control group ($n = 72$). Levels of kynurenine (KYN), kynurenic acid (KYA), xanthurenic acid (XAN), 3-hydroxyanthranillic acid (HAA), quinolinic acid (QA), picolinic acid (PA) and 5-hydroxyindoleacetic acid (HIAA) were determined by HPLC-DAD. A severity of heart occlusion was categorized into four groups, and the relationship was measured with the TRP metabolites. The HIAA and The KYN levels significantly differed ($p < 0.01$) between the CHD group and the control group. Lower levels of QA/XAN, PA/KA, HAA/XAN, KYN/XAN and KYN/TRP were found in the CHD group. However, PA/HAA, PA/HIAA, PA/KYN and XAN/KA values in the CHD group were higher than the control group ($p < 0.05$). This study revealed that the values of PA/KA and PA/HAA provided better choices for a CHD biomarker in postmortem bodies.

Keywords: picolinic acid; tryptophan; tryptophan metabolites; coronary heart disease; sudden unexpected death

---

1. Introduction

Sudden unexpected death (SUD) is defined as a natural, nonviolent, unexpected death occurring within twenty-four hours of the onset of symptoms [1]. A SUD is found in about 56% of medicolegal cases in Thailand [2]. Cardiovascular disease (CVD), including heart and blood vessel disorders, hypertension, coronary heart disease (CHD), cerebrovascular disease, peripheral vascular disease, heart failure, rheumatic heart disease, congenital heart disease and cardiomyopathies, is the major cause of morbidity and mortality worldwide [3]. CHD is the most common cause of SUD [4].

Under the Thai criminal justice system, causes of death in SUD cases are necessary to be identified. Many cases lacked reliable medical documents regarding underlying diseases that could help to explain the causes of death. Both external examination of the heart gross morphology and microscopic findings were appropriate methods for SUD diagnosis.

Cutting the surface of the coronary artery, a type of heart gross morphology examination, is an important procedure for CHD diagnosis [5]. Sometimes, the CHD diagnosis by using this process was not an accurate method and depended on randomized cutting at lesion area. Therefore, the microscopic method helps to confirm the existing CHD. However, in some cases, an autopsy cannot be performed due to different cultural and spiritual believes. In this situation, a cardiac biomarker is an alternative solution for a CHD diagnosis.

Cardiac troponin level in serum has become an increasingly important biomarker for myocardial injury in many cardiovascular diseases, especially in patients with CHD [6,7], and in cardiovascular cases in the forensic field. However, the cardiac troponin might not be specific or suitable enough as a cardiac biomarker in postmortem samples [8].

The kynurenine (KYN) pathway plays an important role in cardio pathophysiology and catabolism pathway is shown in Figure 1. Many studies have indicated changes of KYN and tryptophan (TRP) were found in CHD patients [9–11]. There is an increase of inflammatory cytokines when atherosclerosis occurs, which can induce indoleamine 2,3-dioxygenase (IDO) enzyme, a rate-limiting enzyme in TRP catabolism [12]. The IDO is highly up-regulated by immune activation and inflammation and appears to be important in the pathogenesis of CHD [13]. KYN/TRP value reflects the IDO activity found in CHD patients [14] but in SUD has been less studied.

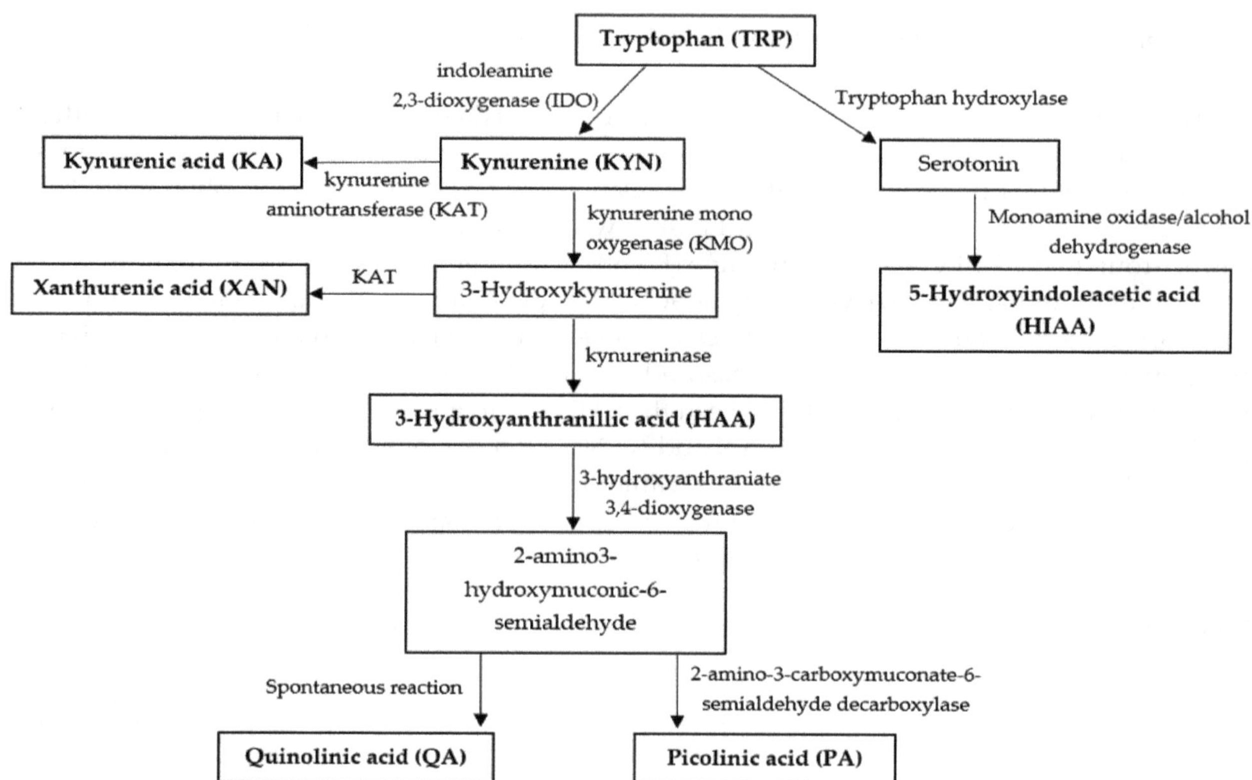

Figure 1. Schematic illustration of tryptophan (TRP) catabolism along with the kynurenine (KYN) and serotonin pathway.

The aim of this study was to determine the downstream of TRP metabolites, both the KYN and serotonin pathways, in order to find out a relation with coronary artery disease in SUDs. The blood concentration levels of TRP and its metabolites including KYN, kynurenic acid (KA), 3-hydroxyanthranillic acid (HAA), xanthurenic acid (XAN), quinolinic acid (QA), picolinic acid (PA) and 5-hydroxyindoleacetic acid (HIAA) in SUDs diagnosed as CHD were compared with those of deaths from noncoronary artery diseases. Furthermore, we compared levels of the metabolites with degree of coronary occlusion.

2. Results

Levels of TRP and its metabolites were found in all subjects, and mean values are shown in Table 1. Mean levels of HIAA and KYN differed between the CHD and the control group. A high level of HIAA was found in the CHD group ($p = 0.018$) but the KYN level was higher than the control group

($p < 0.001$). Mean ratios of PA/HAA, PA/HIAA, PA/KYN and XAN/KA were significantly increased in the CHD group (p-values of 0.043, 0.028, 0.001 and 0.015, respectively). Meanwhile, the QA/XAN, PA/KA, HAA/XAN, KYN/XAN and KYN/TRP levels were significantly higher than those of the control group (p-values of 0.018, 0.044, 0.029, 0.001 and 0.002, respectively). The ratio of TRP and its metabolites reflected the enzyme activities in the TRP catabolism pathway; remarkably, KYN/TRP acting as IDO activity. There were no significant differences in mean levels of QA, PA, HAA, XAN, TRP, KA and other ratios between groups. In this study, the age of the subjects ranged 21–86 years. Mean age in the CHD group (58.16 ± 13.34 years) was similar to the control group (52.89 ± 13.90 years).

Table 1. Blood concentration level of TRP and its metabolites, alongside some significant ratios, compared with the coronary heart disease (CHD) and the control groups.

Metabolites	Range	Total (n = 103)	CHD Group (n = 31)	Control Group (n = 72)	p-Value
TRP (mM)	0.04–0.17	0.06 ± 0.03	0.06 ± 0.02	0.07 ± 0.03	0.076
KYN (mM)	0.70–306.87	71.68 ± 60.88	41.98 ± 47.68	84.47 ± 61.74	<0.001
KA (mM)	0–0.07	0.005 ± 0.01	0.003 ± 0.004	0.007 ± 0.01	0.078
XAN (mM)	0–0.28	0.03 ± 0.04	0.03 ± 0.04	0.02 ± 0.04	0.131
HAA (mM)	0–0.88	0.02 ± 0.09	0.01 ± 0.03	0.02 ± 0.10	0.062
QA (mM)	0.04–4.07	0.61 ± 0.85	0.30 ± 0.23	0.74 ± 0.98	0.124
PA (mM)	0–7.81	0.74 ± 1.11	0.83 ± 1.04	0.70 ± 1.15	0.165
HIAA (mM)	0–364.59	22.75 ± 44.12	27.45 ± 70.41	20.73 ± 26.22	0.018
KYN/XAN ($\times 10^4$)	0–17.83	1.48 ± 2.66	0.73 ± 1.51	1.78 ± 2.97	0.001
KYN/TRP ($\times 10^3$)	0–7.00	1.15 ± 1.08	0.72 ± 0.70	1.34 ± 1.16	0.002
XAN/KA	0–229.84	18.83 ± 36.76	32.22 ± 53.56	13.06 ± 24.85	0.015
HAA/XAN	0–32.33	1.94 ± 3.94	1.17 ± 1.92	2.27 ± 4.52	0.029
QA/XAN ($\times 10^3$)	0–1.30	0.11 ± 0.23	0.05 ± 0.07	0.14 ± 0.26	0.018
PA/HAA ($\times 10^3$)	0–3.33	0.25 ± 0.52	0.33 ± 0.68	0.22 ± 0.44	0.043
PA/HIAA	0–4.37	0.13 ± 0.46	0.29 ± 0.81	0.06 ± 0.14	0.028
PA/KYN	0–0.45	0.03 ± 0.06	0.05 ± 0.09	0.02 ± 0.04	0.001
PA/KA ($\times 10^4$)	0–1.11	0.07 ± 0.13	0.06 ± 0.07	0.07 ± 0.15	0.044
Age (years)	21–86	54.48 ± 13.88	58.16 ± 13.34	52.89 ± 13.90	0.056

The values are presented as means ± SD. A nonparametric Mann–Whitney U-test used for comparing between groups at $p < 0.05$. Abbreviations: QA = quinolinic acid; PA = picolinic acid; HAA = 3-hydroxyanthranillic acid; HIAA = 5-hydroxyindoleacetic acid; KYN = kynurenine; XAN = xanthurenic acid; TRP = tryptophan; KA = kynurenic acid.

Pearson's correlation was used for evaluating a relationship between the TRP metabolite levels and the grade of coronary occlusion. The QA, PA, HAA, KYN, TRP and KA levels and ratio values of the metabolites were significantly correlated with the degree of coronary occlusion; the results are shown in Table 2. The QA, HAA, KYN, TRP and KA levels showed negative correlations ($p = 0.003$, $p = 0.001$, $p < 0.001$, $p < 0.001$, $p = 0.001$, respectively). Only the PA level showed a positive correlation ($p < 0.001$). The ratios of PA/KYN, PA/KA and PA/HAA were more positively correlated than the other ratios, while the ratios of QA/PA and KYN were negatively correlated.

Table 2. Pearson's correlation of TRP and TRP metabolite levels with degree of coronary occlusion.

Metabolites	Correlation Coefficient (r)	p-Value
TRP	−0.356	<0.001
KYN	−0.358	<0.001
KA	−0.322	0.001
HAA	−0.309	0.001
QA	−0.293	0.003
PA	0.361	<0.001
TRP/KA	0.215	0.029
KYN/XAN	−0.275	0.005
KYN/TRP	−0.253	0.01
XAN/KA	0.251	0.01

Table 2. *Cont.*

Metabolites	Correlation Coefficient (*r*)	*p*-Value
HAA/TRP	−0.228	0.02
HAA/XAN	−0.207	0.036
QA/PA	−0.425	<0.001
QA/XAN	−0.202	0.04
QA/TRP	−0.20	0.043
PA/HAA	0.437	<0.001
PA/HIAA	0.383	<0.001
PA/KYN	0.533	<0.001
PA/XAN	0.247	0.012
PA/TRP	0.403	<0.001
PA/KA	0.45	<0.001
HIAA/KYN	0.278	0.004

Statistical significance was determined using a nonparametric Mann-Whitney test at $p < 0.05$.

Box plots revealed the relationship between the grading of occlusion and statistically correlated metabolites (Figure 2). The values of the KYN and KYN/TRP were significantly decreased depending on the degree of coronary artery narrowing. Interestingly, the PA/HAA and PA/KA levels in grades 2, 3 and 4 of occlusion were significantly higher than those in grade 1.

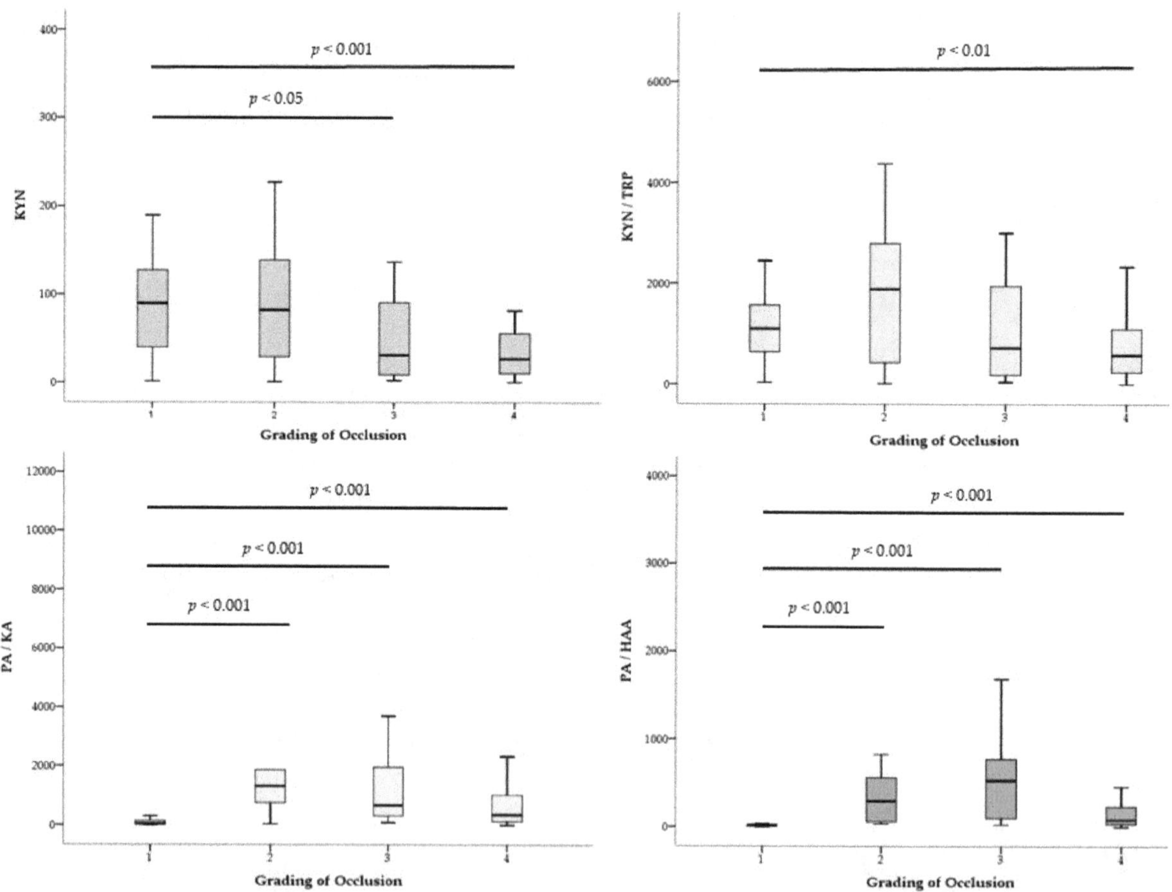

Figure 2. Comparison between blood concentration levels of KYN, KYN/TRP, PA/KA and PA/HAA ratios in each coronary occlusion graded by Mann–Whitney U-test. Statistical differences between the grades are indicated by *p*-value less than 0.05.

Trends of the levels of TRP and its metabolites in terms of degree of coronary artery severity are summarized and shown in Table 3. The levels of XAN, PA and HIAA increased according to degree of coronary artery occlusion; also, the PA level was suitable for indicating occluded coronary artery. While the levels of TRP, KYN, KA, HAA and QA decreased, the TRP and HAA levels were less affected in the CHD group.

Table 3. The trend summary report of TRP, TRP metabolites and significant ratios in the correlation with degree of coronary artery occlusion.

Metabolites	Trend Correlation with Coronary Occlusion Degree
TRP	−
KYN	−
KA	−
XAN	+
HAA	−
QA	−
PA	+
HIAA	+
KYN/TRP	−
PA/KA	+
PA/HAA	+

Results are presented as: (+), indicates the increasing of the metabolite level in the degree of coronary artery occlusion; (−), indicates the decreasing of the metabolite level in the degree of coronary artery occlusion.

3. Discussion

In this work, TRP and its metabolites in blood samples of the 103 males who died from sudden death were investigated. There were different levels of serum TRP and KYN among males and females [14]. We selected only male subjects who had a postmortem interval of within 24 h. To decrease factors affecting TRP metabolism, the subjects who exhibited decomposition, did not have an accurate determination of the time of death or suffered from malignant disease, stroke and tuberculosis were excluded [15,16].

The quantified levels of KA, TRP, and HAA in the SUD sample showed similar ranges compared with normal human serum [17]. The levels of XAN, KYN, HIAA, PA and QA were higher than normal levels in human subjects [18–20]. Levels of TRP metabolites in normal human plasma significantly differed between ethnicities [17]. There have been a few studies about the TRP pathway in Asian ethnicities. Difference in dietary culture [21] and high-TRP diets can influence TRP metabolite levels. At the present, there are still limited data about postmortem blood levels of TRP and its metabolites in all the TRP pathways.

CHD induces oxidative stress in the human body, but physiological defense mechanisms boost antioxidant systems to limit oxidative stress. 2-amino−3-hydroxymuconic-6-semialdehyde is a substrate of both PA and QA [22]. Synthesis of PA, an antioxidant molecule, might affect QA synthesis by competing against the substrate.

Although the PA level was not significantly increased in the CHD group, it had a positive correlation with the occlusion grading. Accumulation of PA coexisted with the reduction of QA downstream catabolism in the severe CHD cases. In Figure 2, the values of PA/HAA and PA/KA in non-occluding coronary artery (grade 1) had the lowest level and significantly differed from the other grades. These ratios could segregate grade 1 from the other grades in the CHD.

Some observed values of 52 ratios reflected enzyme activities in the TRP catabolic pathway for example, KYN/TRP presented as IDO activity and KYN/KA acted as kynurenine amino transferase activity. Not only were the PA/HAA, PA/HIAA, PA/KYN increased in the CHD group but also the PA/HAA, PA/HIAA, PA/KYN, PA/XAN, PA/TRP and PA/KA had positive correlation with the degree of coronary artery occlusion. These findings suggested that PA production might be increased instead of QA production in CHD, leading to the QA/PA having negative correlation. Products ratios in KYN pathway and serotonin pathway were demonstrated in the PA/HIAA value. The positive correlation reflected higher coronary occlusion and might be shifted through the KYN pathway.

In Table 1, no evidence indicates that the QA level was significant among groups, but we found that the QA level correlated with the degree of coronary artery narrowing (Table 2). The decrease of the QA level reflected the severity of coronary occlusion resulting from the negative correlation of the QA/PA. The 2-amino-3-hydroxymuconic-6-semialdehyde might be shifted into the PA pathway in the CHD group. This process was an oxidative stress defense mechanism which decreased pro-oxidant QA level and increased antioxidant PA molecules [23,24]. Normally, the levels of QA and PA are equal [24]. QA plays a main role in neurological disorder, as it is a neuroactive metabolite of HAA and acts as an excitotoxin that is a high-potency agonist of N-methyl-D-aspartate receptors associated with hypertension, myocardial infarction and unstable atherosclerotic plaque [25]. Energetic deficits, behavioral alterations and other neurological diseases are toxic effects of the QA molecule [26].

HAA acts as an antioxidant and anti-inflammatory substance in the oxidative stress process [27]. HAA inhibits atherosclerosis by regulating lipid metabolism [28] and has a significant function in antioxidant systems and the anti-inflammatory process [27]. The decrease of the HAA level in the CHD group was similar to that in the control group, but in the CHD group had a negative correlation with the degree of coronary artery occlusion ($p = 0.001$). Another study showed that the HAA acted as an pro-oxidant since it was catabolized into QA [29]. We found that a decrease of the HAA level in severely occluded coronary artery state occurred to limit the cellular damage response from QA [30]. A protective mechanism might occur via PA synthesis or 2-amino-3-hydroxymuconic-6-semialdehyde production. These phenomena had positive correlations with PA/HAA value.

HIAA is a final product of serotonin pathway. The HIAA level was significantly higher in the CHD group than in the control group. There was no statistically significant correlation between the HIAA level and grading of coronary artery occlusion. The HIAA/KYN value had a positive correlation, which indicated no fluxing through serotonin pathway for the CHD group. The KYN might be catabolized due to the HIAA level not showing statistically significant correlation with the degree of coronary occlusion, and the KYN level was lower than its metabolites level in the CHD group. The HIAA did not correlate with coronary occlusion but it had a significant difference with the CHD group, because pneumonia and sepsis were suggested as causes of death in the control group. Infection state might decrease plasma serotonin, the substrate of HIAA, by inhibiting serotonin transporter in platelets [31].

The XAN level was similar among groups, and no correlation was found with degree of vessel occlusion. Both negative correlation of the QA/XAN and KYN/XAN and positive correlation of the XAN/KA indicated the increase in the XA pathway within the CHD group. The PA/XAN value had a positive correlation, indicating that enzyme activity in XA pathway might be less than in the PA pathway. Under inflammatory condition, kynureninase enzyme was more dominant than KAT enzyme in CHD [32]. However, the XA has remained an obscure pathway in biological systems [33]. A synthesis of XAN is an important process to prevent 3-hydroxykynurenine accumulation, as this is probably a toxic substance [34]. The XAN acted as a potential antioxidant and had an iron-chelating property [35]. However, a study found that the XAN was pro-oxidant and might induce cytotoxicity [36].

KA is a neuroprotective substance and acts as an antagonist to the NMDA receptor [27]. Dysregulation of endogenous KA might cause of hypertension, myocardial infarction and maternal hypertension [37,38]. The KA also acted as a reducing agent and scavenged hydroxyl radicals [39]. The KA levels were not difference between groups, similar to the results of Zuo et al. [33]. The KA level correlated with the degree of coronary occlusion and the ratios of PA/KA, XAN/KA and TRP/KA had a positive correlation. These results suggested that the KA pathway was decreased in severity of vessel narrowing.

The TRP level negatively correlated with the state of occlusion. The TRP level in the CHD group was decreased [26,33,40]. The ratios of QA/TRP and HAA/TRP showed a negative correlation but the TRP/KA was positively correlated. These findings indicated that production rate of the QA, HAA and KA were less than the TRP catabolism rate in the CHD group. The PA/TRP had a positive correlation from increasing flux through PA pathway.

The values of KYN and KYN/TRP in the CHD group were lower than in the control group. The KYN value in the grade 1 occlusion was significantly different with the values in grades 3 and 4. The KYN/TRP significantly differed between grades 1 and 4. The KYN and the KYN/XAN ratio had a negative correlation, while the PA/KYN had a positive correlation. These results demonstrated that decrease of the KYN level depended on the severity of coronary narrowing. Enzymes in the KYN pathway might have lower activity than those in the PA and XAN pathways. Our results revealed that the TRP metabolites in postmortem differed from the CHD patients. The IDO activity is a key enzyme in the TRP metabolism which could be reduced in hypoxia condition and declined in KYN production [41]. Postmortem changes might affect TRP and its metabolites, however this needs to be studied further.

The control group in Table 1 was composed of the occlusion in grades 1 to 3, and grade 4 was only for the CHD group. Thus, mean levels of QA, PA, HAA, TRP and KA in the grades 1 to 3 showed no significant differences compared with the grade 4, but the metabolites still had a correlation with the degree of occlusion.

Many noncommunicable diseases, including type 2 diabetes, nonalcoholic fatty liver disease and obesity, affect the IDO activity in TRP metabolic pathway [10]. Patients with higher TRP level tended to present higher levels of insulin resistance, triglycerides and blood pressure [42]. IDO was up-regulated in older patients and related to increased susceptibility of aged liver to nonalcoholic fatty liver disease development [43]. Therefore, the autopsy cases with diabetes, hypertension and hyperlipidemia should be interpreted as CHD with TRP and its metabolites carefully.

In conclusion, the PA/KA and the PA/HAA were the most suitable for classifying non-CHD out of the CHD in SUDs. The decrease of the QA, HAA, KA, KYN, TRP levels and increase of the PA and XAN levels reflected the degree of occlusion. This is the first study about a prospectively evaluated coronary artery occlusion using the TRP metabolic pathways in postmortem and confirmed by coronary occlusion pathology. The PA/KA and PA/HAA could be used for excluding non-CHD from CHD in SUDs under more than 75% occlusion, graded as level 4 condition. However, our study had several limitations. Firstly, small sample size might cause data misinterpretation. Secondly, the study group was limited to specific geographic area which might not reflect a generalized area. Finally, postmortem changes and other factors might affect TRP and its metabolites.

4. Materials and Methods

4.1. Subjects and Study Design

One hundred three males who died from sudden death and underwent autopsy at Maharaj Nakorn Chiang Mai Hospital, Department of Forensic Medicine, Faculty of Medicine, Chiang Mai University were selected in this study. The subjects who had malignant disease, stroke, tuberculosis disease, age under 15 years and decomposition were excluded. We also excluded subjects who had any evidence of underlying disease such as diabetes, hypertension and hyperlipidemia. Postmortem interval range was specified to be less than 24 h. Thirty-one subjects who were diagnosed with severe occluded coronary artery (occlusion more than 75% of the cut surface, or the cause of death being the CHD group) were included in the study group. The flowchart of the case selection is shown in Figure 3. Written informed consent was obtained from direct relatives. The study protocol was approved by the Research Ethics Committee Faculty of Medicine, Chiang Mai University (FOR-2561-05497).

4.2. Collection and Specimen Preparation

Femoral blood was collected (about 5 mL) in a sodium fluoride tube and stored at −20 °C before analysis. Three milliliters of the blood samples were mixed with acetonitrile (2 mL). The solution was shaken for 5 min and centrifuged at 5500 rpm for 5 min; then, the supernatant was collected. The residues were re-extracted with 2 mL acetonitrile two times. The supernatants were combined and evaporated under nitrogen gas. The residues were reconstituted with 20 mM sodium acetate buffer before analysis with HPLC-DAD.

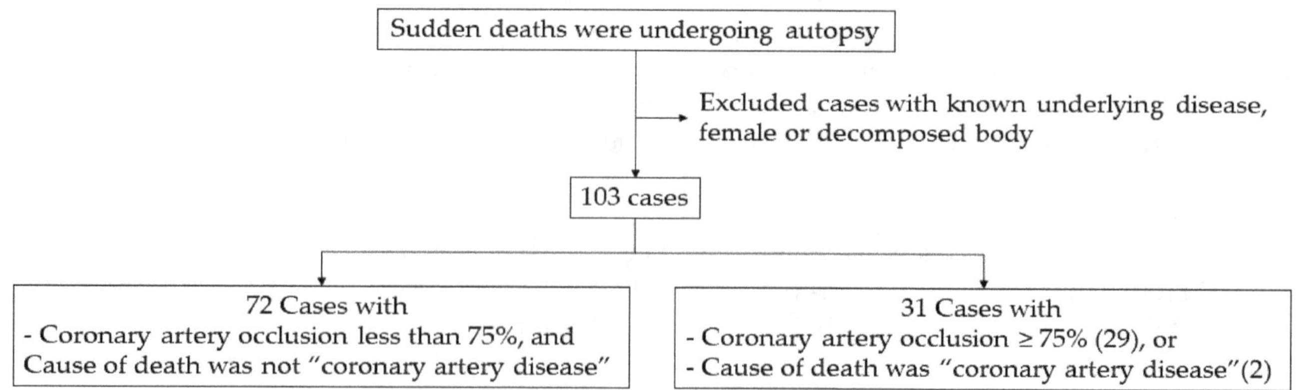

Figure 3. Flowchart of case selection in this study.

4.3. Measurement of Tryptophan and Its Metabolites

The levels of TRP, KYN, KA, XA, HAA, QA, PA and HIAA in plasma were measured by high-performance liquid chromatography with diode array detector (HPLC-DAD) by modified method of Cseh [44]. The sample analysis was performed using an Agilent LC 1260 infinity binary pump system. Gradient elution of two solvents composing a 20 mM sodium acetate buffer pH 6.4 adjusted with acetic acid (A) and acetonitrile (B) was used for detection. The total run time of the program was 16 min. Gradient elution program was begun with 100% of solvent A and was held at this concentration for 0–6 min. This was followed by 95% of solvent A for 6–7 min and then reduced to 80% of solvent A for the next 7–14 min and then increased to 100% of solvent A for the next 14–16 min with flow rate was 0.7 mL/min. An HPLC Chromolith® Performance RP-18e analytical column (100 × 4.6 mm) was used for stationary phase. The spectrums were determined by diode array at 220 to 400 nm for identification or TRP and its metabolites.

4.4. Pathology

Heart tissues were collected and prepared under routine processes of the Department of Pathology, Faculty of Medicine, Chiang Mai University. The heart samples were stained with hematoxylin and eosin (H&E). Percentage of occlusion in heart tissues was calculated by OLYMPUS Cell Sens Standard 2.2 program. Degree of coronary artery occlusion was separated into four grades following percent occlusion: grade 1, occluded less than 25%; grade 2, occluded 25–49%; grade 3, occluded 50–74%; and grade 4, greater than 75%. The grade 1, 2, 3 and 4 samples were from 51, 9, 14 and 29 subjects, respectively. The narrowing could be concentric or eccentric, according to Yang et al.'s method, which indicated that severe narrowing of coronary with less than 25% patency in an area could lead to SUD [13].

4.5. Statistical Analysis

Descriptive statistics were expressed as mean ± S.D. All continuous variables were checked for normal distribution using Shapiro–Wilk normality test. Differences in blood TRP and TRP metabolite levels between the control group and the CHD group were compared using the Mann–Whitney U-test. Correlations between the TRP metabolite levels and degree of coronary occlusion were calculated using Pearson's correlation coefficient. A p-value of less than 0.05 was considered significant.

Author Contributions: The main conceptualization and methodology of the work has been performed by Y.A. and C.J.; sample collection by K.S. and Y.A.; formal analysis and investigation by K.S., T.S., C.J.; data curation by K.S., T.S., C.J.; writing—original draft preparation by K.S.; writing—review and editing by Y.A., T.S. and C.J.;

visualization by K.S., T.S.; supervision by Y.A., C.J.; current project administration by C.J., K.S. All authors have read and agreed to the published version of the manuscript.

Abbreviations

CHD	Coronary heart disease
SUD	Sudden unexpected death
QA	Quinolinic acid
PA	Picolinic acid
HAA	3-Hydroxyanthranillic acid
HIAA	5-Hydroxyindoleacetic acid
KYN	Kynurenine
XAN	Xanthurenic acid
TRP	Tryptophan
KA	Kynurenic acid
IDO	Indoleamine 2, 3-dioxygenase

References

1. Kumar, V.; San, K.P.; Idwan, A.; Shah, N.; Hajar, S.; Norkahfi, M. A study of sudden natural deaths in medico legal autopsies in University Malaya Medical Centre (UMMC), Kuala Lumpur. *J. Forensic Leg. Med.* **2007**, *14*, 151–154. [CrossRef] [PubMed]
2. Udnoon, J.; Chirachariyavej, T.; Peonim, V. Sudden unexpected deaths in different age groups at Ramathibodi Hospital, Bangkok, Thailand: A retrospective autopsy study during 2003–2007. *Southeast Asian J. Trop. Med. Public Health* **2009**, *40*, 162. [PubMed]
3. World Health Organization Cardiovascular Diseases (cvds). Available online: https://www.who.int/en/news-room/fact-sheets/detail/cardiovascular-diseases-(cvds) (accessed on 17 May 2017).
4. Milroy, C.M. Coronary artery disease, sudden death and implications for forensic pathology practice. *Diagn. Histopathol.* **2017**, *23*, 479–485. [CrossRef]
5. Basso, C.; Aguilera, B.; Banner, J.; Cohle, S.; d'Amati, G.; de Gouveia, R.H.; di Gioia, C.; Fabre, A.; Gallagher, P.J.; Leone, O. Guidelines for autopsy investigation of sudden cardiac death: 2017 update from the Association for European Cardiovascular Pathology. *Virchows Arch.* **2017**, *471*, 691–705. [CrossRef]
6. Antman, E.; Bassand, J.-P.; Klein, W.; Ohman, M.; Sendon, J.L.L.; Rydén, L.; Simoons, M.; Tendera, M. Myocardial infarction redefined—A consensus document of the Joint European Society of Cardiology/American College of Cardiology committee for the redefinition of myocardial infarction: The Joint European Society of Cardiology/American College of Cardiology Committee. *J. Am. Coll. Cardiol.* **2000**, *36*, 959–969.
7. Jaffe, A.S.; Ravkilde, J.; Roberts, R.; Naslund, U.; Apple, F.S.; Galvani, M.; Katus, H. It's time for a change to a troponin standard. *Am. Heart Assoc* **2000**, *102*, 1216–1220. [CrossRef]
8. Rahimi, R.; Dahili, N.D.; Zainun, K.A.; Kasim, N.A.M.; Noor, S.M. Post mortem troponin T analysis in sudden death: Is it useful? *Malays. J. Pathol.* **2018**, *40*, 143–148.
9. Wirleitner, B.; Rudzite, V.; Neurauter, G.; Murr, C.; Kalnins, U.; Erglis, A.; Trusinskis, K.; Fuchs, D. Immune activation and degradation of tryptophan in coronary heart disease. *Eur. J. Clin. Investig.* **2003**, *33*, 550–554. [CrossRef]
10. Song, P.; Ramprasath, T.; Wang, H.; Zou, M.-H. Abnormal kynurenine pathway of tryptophan catabolism in cardiovascular diseases. *Cell. Mol. Life Sci.* **2017**, *74*, 2899–2916. [CrossRef]
11. Dehhaghi, M.; Kazemi Shariat Panahi, H.; Guillemin, G.J. Microorganisms, tryptophan metabolism, and kynurenine pathway: A complex interconnected loop influencing human health status. *Int. J. Tryptophan Res.* **2019**, *12*, 1178646919852996. [CrossRef]
12. Ketelhuth, D.F. The immunometabolic role of indoleamine 2, 3-dioxygenase in atherosclerotic cardiovascular disease: Immune homeostatic mechanisms in the artery wall. *Cardiovasc. Res.* **2019**, *115*, 1408–1415. [CrossRef] [PubMed]

13. Yang, K.M.; Lee, S.Y.; Kim, Y.S.; Seo, J.S.; Lee, Y.S.; Seo, J.W. Guidelines for forensic assessment of natural unexpected cardiovascular death. *Basic Appl. Pathol.* **2008**, *1*, 155–163. [CrossRef]
14. Ohashi, H.; Iizuka, H.; Yoshihara, S.; Otani, H.; Kume, M.; Sadamoto, K.; Ichiba, H.; Fukushima, T. Determination of l-tryptophan and l-kynurenine in human serum by using LC-MS after derivatization with (R)-DBD-PyNCS. *Int. J. Tryptophan Res.* **2013**, *6*, IJTR. S11459. [CrossRef]
15. Cheong, J.E.; Sun, L. Targeting the IDO1/TDO2–KYN–AhR pathway for cancer immunotherapy–challenges and opportunities. *Trends Pharmacol. Sci.* **2018**, *39*, 307–325. [CrossRef] [PubMed]
16. Polyzos, K.; Ketelhuth, D. The role of the kynurenine pathway of tryptophan metabolism in cardiovascular disease. *Hamostaseologie* **2015**, *35*, 128–136. [CrossRef] [PubMed]
17. Badawy, A.A.-B.; Dougherty, D.M. Assessment of the human kynurenine pathway: Comparisons and clinical implications of ethnic and gender differences in plasma tryptophan, kynurenine metabolites, and enzyme expressions at baseline and after acute tryptophan loading and depletion. *Int. J. Tryptophan Res.* **2016**, *9*, IJTR. S38189. [CrossRef]
18. Adaway, J.E.; Dobson, R.; Walsh, J.; Cuthbertson, D.J.; Monaghan, P.J.; Trainer, P.J.; Valle, J.W.; Keevil, B.G. Serum and plasma 5-hydroxyindoleacetic acid as an alternative to 24-h urine 5-hydroxyindoleacetic acid measurement. *Ann. Clin. Biochem.* **2016**, *53*, 554–560. [CrossRef]
19. Zuwała-Jagiello, J.; Pazgan-Simon, M.; Simon, K.; Warwas, M. Picolinic acid in patients with chronic hepatitis C infection: A preliminary report. *Mediat. Inflamm.* **2012**, *2012*, 762863. [CrossRef]
20. Basile, A.S.; Saito, K.; Al-Mardini, H.; Record, C.O.; Hughes, R.D.; Harrison, P.; Williams, R.; Li, Y.; Heyes, M.P. The relationship between plasma and brain quinolinic acid levels and the severity of hepatic encephalopathy. *Gastroenterology* **1995**, *108*, 818–823. [CrossRef]
21. Poesen, R.; Mutsaers, H.A.; Windey, K.; van den Broek, P.H.; Verweij, V.; Augustijns, P.; Kuypers, D.; Jansen, J.; Evenepoel, P.; Verbeke, K. The influence of dietary protein intake on mammalian tryptophan and phenolic metabolites. *PLoS ONE* **2015**, *10*, e0140820. [CrossRef]
22. Brundin, L.; Sellgren, C.; Lim, C.; Grit, J.; Pålsson, E.; Landen, M.; Samuelsson, M.; Lundgren, K.; Brundin, P.; Fuchs, D. An enzyme in the kynurenine pathway that governs vulnerability to suicidal behavior by regulating excitotoxicity and neuroinflammation. *Transl. Psychiatry* **2016**, *6*, e865. [CrossRef] [PubMed]
23. Lugo-Huitrón, R.; Ugalde Muñiz, P.; Pineda, B.; Pedraza-Chaverrí, J.; Ríos, C.; Pérez-De La Cruz, V. Quinolinic acid: An endogenous neurotoxin with multiple targets. *Oxidative Med. Cell. Longev.* **2013**, *2013*, 104024. [CrossRef] [PubMed]
24. Grant, R.; Coggan, S.; Smythe, G. The physiological action of picolinic acid in the human brain. *Int. J. Tryptophan Res.* **2009**, *2*, IJTR. S2469. [CrossRef]
25. Leipnitz, G.; Schumacher, C.; Scussiato, K.; Dalcin, K.B.; Wannmacher, C.M.; Wyse, A.T.; Dutra-Filho, C.S.; Wajner, M.; Latini, A. Quinolinic acid reduces the antioxidant defenses in cerebral cortex of young rats. *Int. J. Dev. Neurosci.* **2005**, *23*, 695–701. [CrossRef] [PubMed]
26. Wang, Q.; Liu, D.; Song, P.; Zou, M.-H. Deregulated tryptophan-kynurenine pathway is linked to inflammation, oxidative stress, and immune activation pathway in cardiovascular diseases. *Front. Biosci.* **2015**, *20*, 1116.
27. Liu, G.; Chen, S.; Zhong, J.; Teng, K.; Yin, Y. Crosstalk between tryptophan metabolism and cardiovascular disease, mechanisms, and therapeutic implications. *Oxidative Med. Cell. Longev.* **2017**, *2017*, 1602074. [CrossRef]
28. Zhang, L.; Ovchinnikova, O.; Jönsson, A.; Lundberg, A.M.; Berg, M.; Hansson, G.K.; Ketelhuth, D.F. The tryptophan metabolite 3-hydroxyanthranilic acid lowers plasma lipids and decreases atherosclerosis in hypercholesterolaemic mice. *Eur. Heart J.* **2012**, *33*, 2025–2034. [CrossRef]
29. Giles, G.I.; Collins, C.A.; Stone, T.W.; Jacob, C. Electrochemical and in vitro evaluation of the redox-properties of kynurenine species. *Biochem. Biophys. Res. Commun.* **2003**, *300*, 719–724. [CrossRef]
30. Darlington, L.G.; Forrest, C.M.; Mackay, G.M.; Smith, R.A.; Smith, A.J.; Stoy, N.; Stone, T.W. On the biological importance of the 3-hydroxyanthranilic acid: Anthranilic acid ratio. *Int. J. Tryptophan Res.* **2010**, *3*, IJTR. S4282. [CrossRef]
31. Meier, M.A.; Ottiger, M.; Vögeli, A.; Steuer, C.; Bernasconi, L.; Thomann, R.; Christ-Crain, M.; Henzen, C.; Hoess, C.; Zimmerli, W. Activation of the tryptophan/serotonin pathway is associated with severity and predicts outcomes in pneumonia: Results of a long-term cohort study. *Clin. Chem. Lab. Med. (Cclm)* **2017**, *55*, 1060–1069. [CrossRef]

32. Heyes, M.P.; Saito, K.; Major, E.O.; Milstien, S.; Markey, S.P.; Vickers, J.H. A mechanism of quinolinic acid formation by brain in inflammatory neurological disease: Attenuation of synthesis from L-tryptophan by 6-chlorotryptophan and 4-chloro-3-hydroxyanthranilate. *Brain* **1993**, *116*, 1425–1450. [CrossRef] [PubMed]
33. Zuo, H.; Ueland, P.M.; Ulvik, A.; Eussen, S.J.; Vollset, S.E.; Nygård, O.; Midttun, Ø.; Theofylaktopoulou, D.; Meyer, K.; Tell, G.S. Plasma biomarkers of inflammation, the kynurenine pathway, and risks of all-cause, cancer, and cardiovascular disease mortality: The Hordaland Health Study. *Am. J. Epidemiol.* **2016**, *183*, 249–258. [CrossRef] [PubMed]
34. Gobaille, S.; Kemmel, V.; Brumaru, D.; Dugave, C.; Aunis, D.; Maitre, M. Xanthurenic acid distribution, transport, accumulation and release in the rat brain. *J. Neurochem.* **2008**, *105*, 982–993. [CrossRef] [PubMed]
35. Reyes Ocampo, J.; Lugo Huitrón, R.; González-Esquivel, D.; Ugalde-Muñiz, P.; Jiménez-Anguiano, A.; Pineda, B.; Pedraza-Chaverri, J.; Ríos, C.; Pérez de la Cruz, V. Kynurenines with neuroactive and redox properties: Relevance to aging and brain diseases. *Oxidative Med. Cell. Longev.* **2014**, *2014*. [CrossRef] [PubMed]
36. Murakami, K.; Haneda, M.; Yoshino, M. Prooxidant action of xanthurenic acid and quinoline compounds: Role of transition metals in the generation of reactive oxygen species and enhanced formation of 8-hydroxy-2′-deoxyguanosine in DNA. *Biometals* **2006**, *19*, 429–435. [CrossRef]
37. Konradsson-Geuken, Å.; Wu, H.; Gash, C.; Alexander, K.; Campbell, A.; Sozeri, Y.; Pellicciari, R.; Schwarcz, R.; Bruno, J. Cortical kynurenic acid bi-directionally modulates prefrontal glutamate levels as assessed by microdialysis and rapid electrochemistry. *Neuroscience* **2010**, *169*, 1848–1859. [CrossRef]
38. Zmarowski, A.; Wu, H.Q.; Brooks, J.; Potter, M.; Pellicciari, R.; Schwarcz, R.; Bruno, J. Astrocyte-derived kynurenic acid modulates basal and evoked cortical acetylcholine release. *Eur. J. Neurosci.* **2009**, *29*, 529–538. [CrossRef]
39. Hardeland, R.; Zsizsik, B.; Poeggeler, B.; Fuhrberg, B.; Holst, S.; Coto-Montes, A. Indole-3-pyruvic and-propionic acids, kynurenic acid, and related metabolites as luminophores and free-radical scavengers. In *Tryptophan, Serotonin, and Melatonin*; Springer: Berlin, Germany, 1999; pp. 389–395.
40. Pedersen, E.R.; Tuseth, N.; Eussen, S.J.; Ueland, P.M.; Strand, E.; Svingen, G.F.T.; Midttun, Ø.; Meyer, K.; Mellgren, G.; Ulvik, A. Associations of plasma kynurenines with risk of acute myocardial infarction in patients with stable angina pectoris. *Arterioscler. Thromb. Vasc. Biol.* **2015**, *35*, 455–462. [CrossRef]
41. Schmidt, S.K.; Ebel, S.; Keil, E.; Woite, C.; Ernst, J.F.; Benzin, A.E.; Rupp, J.; Däubener, W. Regulation of IDO activity by oxygen supply: Inhibitory effects on antimicrobial and immunoregulatory functions. *PLoS ONE* **2013**, *8*, e63301. [CrossRef]
42. Chen, T.; Zheng, X.; Ma, X.; Bao, Y.; Ni, Y.; Hu, C.; Rajani, C.; Huang, F.; Zhao, A.; Jia, W. Tryptophan predicts the risk for future type 2 diabetes. *PLoS ONE* **2016**, *11*, e0162192. [CrossRef]
43. Zhou, C.C.; Yang, X.; Hua, X.; Liu, J.; Fan, M.B.; Li, G.Q.; Song, J.; Xu, T.Y.; Li, Z.Y.; Guan, Y.F. Hepatic NAD+ deficiency as a therapeutic target for non-alcoholic fatty liver disease in ageing. *Br. J. Pharmacol.* **2016**, *173*, 2352–2368. [CrossRef] [PubMed]
44. Haruki, H.; Hovius, R.; Pedersen, M.G.; Johnsson, K. Tetrahydrobiopterin biosynthesis as a potential target of the kynurenine pathway metabolite xanthurenic acid. *J. Biol. Chem.* **2016**, *291*, 652–657. [CrossRef] [PubMed]

2

Non-Coding RNAs as Blood-Based Biomarkers in Cardiovascular Disease

Raquel Figuinha Videira [1,2,3], Paula A. da Costa Martins [1,2,3] and Inês Falcão-Pires [3,*]

1 CARIM School for Cardiovascular Diseases, Faculty of Health, Medicine and Life Sciences, Maastricht University, 6229 ER Maastricht, The Netherlands; r.figuinhavideira@maastrichtuniversity.nl (R.F.V.); p.dacostamartins@maastrichtuniversity.nl (P.A.d.C.M.)
2 Department of Molecular Genetics, Faculty of Science and Engineering, Maastricht University, 6229 ER Maastricht, The Netherlands
3 Cardiovascular Research and Development Center, Faculty of Medicine, University of Porto, 4200-319 Porto, Portugal
* Correspondence: ipires@med.up.pt

Abstract: In 2020, cardiovascular diseases (CVDs) remain a leading cause of mortality and morbidity, contributing to the burden of the already overloaded health system. Late or incorrect diagnosis of patients with CVDs compromises treatment efficiency and patient's outcome. Diagnosis of CVDs could be facilitated by detection of blood-based biomarkers that reliably reflect the current condition of the heart. In the last decade, non-coding RNAs (ncRNAs) present on human biofluids including serum, plasma, and blood have been reported as potential biomarkers for CVDs. This paper reviews recent studies that focus on the use of ncRNAs as biomarkers of CVDs.

Keywords: ncRNAs; biomarkers; cardiovascular diseases; diagnosis

---

1. Introduction

Cardiovascular diseases (CVDs) including aortic stenosis, hypertension, myocardial infarction, congenital heart diseases, aortic aneurysms, and right ventricle dysfunction can lead to heart failure (HF) and, ultimately, death. CVDs alone are responsible for more than 17.9 million deaths per year, corresponding to 31% of all deaths globally and being the first cause of morbidity and mortality worldwide (World Health Organization (WHO), data from 2019 [1]). Unfortunately, for most CVDs, treatment efficacy and outcome remain highly compromised by incorrect or late diagnosis. This unpredictability is attributed to the scarcity of obvious symptoms that indicate cardiac dysfunction, thus some CVDs are classified as "silent killers", contributing to a diagnosis that occurs after acute and/or severe symptoms episodes, usually occurring at a stage where reverting cardiac damage is no longer possible (WHO [1]).

Clinical management of CVDs could be facilitated by detection of blood-based biomarkers that reliably reflect the current condition of the heart. The term biomarker arises from the junction of the words "biological" and "marker". Biomarkers are defined by WHO as "any substance, structure, or process that can be measured in the body or its products and influence or predict the incidence of outcome or disease". Later, the definition of a biomarker was extended to "any measurement reflecting an interaction between a biological system and a potential hazard, which may be chemical, physical, or biological" [2].

Ideally, a human biomarker should be of easy access and acquirement, display a high degree of specificity and sensitivity, be stable in its environment (plasma, urine, blood, and saliva, among others), and thus have little or no variability [3]. While it is desirable that a biomarker can be determined by a simple, fast, and low-cost method [3], very few molecules satisfy these criteria and rather just meet a reduced number of these requirements. Up to date, CVD biomarkers are restricted to troponins, natriuretic peptides (namely, atrial natriuretic peptide (ANP) and brain natriuretic peptide (BNP)), matrix metalloproteases, and galectin-3, but other promising factors, such as non-coding RNAs, are slowly being introduced as both prognostic and diagnostic tools in cardiovascular clinical practice [4]. The search for ideal CVD biomarkers has deepened in the past years; however, there is still a long way to go until the golden biomarkers enter clinical practice.

In the recent years, a new class of potential biomarkers, including non-coding RNAs (ncRNAs), has received much attention in the cardiovascular field. Representing almost 60% of cell transcriptome, ncRNAs are functional RNA molecules that, despite lacking a protein-coding region, are essential players in gene regulation and, consequently, in cell function and survival [5]. The discovery of the first ncRNA lin-4, a small RNA able to decrease the translation of another gene, *Lin-14*, by directly binding to lin-14 RNA molecule [6], opened doors to discover many other forms of ncRNAs including microRNAs (miRNAs, miRs), long non-coding RNAs (lncRNAs), and circular RNAs (circRNAs), among others.

MiRNAs are small ncRNA (18–25 nucleotides) that inhibit the expression of their target gene(s) by sequence-specific recognition. The transcript-binding sequence is usually located in the 3′-untranslated region (3′-UTR), whereas the complementary seed sequence is located in the first two to eight nucleotides of the miRNA [7]. The degree of binding complementary between miRNA and mRNA sets the outcome of target transcript expression with high complementary, leading to transcript destabilization followed by degradation in processing bodies (p-bodies) [8]. Meanwhile, a low complementary degree leads to translational repression, as binding to the mRNA cap prevents the translation initiation factor eIF4E, inhibiting the assembly of the ribosomal subunits or even promoting premature ribosomal drop-off and mRNA release from the ribosomal translational complex [9–11]. All of these regulatory mechanisms potentially enable a single miRNA to control hundreds of different target transcripts. Besides these endogenous mechanisms of action, cells can also secrete miRNAs that will be found extracellularly in human biofluids such as saliva, urine, serum, and plasma [12].

Although miRNAs are established as an important and possibly the most described group of ncRNAs, the largest portion of the ncRNA transcriptome is composed of lncRNAs. LncRNAs are a class of non-coding linear transcripts of more than 200 nucleotides in length, which frequently miss an open reading frame (ORF) and influence gene expression in a variety of manners [13]. Notwithstanding, some lncRNAs may display protein-coding functions, and several shared attributes of mRNAs such as 5′ cap, more than one exon, alternative splicing, and poly(A) tails [13]. LncRNAs are commonly classified according to their genomic localization; those entirely transcribed from intronic regions of protein-coding RNA are termed intronic lncRNA, whereas the case wherein a lncRNA is transcribed from an intergenic region is named intergenic lncRNA. Additionally, a lncRNA could also be transcribed from an enhancer region, a regulatory DNA sequence of gene expression that increases promoter's activity, which are named eRNAs [14].

Similar to miRNAs, lncRNAs can also be found in different cellular compartments such as nucleus, cytoplasm, and extracellular space. In the nucleus, lncRNAs will influence transcription by recruiting regulatory factors and catalytic proteins; alternately, eRNAs drive proteins to enhancer regions, anchoring them to DNA in the right position and organizing chromatin interaction [15]. Oppositely, some lncRNAs recruit polycomb repressive complex 1 and 2 (PRC1, PRC2), promoting methylation marks and decreasing transcription [16,17]. In the cytoplasma, lncRNAs may act as miRNA sponges, preventing small ncRNAs from binding to their target transcripts or, alternatively, lncRNAs can serve as scaffolds for nucleoprotein complexes influencing mRNA translation and interfering with mRNA splicing and degradation [18,19]. Despite their many described functions, lncRNAs are still an understudied class, with many lncRNAs remaining to be identified and their functions described. Similar to miRNAs, lncRNAs can also be found in extracellular spaces and fluids, encapsulated in vesicles or bound to other particles, and have, therefore, also been studied as potential biomarkers of CVDs. Unlike protein-coding and other ncRNAs, lncRNAs sequence is poorly conserved among species, despite that the promoter regions of lncRNAs are often conserved, as well as their structure (namely their 3D conformation and shape) and their functionality [13].

A newly found class of ncRNAs is circRNAs, which, in contrast with previously reported ncRNAs, are characterized by a circular form that arises as a consequence of back splicing events [20]. CircRNAs are small, single-stranded RNA sequences with loop structures covalently closed that confer them, unlike linear ncRNAs, protection from degradation by ribonucleases [20]. CircRNAs can act as decoy elements working through protein interaction; regulate mRNA splicing processes by recruiting splicing factors; and, under special conditions, they could be translated into proteins once internal ribosome entry site (IRES) was initiated [21].

Furthermore, circRNAs are conserved among species, with some of them displaying cell-type and spatial-temporal specificity [22]. Emerging evidence suggests a myriad of mechanisms by which circRNAs can influence gene expression, participating in cell function and contributing to pathological processes, including several ones associated with CVDs [23]. Another peculiarity of circRNAs is the presence of multiple miRNA response elements (MERs), which may compete with miRNA targets for binding and, as such, serve as miRNA sponges [23].

CircRNAs can also affect gene transcription of the so-called parent gene, the gene that mRNA gives origin to the circRNA after back splicing, through interaction with RNA polymerase II and regulation of its transcriptional activity [24]. As for other ncRNAs, circRNAs can also be detected in different human biofluids, and their role as biomarkers has been recently reported in cancer [25,26].

Here, we will review the literature on the detection of ncRNAs in human samples of blood, plasma, and serum and conclude on their potential as biomarkers of CVDs.

A variety of cardiac diseases have different etiologies and specific events that can lead to the expression and circulation of cardiac-derived biomarkers

2. Aortic-Related Diseases

2.1. Aortic Valve Stenosis

Aortic valve stenosis (AS) affects more than 5% of the population above 65 years old. It is defined as a narrowing of the aortic valve that progressively imposes resistance to the blood flow from the left ventricle (LV) to the aorta [27]. Unfortunately, as AS symptoms occur at an advanced disease stage, where cardiac damage is no longer reversible, the disease has a dismal prognosis in symptomatic individuals. Currently, there is no pharmacological treatment for AS and the most efficient solutions include surgical aortic valve replacement (SAVR) or trans-catheter aortic valve replacement (TAVR). However, valve replacement has been associated with risk of vascular access-site bleeding, blood transfusion-related infections, stroke, para-valvular leaks, and heart block, which also increase the risk of HF and death following valve replacement [28].

ncRNAs have been studied as prospective biomarkers of AS thanks to their potential to reflect AS pathogenesis and to be detected at an earlier AS stage. Blood-based ncRNA biomarkers could aid in patient's risk stratification and decision making, such as the timing and type of intervention (SAVR vs. TAVR), as well as in predicting AS progression.

Clinically, AS is associated with LV hypertrophy and cardiac fibrosis. In fact, a study measuring the plasma levels of miR-1, miR-133, and miR-378 in AS patients suggested that all three miRNAs were downregulated [29]. Yet, miR-378 is even lower expressed in patients with LV hypertrophy in comparison with those without hypertrophy, which indicates a strong negative correlation between miR-378 and LV mass and placing miR-378 as an independent predictor of LV hypertrophy in AS [29]. In a similar cohort of AS patients, circulating miR-210 was shown to be increased and to inversely correlate with LV end diastolic dimensions, cardiac parameters affected in AS [30]. This miRNA may also predict mortality as higher levels of miR-210 were found in patients with a high risk of mortality in follow-up studies. Although miR-210 is not established as an AS-specific marker, the results reported are comparable to data obtained for the N-Terminal fragment of BNP levels and, when combined with other cardiovascular (CV) parameters, could help predict CV risk associated with AS [30].

Another study showed the presence of myocardial fibrosis in severe AS patients with LV preserved ejection fraction (EF). Interestingly, fibrosis directly associates with miR-21 plasma levels, suggesting that miR-21 levels reflect the degree of myocardial fibrosis [31]. Furthermore, plasma miR-21 levels provided more accuracy, sensitivity, and specificity to distinguish myocardial fibrosis when compared with common AS parameters such as global longitudinal strain and BNP levels [31]. Similar results were found by Villar et al., unravelling that not only is circulating miR-21 increased in AS patients compared with healthy controls, but also an increase in circulating miR-21 increase is proportional to an increment in myocardial miR-21 expression as well as of cardiac fibrotic genes [32].

Analysis of peripheral blood collected from AS patients demonstrated that serum miR-19b levels are abnormally decreased and inversely correlated with LV stiffness and collagen cross-linking when matched to age and gender healthy controls [33]. Previously, members of the miR-17-92 cluster, to which miR-19 belongs, were reported to regulate myocardial fibrosis and angiogenesis [34]. However, the role of angiogenesis is still unclear, with some studies reporting that the degree of myocardial angiogenesis is accompanied by increased hypertrophy, worsening of systolic function, and severe AS [35,36]. On the other hand, a study demonstrated that increased angiogenesis and cardiomyocytes proliferation prevent maladaptive remodeling in a model of LV pressure-overload [37].

Interestingly, a number of different miRNAs have been related to different phenotypes of AS [38]. For example, AS patients with a low flow condition display high levels of miR-1, miR-21, and miR-133, whereas higher levels of miR-133 reflect LV hypertrophy [38]. In fact, patients with severe AS and reduced EF demonstrated increased levels of miR-1, miR-29, and miR-133 [38]. Curiously, in conditions of pressure-overload such as AS, miR-29 levels were clinically different among males and females [39]. Above the age of 50 and compared with control healthy women, women with AS showed a significant enrichment of miR-29 that is associated with increased LV mass and concentricity [39].

Despite certain circRNAs showing aortic valvular tissue specificity, and several associations that have been suggested between lncRNAs and AS pathology, to date, no studies have reported the association of AS with either plasma circRNAs or lncRNAs [40,41].

2.2. *Aortic Aneurysm*

Aortic aneurysm (AA) represents an important cause of death. AA is clinically characterized by an enlargement of at least 50% of an aortic segment compared with the same segment in healthy individuals and can be subdivided in thoracic aortic aneurysm (TAA) or abdominal aortic aneurysm (AAA), the latter being the most frequent [42]. AA is accompanied by progressive degeneration of the aortic wall [42]. Initially, a bulge-like dilation of a segment of the aortic wall tends to expand and increase the risk of rupture [42].

AA incidence and prognosis is associated with patient's sex and age, typically men and elderly populations are more affected by AA and demonstrate worse outcomes [42]. To date, there are no efficient pharmacological therapies against AA; therefore, when an AA progresses to a severe stage, surgery procedures are required [42].

An early and correct diagnosis could avoid surgery and improve patient's outcome. As nearly all patients are asymptomatic, an early diagnosis becomes difficult [43]. Most of the cases are detected during screenings using imaging techniques such as computerized tomography angiogram (CTA), ultrasound sonography (US), and magnetic resonance imaging (MRI) [42]. However, these techniques are expensive and incur hazards, thus new markers are needed, which encourages the exploration of ncRNAs' potential candidates. Recently, blood-based biomarkers such as tenascin-C, C-reactive protein, cystatin C, cathepsin, iron, immune system cells (lymphocytes and monocytes), genetic markers, and ncRNAs have emerged as attractive alternatives to help in AA diagnosis [44].

Among ncRNAs, miRs continue in the front of the biomarkers run as the most well described and studied ncRNAs. Therefore, it is not surprising that most AA related studies on ncRNAs focus on miRs.

In 2020, a small study described seven circulating miRs with an altered expression in AAA condition ($n = 16$) when compared with the control (miR-103a-3p, miR-27b-3p, miR-99a-5p, miR-375, miR-221-3p, miR-146a-5p, and miR-1260) [45]. After variable adjustment, only miR-221-3p and miR-27b-3p remained significantly overexpressed in AAA plasma, suggesting its potential as AAA biomarkers [45].

A work from *Wanhainen* et al. analyzed the circulating miRNA profile of 169 AAA patients and contrasted it against the profile of 48 healthy age and sex-matched individuals [46]. Of a predefined panel composed of the 172 most expressed miRs in plasma, 103 were found to be differentially expressed in the plasma samples of AAA patients relative to the plasma samples of healthy individuals [46]. The top altered miRs included miR-10b-5p, which displayed a specificity of 70% and a sensitivity of 60%, but, by adding let-7i-5p to the analysis, a specificity of 71% at a sensitivity of 90% was reached, allowing the discrimination between controls and AAA patients [46]. Despite improved sensitivity after combining different miRs, this result is still disappointing when compared with other studies and biomarkers.

On the other hand, lncRNAs were also reported as potential biomarkers for TAA [47]. In fact, TAA patients revealed decreased LUCAT1 and SMILR plasma levels when compared with a control group [47]. However, only LUCAT1 demonstrated an area under curve (AUC) higher than 0.65, indicating a modest potential diagnostic value for TAA [47].

More promising results were obtained by Tian et al., who investigated the potential role of plasma circMARK3 to identify an advanced stage of aortic aneurysms, such as aortic dissection (when the inner aortic wall becomes tore), particularly acute aortic dissection -Standford type A (AAAD) [48]. The results showed that 506 circulating circRNAs were significantly dysregulated in AAAD cohort group compared with controls, including circRNAs that were 320 were significantly increased and 186 circRNAs that were significantly decreased [48]. From these, circMARK3 was chosen for further validation as a biomarker because of its high expression on AAAD [48]. After receiver operating characteristic (ROC) analysis, serum circMARK3 was characterized by an AUC of 0.9344 (using a cutoff value of 1.497), a sensitivity of 90.0%, and specificity of 86.7% [48]. Further combination of serum circMARK3 and miR-1273-3p revealed even improved results, namely, sensitivity and specificity were increased to 93.3% and 86.7%, respectively. The AUC of the combined ncRNAs was 0.9644 when using a cutoff value of 0.4807 [48].

Together, the results obtained by Tian et al. are very encouraging and highly suggest serum circMARK3 and miR-1273-3p as potential biomarkers for the AAAD condition.

3. Coronary Artery Disease

Often viewed as an inflammatory disorder, coronary artery disease (CAD) occurs when vessels that supply blood to the heart (coronary arteries) become damaged [49]. Artery plaque buildup due to atherosclerosis is a frequent cause of CAD, resulting in the narrowing of coronary arteries followed by myocardial ischemia and, ultimately, thrombosis and HF [49]. As the presence of plaques is influenced by age, smoking, and an unhealthy lifestyle, CAD affects mainly adults and elderly populations, displaying worse prognosis in developing countries [49]. Current therapeutic strategies are focused on pharmacological interventions to reduce the risk of atherosclerotic complications (decrease low density lipoprotein (LDL) levels, anti-thrombotic drugs) and symptoms (beta blockers and ranolazile, a drug that prevents late phase of the inward sodium current contributing to cardiac relaxation during diastole) [49]. At an advanced disease stage, mechanical interventions such as angioplasty, percutaneous coronary intervention (PCI) or coronary bypass surgery are needed to vascularize the blocked artery and to re-establish blood flow [49]. Although early CAD diagnosis is imperative to prevent plaque rupture and further associated complications, the existing methods, such as computed tomography, electrocardiogram (ECG), and echocardiography, may not be applied to the broad population owing to limited equipment availability, operated-dependent results, time constraints, and costs.

As CAD pathology is directly influenced by endothelial dysfunction, is it feasible to assume that endothelial-related miRNAs could constitute reliable biomarkers of CAD. Accordingly, miR-17 described as a negative regulator of tumor angiogenesis is highly expressed in plasma from patients with severe CAD and is a potential biomarker candidate [50]. Other miRNAs have been portrayed as potential biomarkers in plasma of CAD patients when compared with healthy control groups. Such is the case of plasma increased levels of miR-33, miR-208b, and miR-499, as well as decreased expression of miR-155, miR-145, and let-7c [51–53].

Notwithstanding, the levels of circulating miRNAs are not only capable of indicating the presence of CAD lesion, but also can differentiate and correlate with CAD severity, as shown for miR-206 [54]. Patients with major blocked coronary arteries or with a higher number of blocked coronary arteries have higher levels of miR-206 when compared with patients with less severe lesions or healthy controls [54]. As such, miR-206 is upregulated in individuals with three blocked coronary arteries when compared with individuals two blocked coronary arteries, and those showed enhanced levels of miR-206 when compared with individuals with only one blocked coronary artery.

Analysis of atherosclerosis- and cardiac-related lncRNAs levels in peripheral blood mononuclear cells (PBMCs) from CAD patients and healthy individuals revealed that three lncRNAs, KCNQ1OT1, HIF1A-AS2, and APO1, are significantly increased in patients when compared with the healthy controls [55]. Of the three, APO1 revealed the best diagnostic value with a sensitivity of 100% and a specificity of 80% [55]. The combination of these three lncRNAs improved the diagnostic score by increasing the specificity to 90% and maintaining the sensitivity at 100%. These results place KCNQ1OT1, HIF1A-AS2, and APO1 at the top of potential CAD biomarkers to be used in the clinics [55]. Another study revealed HOTAIR, an lncRNA reported to be involved in vascular inflammation and age-associated-CVDs, as being upregulated in both plasma and PBMCs samples of CAD patients when compared with non-CAD patients [56]. Assessment of lncRNA expression profiles in plasma samples of both groups detected several differentially expressed lncRNAs, including lncRNAs GAS5 [57]. Although previously associated with several CVDs such as diabetes mellitus, hypertension, and valvular disease, a recent study has reported GAS5 to be significantly downregulated in CAD and diabetes mellitus, but not altered in other cardiovascular diseases such as hypertension, abnormal aortic aneurysm, viral myocarditis, atrial fibrillation, valvular disease, dilated cardiomyopathy, and peripheral artery disease [57].

A similar approach was taken by *Vilades* and colleagues, who categorize CAD patients according to the levels of plasma circ_0001445 (circSMARCA5), whose expression inversely correlated to coronary atherosclerosis extension and severity [58]. In fact, augmented circSMARCA5 levels are associated with a decreased segment stenosis score as well as with decreased cardiovascular risk [58]. Furthermore, RNA sequencing from plasma exosomes of CAD and non-CAD patients identified 335 exosomal circRNAs to be differentially expressed among the two groups [59]. After adjusting for risk factors, circ0005540 was upregulated in CAD patients, and displayed high sensitivity and specificity for identifying CAD patients, suggesting its potential as a CAD biomarker [59]. Similarly, circZNF609 also seems to be a promising biomarker for CAD [60]. CirZNF609 expression in peripheral blood leucocytes is decreased in CAD patients when compared with the control cohort [60]. Despite the different etiologies of CAD, overall, circZNF609 featured a specificity of 0.765 (76.5%) and a sensitivity of 0.804 (80.4%), indicating a moderate predicting value to identify CAD patients [60]. Furthermore, a microarray analysis of CAD and control PBMCs detected upregulation of circ_0001879 and circ_0004104 in CAD patients and these levels were associated not only with standard CAD biomarkers, but also with CAD risk factors [61]. Whereas both circRNAs can be individually used as biomarkers, combining both only showed an improved diagnostic value when combined with conventional CVD markers such as serum creatinine and CVD risk factors as hypertension, high LDL, smoking, and drinking, among others [61].

4. Myocardial Infarction

One of the consequences of CAD is the formation of a blood clot that, among other causes, occludes coronary arteries, resulting in ischemia and myocardial infarction (MI, also known as heart attack). In fact, a correlation between CAD and MI was previously established, namely on how well plasma miRNAs can predict CAD progression towards acute MI. A higher number of stenosed coronary vessels is associated with lower plasma miR-99a levels in MI patients [62]. Following PCI, miR-99 expression levels were re-established to comparable levels as observed in healthy volunteers. In MI, lower plasma miR-99 levels negatively correlated with those of cardiac troponin I and creatinine kinase (markers of cardiac dysfunction), suggesting that miR-99 expression might be necessary for proper cardiac function [62]. Similarly, miR-181a was also suggested to be a biomarker for MI as its increased plasma concentration is proportional to the severity of coronary stenotic lesions as well as deterioration of LV function [63]. Accordingly, miR-181a levels were positively correlated with creatinine kinase levels, and reduced 48 h after PCI [62,63].

Data from Centers for Disease Control and Prevention (CDC), a U.S. national public health institute, respective to the U.S. population, reported that, every 40 s, someone dies from a heart attack, and for every five occurrences, one is silent, meaning that no symptoms are recognized by the patient. Commonly, MI is diagnosed by combining an ECG test and analysis of biomarkers such as cardiac troponin I and T levels. However, ECG can only detect 30–70% of MI cases, highlighting the need for more accurate and sensitive biomarkers [64].

Various plasma miRNAs have been described as potential indicators of myocardial infarction, likely the most studied and described event among all cardiovascular diseases. Hence, miR-1, miR-126, miR-30a, miR-195, miR-26a-1, miR-146a, and miR-199a-1 were revealed to be upregulated in individuals diagnosed with acute MI (AMI) [65–67], with some of them, that is, miR-1, miR-126, miR-30a, and miR-195, reaching their maximal expression 8 h after the onset of symptoms [65,67,68]. In contrast, let-7b and miR-132-5p levels were decreased in acute MI patients when compared with control subjects [65]. AUC of ROC analysis only granted a modest individual value of sensitivity and specificity (below 90%), suggesting that each miRNA has moderate potential in the diagnosis of AMI patients. However, clustering of different miRNAs was more encouraging as an AUC of 0.913 was obtained when grouping miR-26a-1, miR-146a, and miR-199a-1 [66]. Other miRNAs such as miR-22-5p and miR-150-3p were also increased in MI by 36.47- and 4.09-fold, respectively, and even though they continued to be elevated for 72 h, the peak was reached at the onset of symptoms [69]. The sensitivity and specificity of the different miRNAs were calculated at different time points. Despite the fact that individual miRNAs showed a moderate power, when combined together, miR-132-5p, miR-22-5p, and miR-150-3p presented a better diagnostic value to distinguish AMI patients [69].

Microarray analysis in plasma samples of a small group of AMI patients identified 33 differentially expressed miRNAs, from which miR-30d-5p and miR-125-5p were selected for validation in a larger study population composed of 230 AMI patients and 79 healthy controls [70]. Despite the notable diagnostic value (namely specificity and sensitivity) of cardiac troponin I, the results obtained for miR-30d-5p surpassed the performance of cardiac troponin I by displaying an AUC of 0.915 [70] and highlighting the potential diagnostic use of miR-30d-5p and miR-125-5p in patients suspected of developing AMI [70].

Less promising results were reported for miR-221-3p, which, despite being upregulated by 3.89-fold in AMI [71], and an AUC of 0.881, did not reach the values of the standard marker troponin and neither improved the AUC levels when combined with troponin [71]. In line, miR-486 and miR-150 were also described as "exhibiting strong differentiation power" between healthy controls and AMI patients. However, the combination of both miR-486 and miR-150 only showed a moderated predictive power with an AUC of 0.731 [72]. Nevertheless, these two miRNAs were able to modestly classify

AMI patients into ST elevation MI (STEMI) and non-ST elevation MI (NSTEMI) [72]. Typically, STEMI is associated with a more severe condition and worse prognosis.

Interestingly, even after pharmacological treatment, progression towards maladaptive remodeling occurs in approximately 30% of AMI patients [73]. A total of 14 plasma miRNAs and 16 serum miRNAs were found to be dysregulated in samples from AMI subjects [74]. Following cross data and validation (in different cohorts), only miR-30a-5p was significantly upregulated in patients with (HF) after an MI episode. Interestingly, miR-30a-5p levels at the onset of AMI negatively correlate with LVEF six months after AMI, suggesting a prognostic value for miR-30a-5p, despite that it might also represent a marker of myocardial ischemia. The discriminatory power of miR-30a-5p to identified HF versus non-HF patients after MI was assessed by AUC calculation, resulting in an AUC of 75% [74].

As mentioned previously, one mechanism of action of lncRNAs is by competitively binding to miRNAs' target binding site, which prevents the attachment of mRNA–miRNA, thus inhibiting miRNA action. For example, lncRNA HOTAIR has a sponge like effect on miR-1, an miRNA upregulated in AMI cases [75]. HOTAIR is decreased in serum from subjects with AMI, reaching its lower expression 6 to 12 h after the onset of the first symptoms and negatively correlating with its target, miR-1 and cardiac troponin I [75]. Three days after the AMI episode, miR-1, cardiac troponin I, and HOTAIR levels are re-established [75]. Additionally, a study in mice subjected to hypoxia demonstrated that HOTAIR is myocardium-specific and that plasma HOTAIR in mice behaves similar to what was observed in humans, suggesting its myocardial origin [75].

Another myocardial enriched lncRNA is UCA1, which, similar to HOTAIR, is also decreased in the plasma of AMI individuals [76]. By clustering AMI patients according to the time from initial symptoms, it was possible to analyze the time course expression of UCA1 following an MI event [76]. While the lowest levels were reached between 6 and 12 h and remained low up to 48 h after AMI, from this point on, UCA1 levels increased and, at 96 h post-AMI, they were higher in AMI patients compared with the controls [76]. Interestingly, UCA1 also negatively correlates with miR-1 expression, but no mechanism has yet been described associating the two ncRNAs [76]. Although the predictive value of UCA1 alone is not as potent as standard biomarkers, the overall predictive power of UCA1 for AMI was increased to 0.983 AUC when combined with creatinine kinase [76].

Other lncRNAs have been attributed biomarker potential when screening for differentially expressed lncRNAs in plasma of 46 STEMI patients. While aHIF, KCNQ1OT1, and LIPCAR were found to be increased, six others, including HOTAIR, UCA1, MIAT, MALAT1, ANRIL, and CPNE3, were decreased in these patients [77]. The most promising diagnostic values were revealed for LIPCAR, with a sensitivity of 82% and a specificity of 75% in distinguishing STEMI subjects, and with LIPCAR levels positively correlating with cardiac troponin I and creatinine kinase and inversely with LV ejection fraction [77]. Notably, the increased levels of LIPCAR observed upon an STEMI event were decreased shortly after PCI [77].

Despite the relatively new role of circRNAs as biomarkers of AMI, Deng et al. found 160 circRNAs to be differentially expressed in AMI patients, with 87 of them being increased and 73 decreased when compared with healthy controls [78]. Among the most downregulated was circRNA_081881, showing a 12.5-fold change compared with the control group [78]. Currently, the most studied circRNA in MI is the myocardial infarction-associated circular RNA (MICRA) [79,80], which, by being decreased in plasma of MI patients, positively correlates with LV ejection fraction and accentuates the risk of LV dysfunction [79].

5. Congenital Heart Defects

In the past decade, prenatal testing made crucial advances and increased the survival rate up to 87% in the first year. Currently, neonatal congenital heart defects (CHDs) have an incidence of 4–8 per 1000 births and their manifestations range from minor defects (such as small intracavitary communications) to severe defects that can even lead to prenatal lethality (CDC data, September 2020). The most common include tetralogy of fallot (TOF), atrial septal defect (ASD), ventricular septal defect

(VSD) single ventricle (SV), persistent truncus arteriosus (PTA), and bicuspid aortic valve disease (BAV) [81]. A favorable CHD prognosis and reduced mortality is associated with early and correct diagnosis. However, the standard diagnostic method to detect CHD usually includes echocardiography and has an efficiency rate up to 35%, which is considerably low [82]. Additionally, some CHDs are diagnosed only after birth, during infancy, or even during adulthood. During pregnancy, several cardiogenesis-associated ncRNAs are potentially secreted by the fetus and enter into the maternal bloodstream, where they can be detected by blood analysis and used as biomarkers for CHD [83]. Multiple studies have also linked specific CHDs with an altered miRNA expression profile. In particular, children with ASD present a significant upregulation of let-7a and miR-486 and, although not statistically significant, an increase in hsa-let-7b levels when compared with healthy children [84]. Interestingly, mothers of ASD children express a similar miRNA expression pattern. In fact, because let-7a expression levels positively correlated between mothers and their offspring [84], its levels in the mother could predict ASD in children with a sensitivity of 82% and a specificity of 91%, indicating a significant diagnostic value of this miRNA in detecting ASD in children [84].

Bicuspid aortic valve disease (BAV), the most common anomaly of the human heart, results from an anomaly during valvulogenesis that is characterized by no splitting between two adjacent cusps, and it is frequently accompanied by dilation of the ascending aorta [85]. The most prominent miRNAs in adult BAV patients seem to be miR-122, miR-130a, and miR-486, and miR-718, with the latter being altered in BAV patients and inversely correlating with the diameter of the ascending aorta and, therefore, suggested as a potential biomarker of aortic dilation [86].

Overall, CHDs can be distinguished from non-CHDs through specific alterations in miRNA expression patterns [87]. Namely, miR-125b-2-3p, miR-1284, miR-142-5p, miR145-3p, miR-4426, miR-4666a-3p, and miR-4681 are downregulated, while miR-1275, miR-3664-3p, and miR4796-3p are upregulated in women pregnant with a CHD child compared with women pregnant with a non-CHD child [87]. Notably, such differences are no longer observed 24 h after delivery, supporting the hypothesis that the above miRNAs are pregnancy-related. ROC analysis demonstrated miR-142-5p to have the highest diagnostic accuracy with an AUC of 0.804 [87]. Indeed, the combination of the top four miRNAs (miR-142-5p, miR-1275, miR-4666a-3p, and miR-3664-3p) improved the accuracy in discriminating CHD from controls [87]. Interestingly, specific miRNAs can also be related to a particular CHD phenotype. For example, VSD revealed changes in miR-142-5p, miR-1275, miR-4666a-3p, and miR-3664-3p; TOF related to dysregulation of miR142-5p, miR-4666a-3p, and miR-3664-3p, while both SV and PTA were linked to miR-142-5p and miR-3664-3p differential expression [87].

A relatively small study, including 22 pregnant CHD-positive and 17 CHD-free controls, suggested miR-99a to be upregulated in the peripheral blood of the CHD-positive pregnant women when compared with the control group [88]. However, no diagnostic value was determined for this miRNA.

Yu et al. also suggested that a different group of miRNAs could identify CHDs such as ventricular septal defect (VSD), atrial septal defect (ASD), and tetralogy of fallot (TOF) [83]. The group composed of miR-19b, miR-22, miR-29c, and miR-375 is upregulated in maternal serum of CHD fetuses when compared with maternal serum of non-CHD fetuses [83]. When miRNAs were clustered according to the disease phenotype, all miRNAs were significantly upregulated in TOF, whereas only miR-19b and miR-29c were significantly increased in VSD and miR-19b, miR-29c, and miR-375 were increased in ASD [83]. Although all the miRNAs demonstrated a significant discriminatory value, and thus could be used as a disease biomarker for the detection of fetal CHD, the combination of all four miRNAs proved to be a more efficient diagnostic strategy.

Regarding lncRNAs in CHDs, HOTAIR was found to be upregulated in both myocardial tissue and plasma samples of ASD, VSD, and patent ductus arteriosus (PDA) patients when compared with healthy subjects, and thus was indicated as a potential biomarker for CHD [89]. HOTAIR seems to work through recruitment of PRC2 and inducing epigenetic modifications during embryonic heart development [89].

From a microarray-based strategy, 17,603 lncRNAs were found to be differentially present in the plasma of fetal CHD pregnant women [82]. From these, 3694 lncRNAs were significantly upregulated and 3919 were downregulated. Subsquently, this subgroup was subjected to gene ontology (GO) analysis to describe their association with specific biological processes, cellular components, and molecular functions through. GO analysis recognized 26 CHD-related lncRNAs, among which four were differentially altered in VSD, as well as another four in TOF, and two others were significantly different in ASD [82]. Overall, pregnant women with fetal CHD revealed alterations in ENST00000436681, ENST00000422826, AA584040, AA709223, and BX478947, when compared with the control group [82], all of them showing a moderated discriminating effect; therefore, it was suggested as potential lncRNA biomarkers to predict fetal CHD.

More recently, the possible value of circRNAs in the diagnosis of CHD has also been addressed. A study including 40 children with CHD (namely VSD and ASD) and 40 healthy children identified 10 upregulated and 157 downregulated circRNAs in the plasma of the CHD group. Validation by qPCR demonstrated three circRNAs, hsa_circRNA_004183, hsa_circRNA_079265, and hsa_circRNA_105039, to be significantly decreased in the affected group [90]. Hsa_circRNA_105039 presented the best diagnostic value with a sensitivity of 80%, a specificity of 100%, and AUC of 0.907, but altogether, the three circRNAs had an AUC of 0.965, suggesting a combinatorial approach to be effective in the diagnosis of CHD [90].

6. Right Ventricle Dysfunction

The right ventricle (RV) is responsible for pumping venous blood into the pulmonary vascular bed on the way to the LV, thereby contributing to left ventricular filling and cardiopulmonary function. Its thin walls and the direct connection with low impedance pulmonary circulation make the RV more sensitive to pressure than to volume overload [91]. Pulmonary hypertension (PH), pulmonary embolism, RV infarction, and cardiomyopathies are among the main causes of RV dysfunction and, consequently, failure [92]. Despite its critical contribution to heart function, the RV has been somewhat neglected, with only a few studies having specifically focused on RV failure. The limited knowledge of RV biology and function contributes to the poor prognosis of RV failure (RVF) patients, with both treatment and diagnosis of RVF remaining challenging. Conventional diagnostic approaches are based on ECG, 3D-echocardiography and strain imaging, magnetic resonance imaging, and blood marker analysis such as lactate and BNP levels [93]. Although ncRNAs also recently started receiving attention in the RV field, there is still a scarce number of studies reporting on ncRNAs as biomarkers on RVF.

Arrhythmogenic cardiomyopathy (ACM) is a life-threating genetic disease where RV myocardial tissue is replaced by fibro-fatty tissue, leading to arrhythmias and, eventually, HF [94]. ACM is particularly challenging to detect because of variance expression and penetrance of the mutated gene, and as a consequence, genetics tests can result in inconclusive diagnostics [94]. miRNA profiling studies revealed miR-320a to be downregulated in ACM patients, when compared with healthy controls [94]. Intermediate values of sensitivity and specificity obtained for miR-320a were increased when combined with EGC analysis, thus improving its diagnostic potential [94]. Despite these promising results, so far, no correlation between miR-320a levels and disease severity has been found [94].

PH is a multifactorial disease, with several subgroups being characterized by an increase in RV afterload that can precede (right) HF and, eventually, death. The first report on PH-associated circulating miRNAs analyzed plasma samples from PH patients undergoing right heart catheterization [95]. MiRNAs such as miR-1, miR-26a, miR-29c, miR-34b, miR-451, and miR-1246 were found to be downregulated, whereas miR-130a, miR-133b, miR-191, miR-204, and miR-208b were profoundly upregulated in PH subjects when compared with control subjects. From all these, only miR-208b and miR-130 could be correlated with PH severity [95].

Another similar study revealed miR-451 as being significantly decreased in PH patients compared with non-PH patients (individuals diagnosed with other conditions) [96]. Although the diagnostic value of miR-451 was as moderate as the conventional Doppler-echo, combing both improved the diagnostic value of miR-451 in PH [96]. More recently, miR-424 was also linked to PH and found to be upregulated in plasma of PH patients [97], with patients with severe PH clearly displaying higher miR-424 levels when compared with individuals with less severe PH [97]. As miR-424 inversely correlates with cardiac output parameters in PH patients, it has been suggested has a potential marker of PH [97].

7. Pathological Reverse Remodeling

Cardiac pathological remodeling associated with the above-mentioned different cardiovascular diseases can lead to HF and, eventually, death. The severity of cardiac pathological remodeling frequently predicts treatment outcome and patient response [98]. In light of the current findings, such remodeling can be reversed and result in improved of cardiac function and, consequently, better patient prognosis and survival [99–101]. Reverse remodeling (RR) can be defined by any functional, structural, cellular, and/or molecular changes, resulting in improved heart function following pathological remodeling [99]. Factors contributing to the process include both pharmacological angiotensin-converting enzyme inhibitors, beta-blockers, and mechanical therapy such as cardiac resynchronization therapy (CRT), PCI, left ventricle assist device implantation (LVAD), and AVR surgery, among others [99]. Unfortunately, a fraction of patients undergoing cardiac therapy do not develop a favorable clinical response; do not show improved cardiac function; and, in some cases, cardiac condition is worsened after treatment [99,102]. Such patients, with incomplete reverse remodeling, are classified as non-responders, while patients with improved cardiac function and complete reverse remodeling are categorized as responders [99].

Understanding the features of cardiac pathological remodeling and the cardiac response to therapy has become a major objective towards better care of CVD patients. In line, biomarkers, and more specifically ncRNAs, are claiming a greater role towards establishing reverse remodeling and predicting patient outcome upon specific therapies.

Presently, the only therapy that consistently increases survival of AS patients is AVR surgery. However, the persistence of hypertrophy after AVR surgery is a main limiting factor for patient survival and positive outcomes. Circulating miR-133a levels prior to AVR surgery are a positive predictor of LV mass normalization and subsequent decrease of cardiac hypertrophy up to one year after surgery. When combined with other clinical parameters, miR-133a yielded an AUC of 0.89 [103] and is currently considered one of the most promising biomarkers to predict LV normalization in AS patients after AVR [103].

A negatively patient outcome after mechanical therapy such as coronary artery bypass graft or AVR due to CAD and AS, respectively, is associated with high levels of serum miR-423-3p [104]. Although this is specifically significant in patients with unstable angina, when compared with individuals with stable angina or AS, the reason that miR-423-3p is particularly elevated in these patients is inconclusive [104].

Another study collectively addressed miRNA expression in the Pro-BNP Outpatient Tailored CHF Therapy (PROTECT) cohort to predict left ventricle reverse remodeling (LVRR) based on miRNAs that have been involved in human HF phenotypes or known to influence common HF signaling pathways [105]. Only 41% of the participants exhibited complete RR, considered as more than 15% reduction in LV end-systolic volume index [105]. Not only PCA analysis identified miR-423-5p and miR-212-5p as dysregulated in the plasma of systolic HF patients, they were also associated with LVRR and shared 14 target genes related to HF [105]. Together with the fact that miR-423-5p and miR-212-5p are also upregulated in myocardium tissue of end-stage HF in mice, these findings support the prospective role of miRNAs in discriminating LVRR [105].

Aside from the merit of circulating miRNAs, lncRNAs such as LIPCAR, H19, ANRIL, and MHRT have also emerged as potential biomarkers for LVRR. For example, higher plasma levels of LIPCAR and H19 in CAD patients are associated with chronic HF [106]. In HF patients, higher levels of LIPCAR are associated with a higher risk of hospitalization and mortality due to HF when compared with HF patients with lower LIPCAR levels [107]. Similarly, plasma MHRT is significantly lower in patients with HF and is able to distinguish HF from healthy subjects by presenting an AUC of 0.925 [108]. Among HF patients, lower levels of plasma MHRT significantly correlate with a lower survival rate when compared with HF patients displaying higher MHRT levels.

As previously mentioned, one treatment for CAD is coronary intervention by the use of a stent; however, 12% of patients with stent therapy showed angiographic restenosis, in-sent restenosis (ISR) [109]. ISR is defined as a "narrowing of a coronary artery at the stented segment", and is associated with increased plasma levels of ANRIL, when compared with CAD patients without restenosis [110]. To note, ANRIL was found as an independent risk factor for ISR incidence, with a modest diagnostic value demonstrated by an AUC of 0.749. In addition, ANRIL demonstrated a specificity of 75% and sensitivity of 68.4% after a cutoff value of 1.34 [110].

Finally, plasma circRNA MICRA was found to be a strong predictor of LV dysfunction 3 to 4 months after an AMI episode, and lower MICRA levels in MI patients are at higher risk of LV dysfunction [80].

8. Conclusions

Misdiagnosed CVDs have severe consequences on a patient's life quality and associated survival rate. The use of standard biomarkers for CVDs as the quantitative assessment of circulating cardiac troponins and natriuretic peptides levels it is still not specific and neither sensitive enough for early detection. Moreover, the complexity of many biological and molecular mechanisms observed on the different CVDs makes the use of a single biomarker insufficient for a correct diagnosis. Currently, circulating ncRNAs display great potential as biomarkers owing to their high abundance and stability in the blood, and ncRNAs can provide a valuable measure of heart health condition. Therefore, ncRNAs have been portrayed as potential non-invasive tools and might help on CVDs' diagnosis and prognosis, allowing tailored healthcare to each individual and a reduction of the associated societal and economic burden. However, the expression profile of ncRNAs could be influenced by age, sex, and medical drugs, which might add more complexity to our understanding of ncRNAs in CVDs. Furthermore, up to date, only a scarce number of works reported a higher individual diagnostic value of ncRNAs when compared with standard CVD markers; however, frequently, this value is improved when a set of ncRNAs is used or combined with standard CVD markers. The majority of the studies are characterized by a smaller sample size, with some possible cofounders associated (region, ethnicity, age, social status), and a short-term follow-up thwarts the hunting for the ideal biomarker. Interestingly, some ncRNAs such as muscle specific miR-1 and lncRNA HOTAIR are reported in several diseases (Table 1), suggesting a feature of a general CVD biomarker, while others appear to have disease-specificity (Figure 1 and Supplementary Table S1). New findings on ncRNAs and their role as blood-based biomarkers are reported frequently, such as the study of Viereck, who performed an extensive review on this topic [111]. Despite the vast amount of data on CVDs and plasma ncRNAs, their inclusion in medical guidelines is still far off in the upcoming years. Thus, we recommend researchers who aim to validate potential biomarkers in big cohorts to rely on the candidates derived from studies that include the largest sample sizes, on biomarkers that have the high sensitivity and specificity, and on biomarkers that show a significant correlation with cardiac parameters associated with the specific cardiovascular disease.

Table 1. List of non-coding RNAs (miRNAs, lncRNAs, and circRNAs) involved in multiple cardiovascular diseases. AS, aortic valve stenosis; MI, myocardial infarction; PH, pulmonary hypertension; TOF, tetralogy of fallot; VSD, ventricular septal defect; ASD, atrial septal defect; PDA, patent ductus arteriosus; BAV, bicuspid aortic valve disease; CAD, coronary artery disease. Arrows indicate the direction of miRNA variation: ↓ and ↑ correspond to a under-expression and over-expression of the miR.

NcRNA	Disease	Variation	Reference
miR-1	AS	↓	[29]
	MI	↑	[68]
	PH	↓	[95]
miR-150	MI	↑	[69]
	MI	↑	[72]
miR-19b	TOF	↑	[83]
	VSD	↑	[83]
	ASD	↑	[83]
	AS	↓	[34]
miR-208b	CAD	↑	[52]
	PH	↑	[95]
miR-29c	TOF	↑	[83]
	ASD	↑	[83]
	PH	↓	[95]
	VSD	↑	[83]
miR-375	TOF	↑	[83]
	ASD	↑	[83]
miR-486	MI	↑	[72]
	ASD	↑	[84]
	BAV	↑	[86]
miR-99	CAD	↓	[62]
	MI	↓	[62]
NcRNA	Disease	Variation	Reference
HOTAIR	CAD	↑	[56]
	ASD	↑	[89]
	VSD	↑	[89]
	PDA	↑	[89]
	MI	↓	[77]
	MI	↓	[75]
KCNQ1OT1	CAD	↑	[55]
	MI	↑	[77]
UCA	MI	↓	[76]
	MI	↓	[77]
NcRNA	Disease	Variation	Reference
circRNA_004183	ASD	↓	[90]
	VSD	↓	[90]
circRNA_079265	ASD	↓	[90]
	VSD	↓	[90]
circRNA_105039	ASD	↓	[90]
	VSD	↓	[90]
circRNA MICRA	MI	↓	[79]
circRNA MICRA	MI	↓	[80]

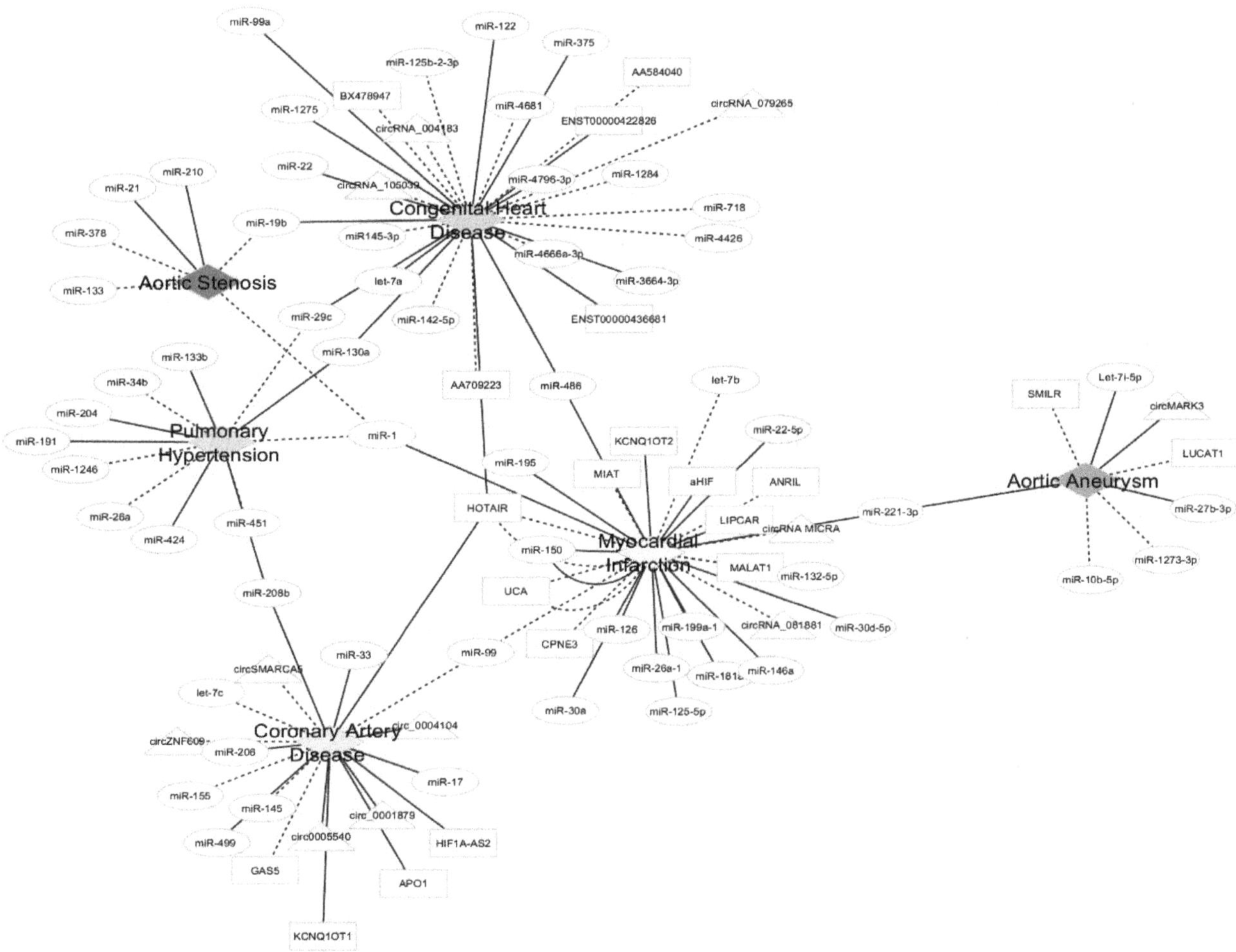

Figure 1. Illustrative cytoscape network combining the studies reported within this review. Aortic valve stenosis (red), congenital heart disease (pink), coronary artery disease (green), myocardial infarction (yellow), aortic aneurism (orange), and pulmonary hypertension (blue) are the five central nodes (diamond shape) and specific associations to ncRNAs are denoted by edges. The different ncRNAs are represented by different edges shapes: miRNAs are in circular shape, lncRNAs are in rectangular shape, and circRNAs are in triangular shape. Dashed lines represent upregulated plasma ncRNAs, while solid lines represent downregulated ncRNAs in plasma.

Author Contributions: R.F.V. drafted manuscript and drew the figure; P.A.d.C.M. and I.F.-P. approved the final version of manuscript; P.A.d.C.M. and I.F.-P. edited and revised the manuscript. All authors have read and agreed to the published version of the manuscript.

References

1. Zhao, Y.; Henein, M.Y.; Mörner, S.; Gustavsson, S.; Holmgren, A.; Lindqvist, P. Residual compromised myocardial contractile reserve after valve replacement for aortic stenosis. *Eur. Heart J. Cardiovasc. Imaging* **2011**, *13*, 353–360. [CrossRef] [PubMed]

2. Strimbu, K.; Tavel, J.A. What are biomarkers? *Curr. Opin. HIV AIDS* **2010**, *5*, 463–466. [CrossRef] [PubMed]
3. Verma, M.; Patel, P.; Verma, M. Biomarkers in Prostate Cancer Epidemiology. *Cancers* **2011**, *3*, 3773–3798. [CrossRef] [PubMed]
4. Wang, J.; Tan, G.-J.; Han, L.-N.; Bai, Y.-Y.; He, M.; Liu, H.-B. Novel biomarkers for cardiovascular risk prediction. *J. Geriatr. Cardiol.* **2017**, *14*, 135–150. [PubMed]
5. Djebali, S.; Davis, C.A.; Merkel, A.; Dobin, A.; Lassmann, T.; Mortazavi, A.; Tanzer, A.; Lagarde, J.; Lin, W.; Schlesinger, F.; et al. Landscape of transcription in human cells. *Nature* **2012**, *489*, 101–108. [CrossRef] [PubMed]
6. Lee, R.C.; Feinbaum, R.L.; Ambros, V. The C. elegans heterochronic gene lin-4 encodes small RNAs with antisense complementarity to lin-14. *Cell* **1993**, *75*, 843–854. [CrossRef]
7. Li, Z.; Rana, T.M. Therapeutic targeting of microRNAs: Current status and future challenges. *Nat. Rev. Drug Discov.* **2014**, *13*, 622–638. [CrossRef]
8. O'Brien, J.; Hayder, H.; Zayed, Y.; Peng, C. Overview of MicroRNA Biogenesis, Mechanisms of Actions, and Circulation. *Front. Endocrinol.* **2018**, *9*, 402. [CrossRef]
9. Chen, S.; Gao, G. MicroRNAs recruit eIF4E2 to repress translation of target mRNAs. *Protein Cell* **2017**, *8*, 750–761. [CrossRef]
10. Petersen, C.P.; Bordeleau, M.E.; Pelletier, J.; Sharp, P.A. Short RNAs repress translation after initiation in mammalian cells. *Mol. Cell* **2006**, *21*, 533–542. [CrossRef]
11. Humphreys, D.T.; Westman, B.J.; Martin, D.I.K.; Preiss, T. MicroRNAs control translation initiation by inhibiting eukaryotic initiation factor 4E/cap and poly(A) tail function. *Proc. Natl. Acad. Sci. USA* **2005**, *102*, 16961–16966. [CrossRef] [PubMed]
12. Tzimagiorgis, G.; Michailidou, E.Z.; Kritis, A.; Markopoulos, A.K.; Kouidou, S.; Kritis, A. Recovering circulating extracellular or cell-free RNA from bodily fluids. *Cancer Epidemiol.* **2011**, *35*, 580–589. [CrossRef] [PubMed]
13. Ulitsky, I.; Bartel, D.P. lincRNAs: Genomics, Evolution, and Mechanisms. *Cell* **2013**, *154*, 26–46. [CrossRef] [PubMed]
14. Ma, L.; Bajic, V.B.; Zhang, Z. On the classification of long non-coding RNAs. *RNA Biol.* **2013**, *10*, 924–933. [CrossRef]
15. Kim, T.K.; Hemberg, M.; Gray, J.M.; Costa, A.M.; Bear, D.M.; Wu, J.; Harmin, D.A.; Laptewicz, M.; Barbara-Haley, K.; Kuersten, S.; et al. Widespread transcription at neuronal activity-regulated enhancers. *Nature* **2010**, *465*, 182–187. [CrossRef]
16. Gupta, R.A.; Shah, N.; Wang, K.C.; Kim, J.; Horlings, H.M.; Wong, D.J.; Tsai, M.-C.; Hung, T.; Argani, P.; Rinn, J.L.; et al. Long non-coding RNA HOTAIR reprograms chromatin state to promote cancer metastasis. *Nat. Cell Biol.* **2010**, *464*, 1071–1076. [CrossRef]
17. Colognori, D.; Sunwoo, H.; Kriz, A.J.; Wang, C.-Y.; Lee, J.T. Xist Deletional Analysis Reveals an Interdependency between Xist RNA and Polycomb Complexes for Spreading along the Inactive X. *Mol. Cell* **2019**, *74*, 101–117.e10. [CrossRef]
18. Shan, Y.; Ma, J.; Pan, Y.; Hu, J.; Liu, B.; Jia, L. LncRNA SNHG7 sponges miR-216b to promote proliferation and liver metastasis of colorectal cancer through upregulating GALNT1. *Cell Death Dis.* **2018**, *9*, 1–13. [CrossRef]
19. Zhang, X.; Wang, W.; Zhu, W.; Dong, J.; Cheng, Y.; Yin, Z.; Shen, F. Mechanisms and Functions of Long Non-Coding RNAs at Multiple Regulatory Levels. *Int. J. Mol. Sci.* **2019**, *20*, 5573. [CrossRef]
20. Greene, J.; Baird, A.-M.; Brady, L.; Lim, M.; Gray, S.G.; McDermott, R.; Finn, S.P. Circular RNAs: Biogenesis, Function and Role in Human Diseases. *Front. Mol. Biosci.* **2017**, *4*, 38. [CrossRef]
21. Pamudurti, N.R.; Bartok, O.; Jens, M.; Ashwal-Fluss, R.; Stottmeister, C.; Ruhe, L.; Hanan, M.; Wyler, E.; Perez-Hernandez, D.; Ramberger, E.; et al. Translation of CircRNAs. *Mol. Cell* **2017**, *66*, 9–21.e7. [CrossRef] [PubMed]
22. Zaiou, M. circRNAs Signature as Potential Diagnostic and Prognostic Biomarker for Diabetes Mellitus and Related Cardiovascular Complications. *Cells* **2020**, *9*, 659. [CrossRef] [PubMed]
23. Li, H.; Xu, J.-D.; Fang, X.-H.; Zhu, J.-N.; Yang, J.; Pan, R.; Yuan, S.-J.; Zeng, N.; Yang, Z.-Z.; Yang, H.; et al. Circular RNA circRNA_000203 aggravates cardiac hypertrophy via suppressing miR-26b-5p and miR-140-3p binding to Gata4. *Cardiovasc. Res.* **2019**, *116*, 1323–1334. [CrossRef] [PubMed]
24. Li, Z.; Huang, C.; Bao, C.; Chen, L.; Lin, M.; Wang, X.; Zhong, G.; Yu, B.; Hu, W.; Dai, L.; et al. Exon-intron circular RNAs regulate transcription in the nucleus. *Nat. Struct. Mol. Biol.* **2015**, *22*, 256–264. [CrossRef]

25. Hang, D.; Zhou, J.; Qin, N.; Zhou, W.; Ma, H.; Jin, G.; Hu, Z.; Dai, J.; Shen, H. A novel plasma circular RNA circFARSA is a potential biomarker for non-small cell lung cancer. *Cancer Med.* **2018**, *7*, 2783–2791. [CrossRef]
26. Wang, X.; Lin, Y.K.; Lu, Z.L.; Li, J. Circular RNA circ-MTO1 serves as a novel potential diagnostic and prognostic biomarker for gallbladder cancer. *Eur. Rev. Med. Pharmacol. Sci.* **2020**, *24*, 8359–8366.
27. Ancona, R.; Comenale, S. Epidemiology of aortic valve stenosis (AS) and of aortic valve incompetence (AI): Is the prevalence of AS/AI similar in different parts of the world? *e-J. Cardiol. Pract.* **2020**, *18*. Available online: https://www.escardio.org/Journals/E-Journal-of-Cardiology-Practice/Volume-18/epidemiology-of-aortic-valve-stenosis-as-and-of-aortic-valve-incompetence-ai (accessed on 14 October 2020).
28. Hu, P.P. TAVR and SAVR: Current Treatment of Aortic Stenosis. *Clin. Med. Insights Cardiol.* **2012**, *6*, 125–139. [CrossRef]
29. Chen, Z.; Li, C.; Xu, Y.; Li, Y.; Yang, H.; Rao, L. Circulating Level of miR-378 Predicts Left Ventricular Hypertrophy in Patients with Aortic Stenosis. *PLoS ONE* **2014**, *9*, e105702. [CrossRef]
30. Røsjø, H.; Dahl, M.B.; Bye, A.; Andreassen, J.; Jørgensen, M.; Wisløff, U.; Christensen, G.; Edvardsen, T.; Omland, T. Prognostic Value of Circulating MicroRNA-210 Levels in Patients with Moderate to Severe Aortic Stenosis. *PLoS ONE* **2014**, *9*, e91812. [CrossRef]
31. Fabiani, I.; Scatena, C.; Mazzanti, C.M.; Conte, L.; Pugliese, N.R.; Franceschi, S.; Lessi, F.; Menicagli, M.; De Martino, A.; Pratali, S.; et al. Micro-RNA-21 (biomarker) and global longitudinal strain (functional marker) in detection of myocardial fibrotic burden in severe aortic valve stenosis: A pilot study. *J. Transl. Med.* **2016**, *14*, 248. [CrossRef] [PubMed]
32. Villar, A.V.; García, R.; Merino, D.; Llano, M.; Cobo, M.; Montalvo, C.; Martín-Durán, R.; Hurlé, M.A.; Nistal, J.F. Myocardial and circulating levels of microRNA-21 reflect left ventricular fibrosis in aortic stenosis patients. *Int. J. Cardiol.* **2013**, *167*, 2875–2881. [CrossRef] [PubMed]
33. Beaumont, J.; López, B.; Ravassa, S.; Hermida, N.; José, G.S.; Gallego, I.; Valencia, F.; Gómez-Doblas, J.J.; De Teresa, E.; Díez, J.; et al. MicroRNA-19b is a potential biomarker of increased myocardial collagen cross-linking in patients with aortic stenosis and heart failure. *Sci. Rep.* **2017**, *7*, 40696. [CrossRef] [PubMed]
34. Iaconetti, C.; Polimeni, A.; Sorrentino, S.; Sabatino, J.; Pironti, G.; Esposito, G.; Curcio, A.; Indolfi, C. Inhibition of miR-92a increases endothelial proliferation and migration in vitro as well as reduces neointimal proliferation in vivo after vascular injury. *Basic Res. Cardiol.* **2012**, *107*, 1–14. [CrossRef] [PubMed]
35. Lee, S.-P.; Kim, H.-K.; Kim, Y.-J.; Oh, S.; Sohn, D.-W. Association of Myocardial Angiogenesis with Structural and Functional Ventricular Remodeling in Aortic Stenosis Patients with Normal Ejection Fraction. *J. Cardiovasc. Ultrasound* **2014**, *22*, 72–79. [CrossRef]
36. Selvam, S.N.; Bowman, M.; Inglis, M.; Kloosterman, R.; Grabell, J.; Casey, L.; Johri, A.M.; James, P.D. Patients with aortic stenosis have von Willebrand factor abnormalities and increased proliferation of endothelial colony forming cells. *J. Thromb. Haemost.* **2020**, *18*, 593–603. [CrossRef]
37. Mohammadi, M.M.; AbouIssa, A.; Isyatul, A.; Xie, Y.; Cordero, J.; Shirvani, A.; Gigina, A.; Engelhardt, M.; Trogisch, F.A.; Geffers, R.; et al. Induction of cardiomyocyte proliferation and angiogenesis protects neonatal mice from pressure overload & ndash; associated maladaptation. *JCI Insight* **2019**, *4*, 5. [CrossRef]
38. Fabiani, I.; Pugliese, N.R.; Calogero, E.; Conte, L.; Mazzanti, M.C.; Scatena, C.; Scopelliti, C.; Tantillo, E.; Passiatore, M.; Angelillis, M.; et al. MicroRNAs distribution in different phenotypes of Aortic Stenosis. *Sci. Rep.* **2018**, *8*, 1–10. [CrossRef]
39. García, R.; Salido-Medina, A.B.; Gil, A.; Merino, D.; Gómez, J.; Villar, A.V.; González-Vilchez, F.; Hurlé, M.A.; Nistal, J.F. Sex-Specific Regulation of miR-29b in the Myocardium Under Pressure Overload is Associated with Differential Molecular, Structural and Functional Remodeling Patterns in Mice and Patients with Aortic Stenosis. *Cells* **2020**, *9*, 833. [CrossRef]
40. Chen, J.; Wang, J.; Jiang, Y.; Gu, W.; Ni, B.; Sun, H.; Gu, W.; Chen, L.; Shao, Y. Identification of circular RNAs in human aortic valves. *Gene* **2018**, *642*, 135–144. [CrossRef]
41. Wang, J.; Wang, Y.; Gu, W.; Ni, B.; Sun, H.; Yu, T.; Gu, W.; Chen, L.; Shao, Y. Comparative Transcriptome Analysis Reveals Substantial Tissue Specificity in Human Aortic Valve. *Evol. Bioinform.* **2016**, *12*, EBO.S37594-84. [CrossRef]
42. Mathur, A.; Mohan, V.; Ameta, D.; Gaurav, B.; Haranahalli, P. Aortic aneurysm. *J. Transl. Intern. Med.* **2016**, *4*, 35–41. [CrossRef] [PubMed]
43. Spin, J.M.; Li, D.Y.; Maegdefessel, L.; Tsao, P.S. Non-coding RNAs in aneurysmal aortopathy. *Vasc. Pharmacol.* **2019**, *114*, 110–121. [CrossRef] [PubMed]

44. Moris, D.; Mantonakis, E.; Avgerinos, E.D.; Makris, M.; Bakoyiannis, C.; Pikoulis, E.; Georgopoulos, S. Novel Biomarkers of Abdominal Aortic Aneurysm Disease: Identifying Gaps and Dispelling Misperceptions. *BioMed Res. Int.* **2014**, *2014*, 1–13. [CrossRef] [PubMed]
45. Plana, E.; Gálvez, L.; Medina, P.; Navarro, S.; Fornés-Ferrer, V.; Panadero, J.; Miralles, M. Identification of Novel microRNA Profiles Dysregulated in Plasma and Tissue of Abdominal Aortic Aneurysm Patients. *Int. J. Mol. Sci.* **2020**, *21*, 4600. [CrossRef]
46. Wanhainen, A.; Mani, K.; Vorkapic, E.; De Basso, R.; Björck, M.; Länne, T.; Wågsäter, D. Screening of circulating microRNA biomarkers for prevalence of abdominal aortic aneurysm and aneurysm growth. *Atherosclerosis* **2017**, *256*, 82–88. [CrossRef]
47. Patamsytė, V.; Žukovas, G.; Gečys, D.; Žaliaduonytė, D.; Jakuška, P.; Benetis, R.; Lesauskaitė, V. Long Noncoding RNAs CARMN, LUCAT1, SMILR, and MALAT1 in Thoracic Aortic Aneurysm: Validation of Biomarkers in Clinical Samples. *Dis. Markers* **2020**, *2020*, 1–6. [CrossRef]
48. Tian, C.; Tang, X.; Zhu, X.; Zhou, Q.; Guo, Y.; Zhao, R.; Wang, D.; Gong, B. Expression profiles of circRNAs and the potential diagnostic value of serum circMARK3 in human acute Stanford type A aortic dissection. *PLoS ONE* **2019**, *14*, e0219013. [CrossRef]
49. Boudoulas, K.D.; Triposkiadis, F.; Geleris, P.; Boudoulas, H. Coronary Atherosclerosis: Pathophysiologic Basis for Diagnosis and Management. *Prog. Cardiovasc. Dis.* **2016**, *58*, 676–692. [CrossRef]
50. Chen, J.; Xu, L.; Hu, Q.; Yang, S.; Zhang, B.; Jiang, H. MiR-17-5p as circulating biomarkers for the severity of coronary atherosclerosis in coronary artery disease. *Int. J. Cardiol.* **2015**, *197*, 123–124. [CrossRef]
51. Faccini, J.; Ruidavets, J.-B.; Cordelier, P.; Martins, F.; Maoret, J.-J.; Bongard, V.; Ferrières, J.; Roncalli, J.; Elbaz, M.; Vindis, C. Circulating miR-155, miR-145 and let-7c as diagnostic biomarkers of the coronary artery disease. *Sci. Rep.* **2017**, *7*, srep42916. [CrossRef] [PubMed]
52. Wang, W.; Li, T.; Gao, L.; Li, Y.; Sun, Y.; Yao, H.-C. Plasma miR-208b and miR-499: Potential Biomarkers for Severity of Coronary Artery Disease. *Dis. Markers* **2019**, *2019*, 1–7. [CrossRef] [PubMed]
53. Reddy, L.L.; Shah, S.A.V.; Ponde, C.K.; Rajani, R.M.; Ashavaid, T.F. Circulating miRNA-33: A potential biomarker in patients with coronary artery disease. *Biomarkers* **2018**, *24*, 36–42. [CrossRef] [PubMed]
54. Zehtabian, S.H.; Alibakhshi, R.; Seyedena, S.Y.; Rai, A.R. Relationship between microRNA-206 plasma levels with the severity of coronary artery conflicts in patients with coronary artery disease. *Bratisl. Med. J.* **2019**, *120*, 581–585. [CrossRef]
55. Zhang, Y.; Zhang, L.; Wang, Y.; Ding, H.; Xue, S.; Yu, H.; Hu, L.; Qi, H.; Wang, Y.; Zhu, W.; et al. KCNQ1OT1, HIF1A-AS2 and APOA1-AS are promising novel biomarkers for diagnosis of coronary artery disease. *Clin. Exp. Pharmacol. Physiol.* **2019**, *46*, 635–642. [CrossRef]
56. Avazpour, N.; Hajjari, M.; Yazdankhah, S.; Sahni, A.; Foroughmand, A.M. Circulating HOTAIR LncRNA Is Potentially Up-regulated in Coronary Artery Disease. *Genomics Inform.* **2018**, *16*, e25. [CrossRef]
57. Yin, Q.; Wu, A.; Liu, M. Plasma Long Non-Coding RNA (lncRNA) GAS5 is a New Biomarker for Coronary Artery Disease. *Med. Sci. Monit.* **2017**, *23*, 6042–6048. [CrossRef]
58. Vilades, D.; Martínez-Camblor, P.; Ferrero-Gregori, A.; Bär, C.; Lu, D.; Xiao, K.; Vea, À.; Nasarre, L.; Vega, J.S.; Leta, R.; et al. Plasma circular RNA hsa_circ_0001445 and coronary artery disease: Performance as a biomarker. *FASEB J.* **2020**, *34*, 4403–4414. [CrossRef]
59. Wu, W.-P.; Pan, Y.-H.; Cai, M.-Y.; Cen, J.-M.; Chen, C.; Zheng, L.; Liu, X.; Xiong, X.-D. Plasma-Derived Exosomal Circular RNA hsa_circ_0005540 as a Novel Diagnostic Biomarker for Coronary Artery Disease. *Dis. Markers* **2020**, *2020*, 1–7. [CrossRef]
60. Liang, B.; Li, M.; Deng, Q.; Wang, C.; Rong, J.; He, S.; Xiang, Y.; Zheng, F. CircRNA ZNF609 in peripheral blood leukocytes acts as a protective factor and a potential biomarker for coronary artery disease. *Ann. Transl. Med.* **2020**, *8*, 741. [CrossRef]
61. Wang, L.; Shen, C.; Wang, Y.; Zou, T.; Zhu, H.; Lu, X.; Li, L.; Yang, B.; Chen, J.; Chen, S.; et al. Identification of circular RNA Hsa_circ_0001879 and Hsa_circ_0004104 as novel biomarkers for coronary artery disease. *Atherosclerosis* **2019**, *286*, 88–96. [CrossRef] [PubMed]
62. Yang, S.-Y.; Wang, Y.-Q.; Gao, H.-M.; Wang, B.; He, Q. The clinical value of circulating miR-99a in plasma of patients with acute myocardial infarction. *Eur. Rev. Med. Pharmacol. Sci.* **2016**, *20*, 5193–5197. [PubMed]
63. Zhu, J.; Yao, K.; Wang, Q.; Guo, J.; Shi, H.; Ma, L.; Liu, H.; Gao, W.; Zou, Y.; Ge, J. Circulating miR-181a as a Potential Novel Biomarker for Diagnosis of Acute Myocardial Infarction. *Cell. Physiol. Biochem.* **2016**, *40*, 1591–1602. [CrossRef] [PubMed]

64. Garvey, J.L.; Zegre-Hemsey, J.; Gregg, R.; Studnek, J.R. Electrocardiographic diagnosis of ST segment elevation myocardial infarction: An evaluation of three automated interpretation algorithms. *J. Electrocardiol.* **2016**, *49*, 728–732. [CrossRef]
65. Long, G.; Wang, F.; Duan, Q.; Yang, S.; Chen, F.; Gong, W.; Yang, X.; Wang, Y.; Chen, C.; Wang, D.W. Circulating miR-30a, miR-195 and let-7b Associated with Acute Myocardial Infarction. *PLoS ONE* **2012**, *7*, e50926. [CrossRef]
66. Xue, S.; Zhu, W.; Liu, D.; Su, Z.; Zhang, L.; Chang, Q.; Li, P. Circulating miR-26a-1, miR-146a and miR-199a-1 are potential candidate biomarkers for acute myocardial infarction. *Mol. Med.* **2019**, *25*, 18. [CrossRef]
67. Hu, H.; Yuan, H.; Li, C.; Yu, H.; Chen, Y. Association of Gene Polymorphisms in the Human MicroRNA-126 Gene with Plasma-Circulating MicroRNA-126 Levels and Acute Myocardial Infarction. *Genet. Test. Mol. Biomarkers* **2019**, *23*, 460–467. [CrossRef]
68. Zhang, R.; Niu, H.; Ban, T.; Xu, L.; Li, Y.; Wang, N.; Sun, L.; Ai, J.; Yang, B. Elevated plasma microRNA-1 predicts heart failure after acute myocardial infarction. *Int. J. Cardiol.* **2013**, *166*, 259–260. [CrossRef]
69. Li, H.; Zhang, P.; Li, F.; Yuan, G.; Wang, X.; Zhang, A.; Li, F. Plasma miR-22-5p, miR-132-5p, and miR-150-3p Are Associated with Acute Myocardial Infarction. *BioMed Res. Int.* **2019**, *2019*, 1–13. [CrossRef]
70. Jia, K.; Shi, P.; Han, X.; Chen, T.; Tang, H.; Wang, J. Diagnostic value of miR-30d-5p and miR-125b-5p in acute myocardial infarction. *Mol. Med. Rep.* **2016**, *14*, 184–194. [CrossRef]
71. Coskunpinar, E.; Cakmak, H.A.; Kalkan, A.K.; Tiryakioglu, N.O.; Erturk, M.; Ongen, Z. Circulating miR-221-3p as a novel marker for early prediction of acute myocardial infarction. *Gene* **2016**, *591*, 90–96. [CrossRef] [PubMed]
72. Zhang, R.; Lan, C.; Pei, H.; Duan, G.; Huang, L.; Li, L. Expression of circulating miR-486 and miR-150 in patients with acute myocardial infarction. *BMC Cardiovasc. Disord.* **2015**, *15*, 51. [CrossRef] [PubMed]
73. Savoye, C.; Equine, O.; Tricot, O.; Nugue, O.; Segrestin, B.; Sautière, K.; Elkohen, M.; Pretorian, E.M.; Taghipour, K.; Philias, A.; et al. Left Ventricular Remodeling After Anterior Wall Acute Myocardial Infarction in Modern Clinical Practice (from the REmodelage VEntriculaire [REVE] Study Group). *Am. J. Cardiol.* **2006**, *98*, 1144–1149. [CrossRef] [PubMed]
74. Maciejak, A.; Kostarska-Srokosz, E.; Gierlak, W.; Dluzniewski, M.; Kuch, M.; Marchel, M.; Opolski, G.; Kiliszek, M.; Matlak, K.; Dobrzycki, S.; et al. Circulating miR-30a-5p as a prognostic biomarker of left ventricular dysfunction after acute myocardial infarction. *Sci. Rep.* **2018**, *8*, 1–11. [CrossRef]
75. Gao, L.; Liu, Y.; Guo, S.; Yao, R.; Wu, L.; Xiao, L.; Wang, Z.; Liu, Y.; Zhang, Y. Circulating Long Noncoding RNA HOTAIR is an Essential Mediator of Acute Myocardial Infarction. *Cell. Physiol. Biochem.* **2017**, *44*, 1497–1508. [CrossRef]
76. Yan, Y.; Zhang, B.; Liu, N.; Qi, C.; Xiao, Y.; Tian, X.; Li, T.; Liu, B. Circulating Long Noncoding RNA UCA1 as a Novel Biomarker of Acute Myocardial Infarction. *BioMed Res. Int.* **2016**, *2016*, 1–7. [CrossRef]
77. Li, M.; Wang, Y.-F.; Yang, X.-C.; Xu, L.; Li, W.-M.; Xia, K.; Zhang, D.-P.; Wu, R.-N.; Gan, T. Circulating Long Noncoding RNA LIPCAR Acts as a Novel Biomarker in Patients with ST-Segment Elevation Myocardial Infarction. *Med. Sci. Monit.* **2018**, *24*, 5064–5070. [CrossRef]
78. Deng, Y.-Y.; Zhang, W.; She, J.; Zhang, L.; Chen, T.; Zhou, J.; Yuan, Z. GW27-e1167 Circular RNA Related to PPARγ Function as ceRNA of microRNA in Human Acute Myocardial Infarction. *J. Am. Coll. Cardiol.* **2016**, *68*, C51–C52. [CrossRef]
79. Salgado-Somoza, A.; Zhang, L.; Vausort, M.; Devaux, Y. The circular RNA MICRA for risk stratification after myocardial infarction. *IJC Heart Vasc.* **2017**, *17*, 33–36. [CrossRef]
80. Vausort, M.; Salgado-Somoza, A.; Zhang, L.; Leszek, P.; Scholz, M.; Teren, A.; Burkhardt, R.; Thiery, J.; Wagner, D.R.; Devaux, Y. Myocardial Infarction-Associated Circular RNA Predicting Left Ventricular Dysfunction. *J. Am. Coll. Cardiol.* **2016**, *68*, 1247–1248. [CrossRef]
81. Xie, N.; Wang, H.; Liu, Z.; Fang, J.; Yang, T.; Zhou, S.; Wang, A.; Qin, J.; Xiong, L. Perinatal outcomes and congenital heart defect prognosis in 53313 non-selected perinatal infants. *PLoS ONE* **2017**, *12*, e0177229. [CrossRef] [PubMed]
82. Gu, M.; Zheng, A.; Tu, W.; Zhao, J.; Li, L.; Li, M.; Han, S.-P.; Hu, X.; Zhu, J.; Pan, Y.; et al. Circulating LncRNAs as Novel, Non-Invasive Biomarkers for Prenatal Detection of Fetal Congenital Heart Defects. *Cell. Physiol. Biochem.* **2016**, *38*, 1459–1471. [CrossRef] [PubMed]

83. Zhu, S.; Cao, L.; Zhu, J.; Kong, L.; Jin, J.; Qian, L.; Zhu, C.; Hu, X.; Li, M.; Guo, X.; et al. Identification of maternal serum microRNAs as novel non-invasive biomarkers for prenatal detection of fetal congenital heart defects. *Clin. Chim. Acta* **2013**, *424*, 66–72. [CrossRef] [PubMed]
84. Song, Y.; Higgins, H.; Guo, J.; Harrison, K.; Schultz, E.N.; Hales, B.J.; Moses, E.K.; Goldblatt, J.; Pachter, N.; Zhang, G. Clinical significance of circulating microRNAs as markers in detecting and predicting congenital heart defects in children. *J. Transl. Med.* **2018**, *16*, 1–11. [CrossRef] [PubMed]
85. Girdauskas, E.; Petersen, J.; Neumann, N.; Naito, S.; Gross, T.; Jagodzinski, A.; Reichenspurner, H.; Zeller, T. Novel Approaches for BAV Aortopathy Prediction—Is There a Need for Cohort Studies and Biomarkers? *Biomolecules* **2018**, *8*, 58. [CrossRef] [PubMed]
86. Martínez-Micaelo, N.; Beltrán-Debón, R.; Baiges, I.; Faiges, M.; Alegret, J.M. Specific circulating microRNA signature of bicuspid aortic valve disease. *J. Transl. Med.* **2017**, *15*, 1–12. [CrossRef] [PubMed]
87. Gu, H.; Chen, L.; Xue, J.; Huang, T.; Wei, X.; Liu, D.; Ma, W.; Cao, S.; Yuan, Z. Expression profile of maternal circulating microRNAs as non-invasive biomarkers for prenatal diagnosis of congenital heart defects. *Biomed. Pharmacother.* **2019**, *109*, 823–830. [CrossRef]
88. Kehler, L.; Biro, O.; Lazar, L.; Rigo, J.; Nagy, B. Elevated hsa-miR-99a levels in maternal plasma may indicate congenital heart defects. *BioMed Rep.* **2015**, *3*, 869–873. [CrossRef]
89. Jiang, Y.; Mo, H.; Luo, J.; Zhao, S.; Liang, S.; Zhang, M.; Yuan, J. HOTAIR Is a Potential Novel Biomarker in Patients with Congenital Heart Diseases. *BioMed Res. Int.* **2018**, *2018*, 1–7. [CrossRef]
90. Wu, J.; Li, J.; Liu, H.; Yin, J.; Zhang, M.; Yu, Z.; Miao, H. Circulating plasma circular RNAs as novel diagnostic biomarkers for congenital heart disease in children. *J. Clin. Lab. Anal.* **2019**, *33*, e22998. [CrossRef]
91. Friedberg, M.K.; Redington, A.N. Right versus left ventricular failure: Differences, similarities, and interactions. *Circulation* **2014**, *129*, 1033–1044. [CrossRef] [PubMed]
92. Lang, I.M. Management of acute and chronic RV dysfunction. *Eur. Heart J. Suppl.* **2007**, *9*, H61–H67. [CrossRef]
93. Ibrahim, B.S. Right ventricular failure. *EJ Cardiol. Pract.* **2016**, *14*, 32.
94. Sommariva, E.; D'Alessandra, Y.; Farina, F.M.; Casella, M.; Cattaneo, F.; Catto, V.; Chiesa, M.; Stadiotti, I.; Brambilla, S.; Russo, A.D.; et al. MiR-320a as a Potential Novel Circulating Biomarker of Arrhythmogenic CardioMyopathy. *Sci. Rep.* **2017**, *7*, 1–10. [CrossRef] [PubMed]
95. Wei, C.; Henderson, H.; Spradley, C.; Li, L.; Kim, I.-K.; Kumar, S.; Hong, N.; Arroliga, A.C.; Gupta, S. Circulating miRNAs as Potential Marker for Pulmonary Hypertension. *PLoS ONE* **2013**, *8*, e64396. [CrossRef]
96. Song, X.-W.; Zou, L.-L.; Cui, L.; Li, S.-H.; Qin, Y.-W.; Zhao, X.-X.; Jing, Q. Plasma miR-451 with echocardiography serves as a diagnostic reference for pulmonary hypertension. *Acta Pharmacol. Sin.* **2018**, *39*, 1208–1216. [CrossRef] [PubMed]
97. Baptista, R.; Marques, C.; Catarino, S.; Enguita, F.J.; Costa, M.C.; Matafome, P.; Zuzarte, M.; Castro, G.; Reis, A.; Monteiro, P.; et al. MicroRNA-424(322) as a new marker of disease progression in pulmonary arterial hypertension and its role in right ventricular hypertrophy by targeting SMURF1. *Cardiovasc. Res.* **2018**, *114*, 53–64. [CrossRef]
98. Puls, M.; Beuthner, B.E.; Topci, R.; Vogelgesang, A.; Bleckmann, A.; Sitte, M.; Lange, T.; Backhaus, S.J.; Schuster, A.; Seidler, T.; et al. Impact of myocardial fibrosis on left ventricular remodelling, recovery, and outcome after transcatheter aortic valve implantation in different haemodynamic subtypes of severe aortic stenosis. *Eur. Heart J.* **2020**, *41*, 1903–1914. [CrossRef]
99. Rodrigues, P.G.; Leite-Moreira, A.; Falcao-Pires, I. Myocardial reverse remodeling: How far can we rewind? *Am. J. Physiol. Circ. Physiol.* **2016**, *310*, H1402–H1422. [CrossRef]
100. Kitai, T.; Grodin, J.L.; Mentz, R.J.; Hernandez, A.F.; Butler, J.; Metra, M.; McMurray, J.J.; Armstrong, P.W.; Starling, R.C.; O'Connor, C.M.; et al. Insufficient reduction in heart rate during hospitalization despite beta-blocker treatment in acute decompensated heart failure: Insights from the ASCEND-HF trial. *Eur. J. Heart Fail.* **2016**, *19*, 241–249. [CrossRef]
101. Schmid, F.; Schlager, O.; Keller, P.; Seifert, B.; Huang, R.; Fröhlich, G.M.; Lüscher, T.F.; Ruschitzka, F.; Enseleit, F. Prognostic value of long-term blood pressure changes in patients with chronic heart failure. *Eur. J. Heart Fail.* **2017**, *19*, 837–842. [CrossRef] [PubMed]
102. Abraham, W.T.; Fisher, W.G.; Smith, A.L.; Delurgio, D.B.; Leon, A.R.; Loh, E.; Kocovic, D.Z.; Packer, M.; Clavell, A.L.; Hayes, D.L.; et al. Cardiac Resynchronization in Chronic Heart Failure. *N. Engl. J. Med.* **2002**, *346*, 1845–1853. [CrossRef] [PubMed]

103. García, R.; Villar, A.V.; Cobo, M.; Llano, M.; Martín-Durán, R.; Hurlé, M.A.; Nistal, J.F. Circulating Levels of miR-133a Predict the Regression Potential of Left Ventricular Hypertrophy After Valve Replacement Surgery in Patients With Aortic Stenosis. *J. Am. Heart Assoc.* **2013**, *2*, e000211. [CrossRef] [PubMed]
104. Miyamoto, S.; Usami, S.; Kuwabara, Y.; Horie, T.; Baba, O.; Hakuno, D.; Nakashima, Y.; Nishiga, M.; Izuhara, M.; Nakao, T.; et al. Expression Patterns of miRNA-423-5p in the Serum and Pericardial Fluid in Patients Undergoing Cardiac Surgery. *PLoS ONE* **2015**, *10*, e0142904. [CrossRef] [PubMed]
105. Shah, R.; Ziegler, O.; Yeri, A.; Liu, X.; Murthy, V.; Rabideau, D.; Xiao, C.Y.; Hanspers, K.; Belcher, A.; Tackett, M.; et al. MicroRNAs Associated With Reverse Left Ventricular Remodeling in Humans Identify Pathways of Heart Failure Progression. *Circ. Heart Fail.* **2018**, *11*, e004278. [CrossRef]
106. Zhang, Z.; Gao, W.; Long, Q.-Q.; Zhang, J.; Lian-Sheng, W.; Liu, D.-C.; Yan, J.-J.; Yang, Z.-J.; Wang, L.-S. Increased plasma levels of lncRNA H19 and LIPCAR are associated with increased risk of coronary artery disease in a Chinese population. *Sci. Rep.* **2017**, *7*, 1–9. [CrossRef] [PubMed]
107. Santer, L.; López, B.; Ravassa, S.; Baer, C.; Riedel, I.; Chatterjee, S.; Moreno, M.U.; González, A.; Querejeta, R.; Pinet, F.; et al. Circulating Long Noncoding RNA LIPCAR Predicts Heart Failure Outcomes in Patients Without Chronic Kidney Disease. *Hypertension* **2019**, *73*, 820–828. [CrossRef]
108. Zhang, L.-E.; Wu, Y.-J.; Zhang, S.-L. Circulating lncRNA MHRT predicts survival of patients with chronic heart failure. *J. Geriatr. Cardiol.* **2019**, *16*, 818–821.
109. Cassese, S.; Byrne, R.A.; Tada, T.; Pinieck, S.; Joner, M.; Ibrahim, T.; King, L.A.; Fusaro, M.; Laugwitz, K.-L.; Kastrati, A. Incidence and predictors of restenosis after coronary stenting in 10 004 patients with surveillance angiography. *Heart* **2014**, *100*, 153–159. [CrossRef]
110. Wang, F.; Su, X.; Liu, C.; Wu, M.; Li, B. Prognostic Value of Plasma Long Noncoding RNA ANRIL for In-Stent Restenosis. *Med. Sci. Monit.* **2017**, *23*, 4733–4739. [CrossRef]
111. Viereck, J.; Thum, T. Circulating Noncoding RNAs as Biomarkers of Cardiovascular Disease and Injury. *Circ. Res.* **2017**, *120*, 381–399. [CrossRef] [PubMed]

3

Growth Differentiation Factor-15 (GDF-15) is a Biomarker of Muscle Wasting and Renal Dysfunction in Preoperative Cardiovascular Surgery Patients

Toshiaki Nakajima [1,*], Ikuko Shibasaki [2], Tatsuya Sawaguchi [1], Akiko Haruyama [1], Hiroyuki Kaneda [1], Takafumi Nakajima [1], Takaaki Hasegawa [1], Takuo Arikawa [1], Syotaro Obi [1], Masashi Sakuma [1], Hironaga Ogawa [2], Shigeru Toyoda [1], Fumitaka Nakamura [3], Shichiro Abe [1], Hirotsugu Fukuda [2] and Teruo Inoue [1]

1. Department of Cardiovascular Medicine, School of Medicine, Dokkyo Medical University, Shimotsuga-gun, Tochigi 321-0293, Japan; tswg0814@gmail.com (T.S.); hal@dokkyomed.ac.jp (A.H.); hirokane1010@gmail.com (H.K.); sho-taka.07@softbank.ne.jp (T.N.); thasegawa6134@gmail.com (T.H.); takuoari@dokkyomed.ac.jp (T.A.); syoutarouobi@yahoo.co.jp (S.O.); masakuma@dokkyomed.ac.jp (M.S.); s-toyoda@dokkyomed.ac.jp (S.T.); abenana@dokkyomed.ac.jp (S.A.); inouet@dokkyomed.ac.jp (T.I.)
2. Department of Cardiovascular Surgery, School of Medicine, Dokkyo Medical University, Shimotsuga-gun, Tochigi 321-0293, Japan; sibasaki@dokkyomed.ac.jp (I.S.); hironaga_0722@yahoo.co.jp (H.O.); fukuda-h@dokkyomed.ac.jp (H.F.)
3. Third Department of Internal Medicine, Teikyo University, Chiba Medical Center, Ichihara, Chiba 299-0111, Japan; fumitaka@med.teikyo-u.ac.jp

* Correspondence: nakat@dokkyomed.ac.jp

Abstract: Frailty and sarcopenia increase the risk of complications and mortality when invasive treatment such as cardiac surgery is performed. Growth differentiation factor-15 (GDF-15) involves various pathophysiological conditions including renal dysfunction, heart failure and cachexia. We investigated the pathophysiological roles of preoperative GDF-15 levels in cardiovascular surgery patients. Preoperative skeletal muscle index (SMI) determined by bioelectrical impedance analysis, hand-grip strength, 4 m gait speed, and anterior thigh muscle thickness (TMth) measured by echocardiography were assessed in 72 patients (average age 69.9 years) who underwent cardiovascular surgery. The preoperative serum GDF-15 concentration was determined by enzyme-linked immunosorbent assay. Circulating GDF-15 level was correlated with age, brain natriuretic peptide, and estimated glomerular filtration rate (eGFR). It was also negatively correlated with SMI, hand-grip strength, and anterior TMth. In multivariate analysis, eGFR and anterior TMth were the independent determinants of GDF-15 concentration even after adjusting for age, sex, and body mass index. Alternatively, the GDF-15 level was an independent determinant of eGFR and anterior TMth. We concluded that preoperative GDF-15 levels reflect muscle wasting as well as renal dysfunction in preoperative cardiovascular surgery patients. GDF-15 may be a novel biomarker for identify high-risk patients with muscle wasting and renal dysfunction before cardiovascular surgery.

Keywords: GDF-15; cardiovascular surgery; operative risk; biomarkers; muscle wasting; sarcopenia; renal dysfunction; chronic kidney disease

---

1. Introduction

As life expectancy has increased, the number of older patients undergoing cardiovascular surgery has also increased, and many such patients have frailty. Frailty is a geriatric syndrome described as decreased reserves when confronted with stressors, which is associated with poor outcomes in both community cohorts and patients [1,2]. In cardiovascular surgery such as transcatheter valve implantation (TAVI), frailty is now identified as an important predictor of adverse outcomes in older patients [1,3,4]. Patients with higher frailty are at increased risk during the postoperative period, with long hospital stays, and postoperative complications such as stroke and death, compared to those with lower frailty [5]. Sarcopenia, the skeletal muscle loss associated with aging, also includes low physical function (hand-grip strength, walking speed) as a component of frailty [6,7]. It is frequently associated with chronic diseases including heart failure, chronic kidney disease (CKD), cancer, wasting, and cachexia [7]. Thus, it is generally accepted that frailty and sarcopenia, as well as physical function are predictors of survival in patients with cardiovascular diseases (CVD), and they increase the risk of complications and mortality when invasive treatments such as cardiovascular operations are performed. Therefore, it is quite important to identify high-risk patients with frailty and sarcopenia before cardiovascular surgery.

Growth differentiation fator-15 (GDF-15) is not highly expressed in most tissues under normal physiological conditions [8,9], but it increases under various pathophysiological conditions such as inflammation [10], oxidant stress [11], and ischemia/reperfusion [12]. Clinical trials reported that GDF-15 is a reliable biomarker of CVD [13–15], and heart failure [16], and it has independent prognostic value in patients with coronary artery bypass grafting (CABG) [17], acute coronary syndromes (ACS) [18,19], and heart failure (HF) [20]. In addition, it has been reported that GDF-15 is a novel serum biomarker of mortality in CKD, and can identify patients at high risk of developing CKD [21–23]. The preoperative GDF-15 level has been also reported to be a novel risk biomarker in association with the EuroSCORE for risk stratification independently of N-terminal pro-B-type natriuretic peptide (NTproBNP) and high-sensitive troponin T [24], and closely related to post-operative morbidity in cardiovascular surgery patients including those undergoing TAVI [25,26]. Furthermore, it has been reported to reflect post-operative acute kidney injury (AKI) in patients undergoing CABG [27] and myocardial injury in patients undergoing off-pump CABG [28]. Thus, GDF-15 appears to be a novel biomarker to identify surgical risk in patients undergoing cardiovascular surgery.

Circulating GDF-15 levels increase with age [20,22], and may partly reflect mitochondrial dysfunction in aging and age-related diseases [29]. Furthermore, several papers showed that GDF-15 may be involved in muscle wasting in a variety of patients including COPD [30], patients undergoing elective high-risk cardiothoracic surgery [31], intensive care unit (ICU) patients [32], and cancer patients [33]. Bloch et al. [31] showed that an elevation of postoperative GDF-15 levels is a potential factor associated with muscle atrophy in patients undergoing cardiovascular surgery. However, the physiological significance of the preoperative GDF-15 level in patients undergoing cardiovascular surgery still remains to be clarified.

Therefore, we investigated the pathophysiological roles of preoperative GDF-15 levels in cardiovascular surgery patients. We provided the first evidence that GDF-15 may be a novel biomarker for identifying high-risk patients with muscle wasting and renal dysfunction, compared with tumor necrosis factor α (TNFα) or insulin growth factor-1 (IGF-1) in cardiovascular surgery patients.

2. Methods

2.1. Participants

A total of 72 preoperative patients (42 males, 30 females) undergoing cardiovascular surgery at Dokkyo Medical Hospital were recruited in this study. The patient characteristics are summarized in Table 1. The mean age was 69.9 ± 13.1 years (23–89 years), and body mass index (BMI) was 24.3 ± 3.9 kg/m^2. Most of the patients had conventional risk factors such as hypertension (HT), diabetes (DM), hyperlipidemia (HL), current smoking, and hemodialysis (HD) as shown in Table 1. The average preoperative New York Heart Association (NYHA) classification was 2.2 ± 1.0. Table 1 also shows the number of patients classified by surgical procedures for cardiovascular disease. The study was approved by the Ethics Committee of the Dokkyo Medical University (No. 27077), and informed consents were obtained from all participants.

Table 1. Patient Characteristics.

Number	72
Male, Female	42, 30
Age, y	69.9 ± 13.1
BMI, kg/m^2	24.3 ± 3.9
Risk factors (percentage)	
Hypertension	75
Diabetes	35
Dyslipidemia	46
Smoking	11
Hemodialysis	8
NYHA classification	2.2 ± 1.0
Coronary artery disease (percentage)	
0-vessel disease	53
1-vessel disease	11
2-vessel disease	6
3-vessel disease	30
Cardiovascular surgery (percentage)	
CABG	26
AVR	21
Other valve replacement/repair (MVR, MVP, TAP, TAR, LAAAC)	17
CABG combined with valve replacement/repair (AVR, MVP, TAP)	8
AVR combined with other valve (MVP, TAP, LAAC) or aortic diseases (TAR)	11
Aortic disease (TAR, TEVAR, et al.)	7
Others	10
Drugs (percentage)	
β-blockers	49
Ca-blockers	38
ACE-I/ARB	58
Diuretics	49
Statins	53
Oral antidiabetic drugs	31
Insulin	8

The mean ± SD values are shown. BMI, body mass index; NYHA, New York Heart Association; CABG, coronary artery bypass grafting; AVR, aortic valve replacement; MVR, mitral valve replacement; MVP, mitral valve plasty; TAP, tricuspid annuloplasty; LAAC, left atrial appendage closure; TAR, total arch replacement; TEVAR, thoracic endovascular aortic repair; ACE-I, angiotensin converting enzyme inhibitors; ARB, angiotensin II receptor blockers; Oral anti-diabetic drugs included α-glucosidase inhibitors, sulfonylurea, biguanide, dipeptidyl peptidase-4 inhibitors, and sodium glucose cotransporter 2 inhibitors.

The biochemical data were analyzed using routine chemical methods in Dokkyo Medical University Hospital clinical laboratory. Hemoglobin A1c (HbA1c), brain natriuretic peptide (BNP), and estimated glomerular filtration rate (eGFR) were measured before the operation. The eGFR was calculated by the following equations:

$$\text{Males: eGFR (mL/min/1.73m}^2\text{)} = 194\ (\text{creatinine}^{-1.094})\ (\text{age}^{-0.287})$$

$$\text{Females: eGFR (mL/min/1.73m}^2\text{)} = 0.739\ \{194(\text{creatinine}^{-1.094})\ (\text{age}^{-0.287})\}$$

The high-sensitivity C-reactive protein (hsCRP) was measured by a latex-enhanced nephelometric immunoassay (N Latex CRP II and N Latex SAA, Dade Behring Ltd., Tokyo, Japan). The homeo-static model assessment of insulin resistance (HOMA-IR), which indicates an index of insulin resistance, was calculated from the fasting blood insulin (immunoreactive insulin (IRI)) concentration and the fasting blood glucose (FBS) level early in the morning, based on the following equation.

$$\text{HOMA-IR} = (\text{IRI})\ (\text{FBS})/405$$

To measure fasting serum GDF-15, TNFα, and IGF-1 levels, peripheral venous blood was drawn into pyrogen-free tubes with and without EDTA on the morning of cardiovascular surgery. Plasma and serum were stored in aliquots at −80 °C for all enzyme linked immunosorbent assay (ELISA).

2.2. Enzyme Linked Immunosorbent Assay (ELISA)

Serum GDF-15 level was measured by a Human Quantikine ELISA Kit (DGD150 for GDF-15, R&D Systems, Minneapolis, MN, USA). Samples, reagents, and buffers were prepared according to the manufacturers' manuals. The detection threshold of GDF-15 was 2.0 pg/mL. The serum concentrations of TNFα were measured by a Human Quantikine HS ELISA Kit (HSTA00E, R&D Systems, Minneapolis, MN, USA), and the detection threshold was 0.022 pg/mL. The serum IGF-1 concentration was measured by a Human Quantikine ELISA Kit (DG100, R&D Systems), and the detection threshold was 0.026 ng/mL.

2.3. Measurement of Gait Speed, Hand-Grip Strength, and Voluntary Isometric Contraction

Maximum voluntary isometric contraction (MVIC) of the hand-grip was measured by using a factory-calibrated hand dynamometer (TKK 5401, TAKEI Scientific Instruments Co., Ltd., Tokyo, Japan). Each patient performed two trials, and the highest value was adopted for analysis. The gait speed was measured as the time needed to walk 4 m at an ordinary pace. MVIC of the knee extensors was measured by using a digital handheld dynamometer (μTas MT-1, ANIMA Co., Ltd., Tokyo, Japan) as described previously [34]. Each subject performed two trials, and the highest score was adopted for analysis.

2.4. Measurements with the Bioelectrical Impedance Analyzer (BIA)

A multi-frequency bioelectrical impedance analyzer (BIA), InBody S10 Biospace device (Biospacte Co, Ltd., Korea/Model JMW140) was used to measure muscle and fat volume as described in detail previously [34]. Thirty impedance measurements were performed using 6 different frequencies (1, 5, 50, 250, 500, and 1000 kHz) at the five segments of the body (right arm, left arm, trunk, right leg, and left leg). The measurements were performed while the subjects rested in the supine position, with their elbows extended and relaxed along their trunk. Body fat volume, body fat percentage, and skeletal muscle volume were measured. Skeletal muscle mass index (SMI; appendicular skeletal muscle mass/height^2, kg/m^2) was also calculated as the sum of lean soft tissue of the two upper limbs and two lower limbs. In this study, sarcopenia was defined according to the Asian Working Group for Sarcopenia (AWGS) [7] criteria (age ≥ 65 years; handgrip < 26 kg or gait speed ≤ 0.8 m/s, and SMI < 7.0 kg/m^2 for males; handgrip < 18 kg or gait speed ≤ 0.8 m/s, and SMI < 5.7 kg/m^2 for females.

2.5. Measurement of Muscle Thickness by Ultrasound

The anterior mid-thigh muscle thickness was measured on the right leg using a real-time linear electronic scanner with a 10.0-MHz scanning head and Ultrasound Probe (L4–12t-RS Probe, GE Healthcare Japan, Tokyo, Japan) and LOGIQ e ultrasound (GE Healthcare Japan), as previously described [34]. From the ultrasonic image, the subcutaneous adipose tissue-muscle interface and the muscle-bone interface were identified. The perpendicular distance from the adipose tissue-muscle interface to the muscle-bone interface was considered to represent the anterior thigh muscle thickness (TMth). The measurement was performed twice in both the supine and standing positions, and the average value was adopted for analysis.

2.6. Statistical Analysis

Data are presented as mean value ± SD. After testing for normality (Kolmogorov-Smirnov), the comparison of means between groups was analyzed by a two-sided, unpaired Student's *t*-test in the case of normally distributed parameters or by the Mann-Whitney-U-Test in the case of non-normally distributed parameters. Associations among parameters were evaluated using Pearson or Spearman correlation coefficients. Multiple linear regression analysis with log (serum GDF-15 concentration), eGFR, or anterior TMth as the dependent variable was performed to identify the independent factors (clinical laboratory data, or physical data) that influenced these dependent variables. Age, sex, and BMI were employed as covariates. When the independent data were not normally distributed, the data were logarithmically transformed to achieve a normal distribution. Receiver operating characteristic (ROC) curves were plotted to identify an optimal cut-off level of the serum concentration of GDF-15 for detecting impaired eGFR. All analyses were performed using SPSS version 24 for Windows (IBM Corp., New York, NY, USA). A p value less than 0.05 was regarded as significant.

3. Results

3.1. Patient Characteristics

All patients had medical treatment including β-blocking agents (49%), calcium-channel blockers (38%), angiotensin receptor blockers (ARB)-/-angiotensin converting enzyme inhibitors (ACEI) (58%), diuretics (49%), statins (53%), and anti-diabetic drugs (31%) (Table 1).

The sex differences of the study patients are shown in Table 2. The mean age of females was significantly higher than that of males ($p < 0.05$). The BMI value was not different between males and females, but body fat percentage (%) in females was significantly higher, compared with that in men ($p < 0.05$).

Table 2. Sex differences in various parameters.

	Total (n = 72)	Male (n = 42)	Female (n = 30)
Age, years	69.9 (13.1)	66.9 (14.4)	73.7 (10.0) *
BMI, kg/m^2	24.3 (3.9)	24.9 (4.5)	24.7 (5.5)
NYHA classification	2.2 (1.0)	2.3 (1.1)	2.1 (0.9)
Gait speed, m/s	0.93 (0.32)	0.99 (0.34)	0.86 (0.28)
Hand-grip strength, kgf	22.8 (8.5)	27.1 (7.9)	16.5 (4.6) ***
Knee extension strength, kgf	20.8 (9.5)	24.4 (9.3)	15.6 (7.1) ***
Body fat percentage, %	32.3 (9.3)	28.4 (7.8)	37.6 (8.7) ***
Skeletal muscle mass index (SMI), kg/m^2	6.5 (1.4)	7.2 (1.3)	5.4 (0.9) ***
Anterior thigh muscle thickness (TMth) (supine), cm	2.28 (0.75)	2.41 (0.80)	2.1 (0.6)
Anterior thigh muscle thickness (TMth) (standing), cm	3.47 (0.95)	3.68 (0.97)	3.2 (0.9) *
HbA1c, %	6.2 (0.9)	6.3 (1.0)	6.0 (0.8)
BNP, pg/mL	355 (570)	399 (673)	268 (345)
eGFR, ml/min/1.73 m^2	58.2 (24.0)	55.7 (26.6)	63.4 (19.3)
Hb, g/dL	12.2 (1.8)	12.3 (1.9)	11.9 (1.7)
HOMA-IR	2.75 (4.20)	3.46 (5.29)	1.64 (1.29)
hsCRP, mg/L	5.9 (12)	7.4 (13.8)	3.3 (7.9)
GDF-15, pg/mL	1676 (1465)	1928 (1655)	1325 (1078)
TNFα, pg/mL	3.5 (2.8)	4.1 (2.9)	2.6 (1.9) *
IGF-1, ng/mL	74.4 (33.4)	77.3 (36.5)	70.4 (28.5)

* $p < 0.05$. *** $p < 0.001$. Males vs. Females hsCRP, high sensitivity C-reactive protein; BNP, brain natriuretic peptide; eGFR, estimate glomerular filtration rate; HOMA-IR, Homeostasis model assessment of insulin resistance; GDF-15, growth differentiation factor-15; TNFα, tissue necrosis factor α; IGF-1, insulin growth factor-1.

The hand-grip strength, knee extension strength, and SMI in females were significantly lower than those in males. The anterior TMth (standing) in males was significantly higher, compared with that in females ($p < 0.05$). The BNP level was not different between males and females (399 ± 673 pg/mL vs. 268 ± 345 pg/mL). The mean eGFR of all the patients was 58.2 ± 24.0 mL/min/1.73 m^2. Furthermore, patients were classified into five groups based on the eGFR levels: normal (eGFR ≥ 90 mL/min/1.73 m^2), low (eGFR 60–89 mL/min/1.73 m^2), moderate (eGFR 30–59 mL/min/1.73 m^2), severe (eGFR 15–29 mL/min/1.73 m^2), and kidney failure (eGFR < 15 mL/min/1.73 m^2). Among total 72 patients, there were 3 patients (normal), 36 patients (low),

25 patients (moderate), 2 patients (severe), and 6 patients (kidney failure). Therefore, the overall prevalence of CKD (eGFR < 60 mL/min/1.73 m^2) was 33 patients out of 72 (44%). The serum TNFα level was 3.5 ± 2.8 pg/mL in all of the patients. It was higher in males than in females (males, 4.1 ± 2.9 pg/mL; females, 2.6 ± 1.9 pg/mL, $p < 0.05$). The serum GDF-15 level did not significantly differ between males and females (males, 1928 ± 1655 pg/mL; females, 1325 ± 1078 pg/mL). The serum IGF-1 concentration also did not significantly differ between males and females (males, 77.3 ± 36.5 ng/mL; females, 70.4 ± 28.5 pg/mL).

3.2. Correlation between Various Parameters and Serum GDF-15, TNFα, and IGF-1 Concentration

The correlations between serum GDF-15, TNFα, and IGF-1 concentrations and the clinical data are shown in Table 3 and Figure 1. Table 3 shows the data obtained from males and females separately, and Figure 1 shows the correlations in all of the patients. The serum GDF-15 level was positively correlated with age in all of the patients ($r = 0.438$, $p < 0.001$, Figure 1Aa), but not TNFα ($r = 0.192$, $p = 0.105$, Figure 1Ba), and serum IGF-1 concentration declined with age ($r = -0.346$, $p = 0.003$, Figure 1Ca). In addition, the serum GDF-15 level was positively correlated with age in both males and females (males, $r = 0.436$, $p = 0.004$; females, $r = 0.637$, $p < 0.001$). The concentration of GDF-15 was positively correlated with BNP in both sexes (males, $r = 0.427$, $p = 0.005$; females, $r = 0.480$, $p = 0.007$), but the serum TNFα level was positively correlated with BNP only in men ($r = 0.465$, $p = 0.002$). The concentration of GDF-15 and TNFα (Figure 1Ab, Figure 1Bb), but not IGF-1 (Figure 1Cb), was negatively correlated with eGFR (Figure 1Ab, GDF-15, $r = -0.768$, $p < 0.001$; Figure 1Bb, TNFα, $r = -0.551$, $p < 0.001$) in all of the patients and both sexes (Table 2). Both GDF-15 and TNFα were negatively correlated with hemoglobin (Hb) in males (GDF-15, $r = -0.560$, $p < 0.001$; TNFα, $r = -0.566$, $p < 0.001$).

Table 3. Correlation matrix between various parameters and serum GDF-15, and TNFα, IGF-1 concentration.

	GDF-15 Males/Females	TNFα Males/Females	IGF-1 Males/Females
Age	0.436 (0.004) **/0.637 (<0.001) ***	0.244 (0.120)/0.261 (0.164)	−0.319 (0.036) */−0.339 (0.066)
BMI	−0.143 (0.367)/−0.062 (0.745)	−0.263 (0.092)/−0.055 (0.772)	0.047 (0.769)/0.194 (0.303)
HbA1C	−0.155 (0.340)/−0.229 (0.223)	−0.154 (0.342)/−0.127 (0.503)	0.261 (0.104)/0.344 (0.063)
BNP	0.427 (0.005) **/0.480 (0.007) **	0.465 (0.002) **/0.214 (0.257)	−0.059 (0.710)/−0.353 (0.055)
eGFR	−0.792 (<0.001) ***/−0.726 (<0.001) ***	−0.642 (<0.001) ***/−0.394 (0.031) *	0.144 (0.363)/0.301 (0.106)
Hb	−0.560 (<0.001) ***/−0.370 (0.044) *	−0.566 (<0.001) ***/−0.065 (0.732)	0.079 (0.617)/−0.006 (0.977)
Body fat percentage	−0.140 (0.403)/0.300 (0.128)	−0.146 (0.382)/0.135 (0.502)	−0.119 (0.479)/0.197 (0.326)
SMI	−0.392 (0.014) */−0.529 (0.005) **	−0.368 (0.021) */−0.189 (0.346)	0.313 (0.053)/0.153 (0.446)
Hand-grip	−0.456 (0.002) **/−0.656 (<0.001) ***	−0.393 (0.010) */−0.298 (0.117)	0.240 (0.126)/0.244 (0.202)
Knee extension	−0.222 (0.169)/−0.541 (0.003) **	−0.431 (0.005) **/−0.192 (0.329)	0.140 (0.390)/0.061 (0.758)
Gait speed	−0.218 (0.165)/−0.558 (0.002) **	−0.190 (0.229)/−0.336 (0.074)	0.256 (0.102)/0.253 (0.186)
Anterior TMth (supine)	−0.636 (<0.001) ***/−0.391 (0.044) *	−0.509 (0.001) **/−0.200 (0.316)	0.429 (0.005) **/0.057 (0.779)
Anterior TMth (standing)	−0.600 (<0.001) ***/−0.557 (0.003) **	−0.434 (0.005) **/−0.267 (0.178)	0.366 (0.020) */0.301 (0.127)
GDF-15	-/-	0.657 (<0.001) ***/0.434 (0.017) *	−0.203 (0.198)/−0.553 (0.002) **
TNFα	0.657 (<0.001) ***/0.434 (0.017) *	-/-	−0.233 (0.137)/−0.479 (0.007) **

* $p < 0.05$ ** $p < 0.01$ *** $p < 0.001$. SMI, skeletal muscle mass index; TMth, thigh muscle thickness.

Table 3 also shows the relationships between serum GDF-15, TNFα, IGF-1 concentrations and the physical data. Figure 2 shows the correlations between serum GDF-15, TNFα, IGF-1 concentrations and the physical data in men. The serum GDF-15 level was negatively correlated with hand-grip strength, SMI, anterior TMth (supine, and standing) in both males and females, as shown in Table 3. As shown in Figure 2, there was a negative correlation between the serum GDF-15 level and both anterior TMth (supine) ($r = -0.636$, $p < 0.001$, Figure 2Aa), and hand-grip strength ($r = -0.456$, $p = 0.002$, Figure 2Ab) in men. Similar results were obtained in females as shown in Table 3. On the other hand, a negative correlation was observed between the serum TNFα level and grip strength, knee extension strength, SMI, and anterior TMth (supine, standing) in males, but not in females (Table 3). A negative correlation between the serum TNFα level and both anterior TMth (supine) ($r = -0.509$, $p = 0.001$, Figure 2Ba), and grip strength ($r = -0.393$, $p = 0.010$, Figure 2Bb) was observed in men. On the other hand, a positive correlation was observed between the serum IGF-1 level and anterior TMth (supine) in men ($r = 0.429$,

$p = 0.005$, Figure 2Ca, Table 3), but not hand-grip strength ($r = 0.240$, $p = 0.126$, Figure 2Cb, Table 3). Furthermore, there were no correlations between the serum IGF-1 level and anterior TMth (supine, and standing) in females.

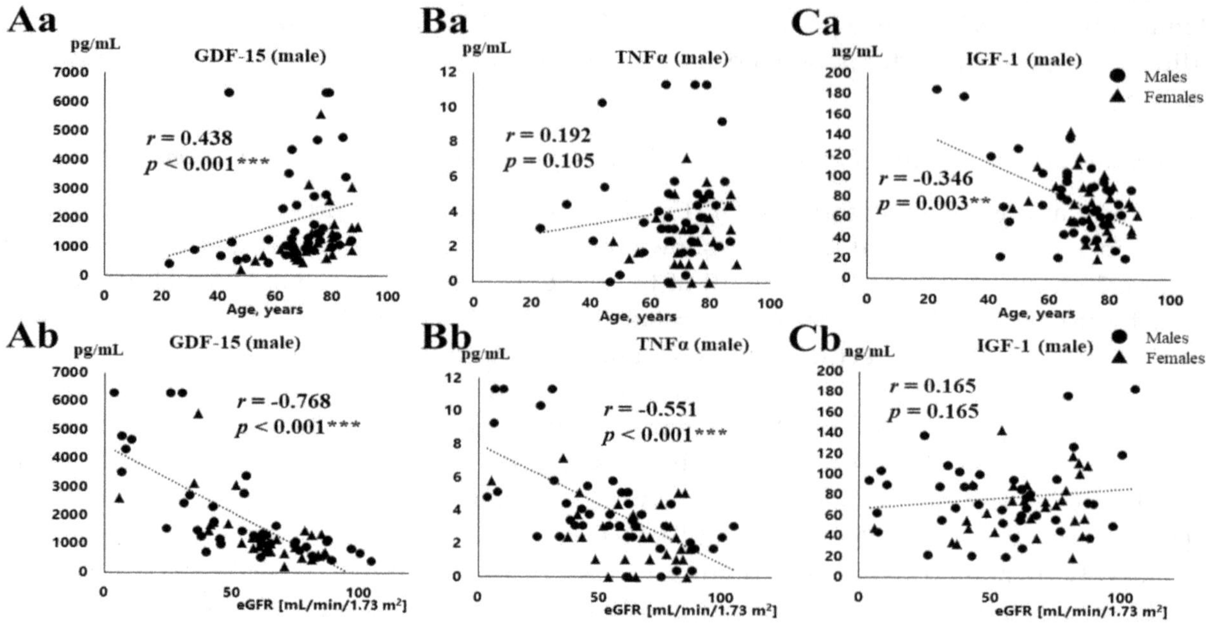

Figure 1. Correlations between clinical data (age, eGFR) and serum concentrations of GDF-15, TNF-α, and IGF-1. Relationships between laboratory data (age (**a**), eGFR (**b**)) and serum concentrations of GDF-15 (**Aa**,**Ab**), TNF-α (**Ba**,**Bb**) and IGF-1 (**Ca**,**Cb**) in males and females. ** $p < 0.01$, *** $p < 0.001$.

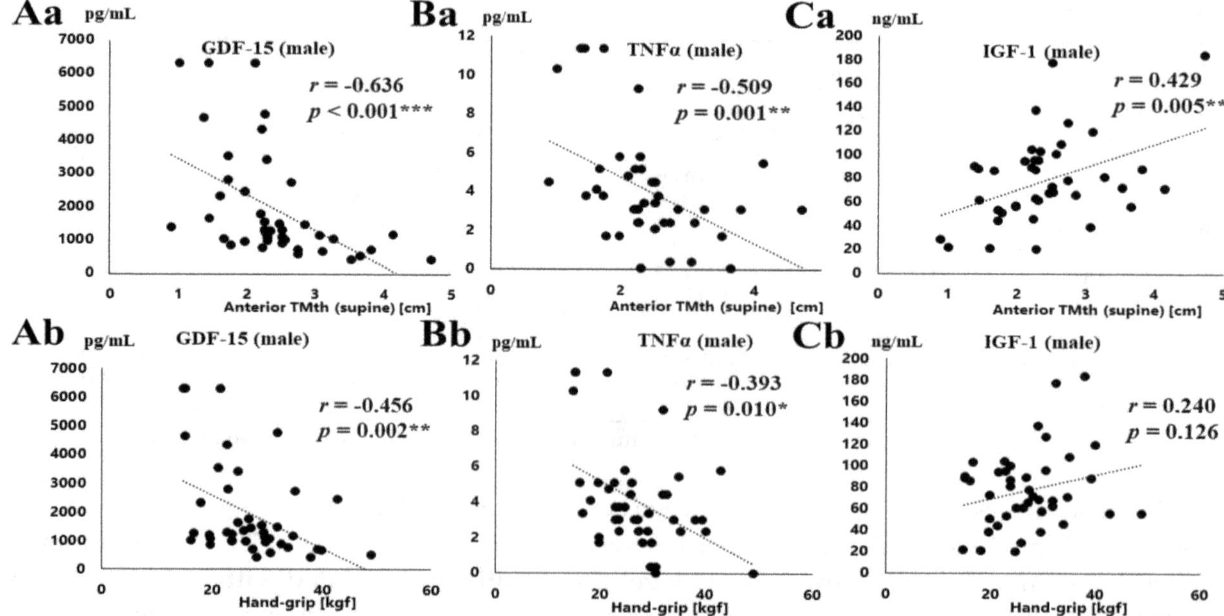

Figure 2. Correlations between the physical data (anterior thigh muscle thickness, grip strength) and serum concentrations of GDF-15, TNF-α, and IGF-1. Relationships between the laboratory data (anterior thigh muscle thickness (TMth, supine) (**a**), grip strength (**b**) and serum concentrations of GDF-15 (**Aa**,**Ab**), TNF-α (**Ba**,**Bb**) and IGF-1 (**Ca**,**Cb**) in males * $p < 0.05$, ** $p < 0.01$, *** $p < 0.001$.

3.3. Relationships among Serum GDF-15, TNFα, and IGF-1 Concentration

Table 3 shows the relationships among the serum GDF-15, TNFα, and IGF-1 concentrations. The serum level of GDF-15 was positively correlated with that of TNFα in both sexes (males, $r = 0.657$,

$p < 0.001$; females, $r = 0.434$, $p = 0.017$). A negative correlation was observed between the serum IGF-1 concentration and GDF-15 ($r = -0.553$, $p = 0.002$) and TNFα ($r = -0.479$, $p = 0.007$) in females, but not males.

3.4. Multiple Regression Analysis of Serum GDF-15 Levels and the Clinical Parameters

The linear regression analysis with serum GDF-15 levels as the dependent variable and clinical data (eGFR, BNP, Hb, SMI, hand-grip strength and anterior TMth (supine) as independent variable were investigated in all of the patients as shown in Table 4A. Univariate regression analysis (Table 4A) showed that eGFR (β = −0.650, $p < 0.001$), and anterior TMth (supine) (β = −0.358, $p = 0.001$) were independent variable to predict serum GDF-15 levels. Multiple regression analysis also showed that eGFR (β = −0.597, $p < 0.001$) and anterior TMth (supine) (β = −0.272, $p = 0.019$) were the independent determinants of GDF-15 concentration after adjusting for age, sex, and body mass index.

Table 4. Multiple linear regression analysis between serum GDF-15 levels and the clinical parameters.

A: Multiple linear regression analysis of GDF15 and the clinical data				
	Dependent variable: log (GDF−15)			
	Model 1	Model 2	Model 3	Model 4
Independent variable.	β-value (*p*)	β-value (*p*)	β-value (*p*)	β-value (*p*)
eGFR	−0.650 (<0.001) ***	−0.655 (<0.001) ***	−0.613 (<0.001) ***	−0.597 (<0.001) ***
BNP (log)	−0.009 (0.929)	−0.011 (0.912)	−0.042 (0.649)	−0.040 (0.663)
Hb	−0.106 (0.257)	−0.110 (0.253)	−0.079 (0.372)	−0.084 (0.343)
SMI	0.036 (0.722)	0.031 (0.771)	−0.171 (0.139)	−0.196 (0.098)
Hand−grip strength	0.106 (0.312)	0.323 (0.104)	−0.105 (0.367)	−0.059 (0.632)
Anterior TMth (supine)	−0.358 (0.001) **	−0.362 (0.001) **	−0.233 (0.033) *	−0.272 (0.019) *
B: Multiple linear regression analysis of anterior thigh muscle thickness (supine) and serum markers				
	Dependent variable: anterior thigh muscle thickness (supine)			
	Model 1	Model 2	Model 3	Model 4
Independent variable	β-value (*p*)	β-value (*p*)	β-value (*p*)	β-value (*p*)
GDF−15 (log)	−0.401 (0.005) **	−0.311 (0.024) *	−0.384 (0.007) **	−0.390 (0.004) **
TNFα (log)	−0.007 (0.955)	−0.054 (0.671)	−0.068 (0.584)	−0.054 (0.644)
IGF−1	0.256 (0.031) *	0.094 (0.456)	0.071 (0.656)	0.078 (0.506)
C: Multiple linear regression analysis of eGFR and the clinical data				
	Dependent variable: eGFR			
	Model 1	Model 2	Model 3	Model 4
Independent variable	β-value (*p*)	β-value (*p*)	β-value (*p*)	β-value (*p*)
BNP (log)	−0.164 (0.070)	−0.149 (0.106)	−0.149 (0.113)	−0.170 (0.070)
hsCRP (log)	−0.070 (0.377)	−0.094 (0.262)	−0.097 (0.257)	−0.085 (0.999)
Hb	0.035 (0.685)	0.005 (0.958)	0.002 (0.984)	0.011 (0.657)
GDF−15 (log)	−0.583 (<0.001) ***	−0.571 (<0.001) ***	−0.577 (<0.001) ***	−0.565 (<0.001) ***
TNFα (log)	−0.177 (0.069)	−0.196 (0.050)	−0.198 (0.050)	−0.197 (0.050)

Model 1, unadjusted; Model 2, adjusted by age; Model 3, adjusted by age and sex; Model 4, adjusted by age, sex, and BMI.

Alternatively, multiple regression analysis showed that GDF-15 (β = −0.390, $p = 0.004$) was the independent determinant of anterior TMth (supine), even adjusting for age, sex, and BMI (Table 4B).

The regression analysis between eGFR and the clinical data (BNP, CRP, Hb, GDF-15, and TNFα) were performed as shown in Table 4C. Multiple regression analysis showed that GDF-15 (β = −0.565, $p < 0.001$) and TNFα (β = −0.197, $p = 0.050$) were the independent variable to predict eGFR after adjusting for age, sex, and BMI. These results suggest that the serum GDF-15 concentration is a predictor for low eGFR. The ROC curves were plotted to identify the optimal cut-off levels of GDF-15, TNFα, and Hb for detecting eGFR lower than 60 mL/min/1.73 m^2, which was approximately the same value as the mean eGFR (58.2 mL/min/1.73 m^2). To construct the ROC curves, different cut-off values of GDF-15, TNFα, and Hb were used to predict eGFR lower than 60 mL/min/1.73 m^2, with true positives plotted on the vertical axis (sensitivity) and false-positives (1-specificity) plotted on the horizontal axis. The area under the curves (AUCs) for GDF-15, TNFα, and Hb were 92.1%, 78.6%, and 67.5%, respectively. Sensitivity and specificity were 88.2% and 82.9% for GDF-15, 81.8% and 61.5% for TNFα, and 45% and 83% for Hb, respectively. The optimal cut-off value of GDF-15 was 1154 pg/mL as shown in Figure 3.

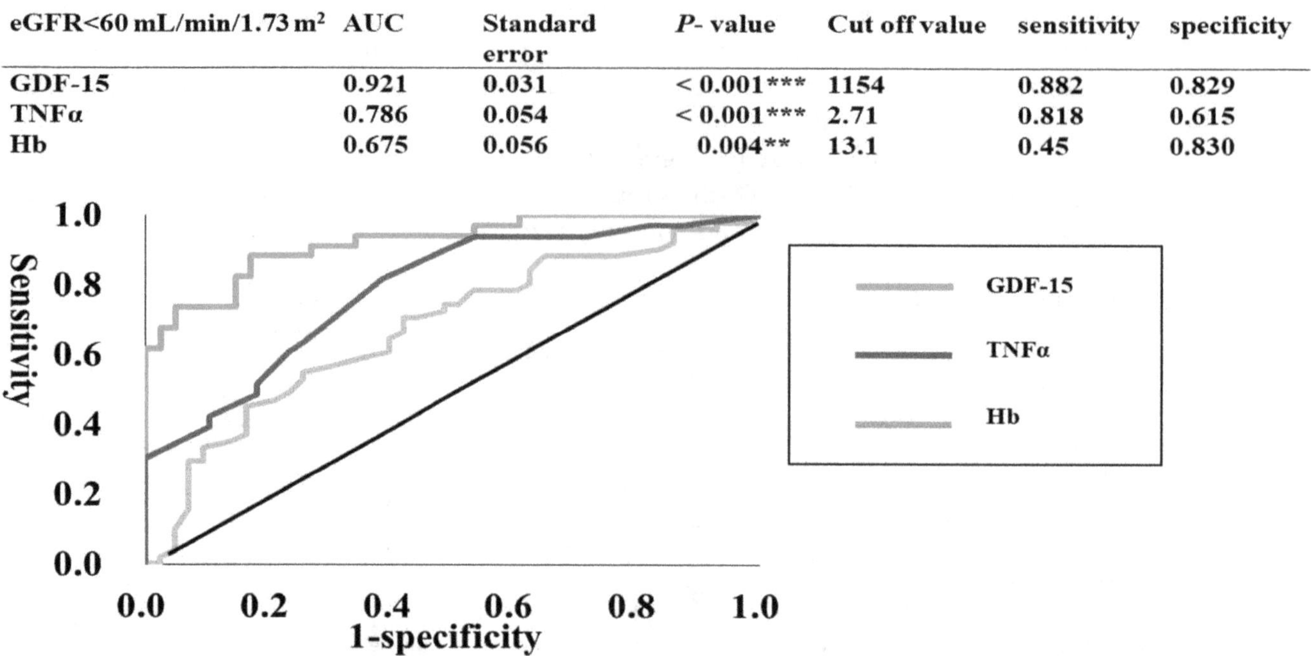

eGFR<60 mL/min/1.73 m²	AUC	Standard error	*P*- value	Cut off value	sensitivity	specificity
GDF-15	0.921	0.031	< 0.001***	1154	0.882	0.829
TNFα	0.786	0.054	< 0.001***	2.71	0.818	0.615
Hb	0.675	0.056	0.004**	13.1	0.45	0.830

Figure 3. ROC curves to identify the optimal cut-off level of GDF-15, TNFα, and Hb for detecting eGFR < 60. In the ROC curves shown, different cut-off values of GDF-15, and TNFα, and Hb were used to predict eGFR < 60, with true positives plotted on the vertical axis (sensitivity) and Figure 1. plotted on the horizontal axis.

3.5. Relationships between Sarcopenia and Serum Concentration of GDF-15, TNFα and IGF-1

Sarcopenia was identified in 24 (36%) of a total of 66 patients evaluated based on the sarcopenia criteria. Serum GDF-15, TNFα and IGF-1 levels were compared in patients with and without sarcopenia (Table 5). Patients with sarcopenia had significantly higher age and BNP levels in both males and females, compared to those without sarcopenia (Table 5). On the other hand, they had significant lower gait speed, hand-grip strength, extension strength, SMI, and anterior TMth (supine, standing). Furthermore, both males and females with sarcopenia had significantly higher GDF-15 levels, compared to those without sarcopenia (males, 1483 ± 1125 pg/mL vs. 3053 ± 2346 pg/m, $p < 0.05$; females, 891 ± 700 pg/mL vs. 1625 ± 1302 pg/mL, $p < 0.05$). The TNFα concentration was significantly higher in males with than without sarcopenia (3.06 ± 1.95 pg/mL vs. 6.07 ± 3.27 pg/mL, $p < 0.01$). IGF-1 levels did not significantly differ between patients with and without sarcopenia in both males and females.

Table 5. Differences in clinical data between the patients with and without sarcopenia.

	Male		Female	
	Sarcopenia (−)	Sarcopenia (+)	Sarcopenia (−)	Sarcopenia (+)
Number	28	11	14	13
Age (years)	63.4 (14.2)	75.6 (10.8) ***	68.9 (10.5)	76.2 (7.3) *
BMI (kg/m^2)	26.0 (4.8)	22.6 (3.0) *	24.9 (3.1)	25.9 (7.3)
Physical capacity				
Gait speed (m/s)	1.08 (0.34)	0.77 (0.28) *	1.01 (0.17)	0.73 (0.32) *
Grip strength (kgf)	30.0 (7.4)	20.2 (4.4) ***	20.1 (3.1)	13.9 (3.5) ***
Knee extension (kgf)	26.9 (8.4)	17.5 (7.3) **	19.2 (7.5)	13.6 (4.8)*
BIA findings				
Body fat percentage (%)	28.8 (7.4)	27.9 (8.9)	35.7 (6.6)	39.8 (10.3)
Skeletal muscle mass index (SMI) (kg/m^2)	7.68 (1.15)	5.90 (0.53) ***	6.05 (0.53)	4.74 (0.63) ***
Muscle thickness				
Anterior TMth (supine) (cm)	2.64 (0.68)	1.65 (0.53) ***	2.45 (0.68)	1.89 (0.48) *
Anterior TMth (standing) (cm)	3.98 (0.88)	2.78 (0.46) ***	3.70 (0.74)	2.77 (0.79) **
HbA1c, %	6.3 (0.9)	6.4 (1.3)	6.12 (0.98)	5.97 (0.60)
BNP, pg/mL	209 (285)	646 (722) **	162 (250)	366 (427) *
eGFR, ml/min/1.73 m^2	59.7 (26.4)	47.9 (26.1)	70.6 (14.4)	56.1 (22.1)
Hb, g/dL	13.0 (1.6)	11.0 (1.7)	12.5 (1.7)	11.5 (1.6)
hsCRP, mg/L	7.1 (12.7)	9.9 (18.5)	4.5 (11.3)	2.0 (2.3)
GDF-15, pg/mL	1483 (1125)	3053 (2346) *	891 (700)	1625 (1302) *
TNFα, pg/mL	3.06 (1.95)	6.07 (3.27) **	2.23 (2.10)	2.92 (1.66)
IGF-1, ng/mL	84.1 (40.0)	62.7 (25.6)	74.7 (23.6)	70.6 (34.6)

* $p < 0.05$. ** $p < 0.01$***. $p < 0.001$. Males vs. Females.

4. Discussion

The major findings of the present study are as follows: (1) In preoperative cardiovascular surgery patients, the circulating GDF-15 level was correlated with age, BNP, and eGFR. It also had a negative correlation with SMI, hand-grip strength, and anterior TMth. The GDF-15 levels were significantly higher in sarcopenia patients. (2) In multivariate analysis, eGFR and anterior TMth were independent determinants of GDF-15 concentration after adjusting for age, sex, and BMI. Furthermore, the GDF-15 level was an independent determinant of eGFR and anterior TMth. These results suggests that an increased GDF-15 level reflects muscle wasting as well as renal dysfunction in preoperative cardiovascular surgery patients. Thus, GDF-15 may be a novel biomarker for identifying high-risk patients with muscle wasting and renal dysfunction in cardiovascular surgery patients.

4.1. Association of Serum GDF-15 Levels with eGFR

The present study showed that the preoperative GDF-15 level in patients undergoing cardiovascular surgery including CABG and AVR was positively associated with age, eGFR, and BNP. This is compatible with the previous paper showing that preoperative GDF-15 levels in patients undergoing CABG were positively associated with age, chronic renal failure, and high NT-proBNP [25]. Clinical studies have also shown that the GDF-15 concentration correlated strongly with age in healthy elderly individuals and patients with coronary artery diseases [20,28]. GDF-15 is expressed in various tissue types such as kidneys, macrophages, cardiomyocytes, and endothelial cells. The expression occurs in response to various stimuli including oxidative and metabolic stress, tissue injury, and inflammation [10–12]. It has been reported that an increase in GDF-15 levels in community-based patients is associated with endothelial dysfunction and subclinical cardiovascular disease [35].

Moreover, clinical trials have shown that GDF-15 can be regarded as a reliable biomarker of CVD [13–15], and chronic heart failure [16]. In addition, GDF-15 is a novel serum biomarker of mortality in CKD and can identify patients at high risk of developing CKD [21,22]. The presence and progression of CVD are often intimately associated with CKD [36,37]. Valvular heart disease, specifically aortic stenosis, is also a well-known complication of renal dysfunction [38,39]. Gibson et al. [40] utilized eGFR in the analysis of outcomes after valve replacement. They showed that a decrease in eGFR of 10 mL/min/1.73 m^2 corresponded to a 31% increase in the risk of postoperative death, and eGFR less than 60 mL/min/1.73 m^2 was the most useful variable in predicting 30 day and midterm mortality. The postoperative GDF-15 value has also been reported to reflect post-operative acute kidney injury (AKI) in CABG patients [27]. In our study, using multivariate analysis, eGFR was an independent determinant of the preoperative GDF-15 level, even after adjusting for age, sex, and BMI. In addition, the GDF-15 level, was an independent determinant of eGFR. In ROC curve analysis, different cut-off levels of GDF-15 were used to predict eGFR lower than 60 mL/min/1.73 m^2, and the AUCs was 92.1% with an optimal cut-off value of 1154 pg/mL. Given that the normal range for human serum GDF-15 level has been reported to be 150-1150 pg/mL [41], and 733-999 pg/mL [42], the cut-off value of 1154 pg/mL shown in our study appears to be a reasonable value for detecting CKD in patients hospitalized for cardiovascular surgery. Thus, GDF-15 appears to be a novel biomarker for identifying surgical risk in patients undergoing cardiovascular surgery. However, further studies using postoperative follow-up are needed to clarify whether the preoperative GDF-15 level can be used as a novel biomarker to identify surgical risk in patients undergoing cardiovascular surgery.

4.2. Association of Serum GDF-15 Levels with Muscle Loss

In cardiac surgery such as TAVI, frailty is identified as a major predictor of adverse outcomes in older surgical patients [1,3–5]. Sarcopenia, the skeletal muscle loss associated with aging, also includes low physical function (grip strength, walking speed) as a component of frailty [6,7]. Sarcopenia is frequently associated with chronic diseases including heart failure, COPD, CKD, cancer, wasting, and cachexia [7]. Thus, frailty and sarcopenia increase the risk of complications and mortality when cardiovascular surgery is performed. We have previously shown that the prevalence of sarcopenia including sarcopenic obesity in CVD patients was 47.5% in males and 60.2% in females [34]. In the present study using preoperative cardiovascular surgery patients, sarcopenia was identified in 36%. In these cardiovascular surgery patients, we found that the circulating GDF-15 level had a negative correlation with SMI, hand-grip strength, and anterior TMth. In multivariate analysis, the GDF-15 level was an independent determinant of anterior TMth, even after correction for age, gender, and BMI. In addition, preoperative GDF-15 levels were significantly higher in those with than without sarcopenia. The results were consistent with previous reports showing that the circulating GDF-15 concentration was negatively correlated with the cross-sectional area of rectus femoris in COPD [30], ICU [32], and cancer patients [33]. Bloch et al. [31] showed that patients who show wasting of the rectus femoris following cardiac surgery are exposed to a more sustained elevation of GDF-15 than those withour muscle wasting. Moreover, several recent papers reported the relationships between GDF-15 levels and physical function such as gait speed, and hand-grip strength in community-dwelling older adults [43,44]. In the present study, a significant relationship between hand-grip strength/knee extension and the GDF-15 level was observed in preoperative cardiovascular surgery patients. From these results, it is very likely that circulating preoperative GDF-15 level may be a biomarker for identifying muscle wasting and sarcopenia in cardiovascular surgery patients.

Several mechanisms underlying GDF-15-induced muscle wasting have been proposed. First, an increase of GDF-15 may cause appetite loss, anorexia, and cachexia as shown in patients with cancer [41,45]. Animal studies also showed that GDF15 causes anorexia/cachexia, and then weight loss through a direct effect on the hypothalamus [46,47]. On the other hand, animal studies showed that local over-expression of GDF-15 in mice causes wasting of the tibialis anterior muscle directly [30], and the in vitro studies using C2C12 myotubes showed that GDF-15 treatment elevates expression of muscle atrophy-related genes, and causes muscle wasting, possibly by a direct effect of GDF-15 on skeletal muscle [32]. Further studies are required to clarify the mechanisms of action of GDF-15 on muscle wasting in patients with CVD including cardiovascular surgery.

4.3. *Relationships between GDF-15 and TNFα, IGF-1 Concentration*

It has been reported that several pro-inflammatory cytokines including TNFα are associated with cachexia and anorexia in both humans and rodents [48,49]. Higher concentrations of TNFα are also associated with a decline in muscle mass and grip strength in older persons [50]. In addition, systemic inflammation and increased circulating TNFα levels have been implicated in various conditions accompanied by muscle atrophy [51]. GDF-15 has been reported to be induced by inflammatory cytokines such as TNFα [10]. In our study, the serum GDF-15 level was positively correlated with the TNFα level, and a correlation was observed between TNFα and muscle mass and grip strength in men. However, multivariate regression analysis showed that that GDF-15, but not TNFα, was the independent determinant of anterior TMth (supine), even adjusting for age, sex, and BMI. These results suggest that GDF-15 is an independent marker of muscle mass, irrespective of TNF-α. Moreover, IGF-1 levels decrease with age and are regarded as a potential mediator of sarcopenia or frailty [52]. Wang et al. [53] showed that GDF-15 inhibits the release of IGF-1 from the liver in children with concomitant disease and failure. In our study, a negative correlation between GDF-15 and IGF-1 concentrations was observed only in females, but not in males. The reason of this sex discrepancy remains unknown. However, whereas the present study showed that IGF-1 was correlated negatively with age and positively with muscle mass, and anterior TMth, there were no significant differences in IGF-1 levels between patients with and without sarcopenia. Furthermore, we found no relationships between IGF-1 levels and hand-grip/extension strength. Thus, the contribution of serum IGF-1 levels to sarcopenia and muscle wasting remains unclear in our cardiovascular surgery patients.

4.4. *Limitations*

This study has several limitations. First, the results do not imply causality, because it was a cross-sectional study. Second, the study had a small number of cardiovascular surgery patients, especially females, and the patients underwent different types of cardiovascular surgery. Therefore, our findings are not necessarily applicable to the general population of cardiovascular surgery patients. Furthermore, most of the subjects had medical treatment. The use of drugs such as β-blockers, ACE-I, and ARB might have affected serum cytokine level. Therefore, the further studies using a large number of patients are required to clarify the pathophysiological roles of GDF-15 in preoperative cardiovascular surgery patients.

5. Conclusions

An elevated GDF-15 level reflects muscle wasting as well as renal dysfunction in preoperative cardiovascular surgery patients. Thus, serum GDF-15 concentration may be a novel biomarker for identifying high-risk patients with muscle wasting and renal dysfunction in cardiovascular surgery patients.

Author Contributions: Conceptualization, T.N. (Toshiaki Nakajima); methodology, A.H.; Resources, T.N. (Toshiaki Nakajima); formal analysis, T.S., T.N. (Toshiaki Nakajima); investigation, H.K., T.N. (Takafumi Nakajima), T.H.; T.A., S.O., S.A., M.S., S.T.; data curation, I.S., H.O.; supervision, F.N., H.F., T.I.; Funding acquisition, T.N. (Toshiaki Nakajima).

Abbreviations

CVD	cardiovascular disease
CABG	coronary artery bypass graft
AVR	aortic valve replacement
MVR	mitral valve replacement
MVP	mitral valve plasty
TVP	tricuspid valve plasty
TAVI	transcatheter valve implantation procedure
TVR	tricuspid valve replacement
TAR	total arch replacement
EVAR	endovascular aneurysm repair
BMI	body mass index
NYHA	New York Heart Association
TNFα	tumor necrosis factor α
GDF-15	growth differentiation factor-15
IGF-1	insulin growth factor 1
TGF-β;	transforming growth factor β
SMI	skeletal muscle mass index
BNP	brain natriuretic peptide
eGFR	estimated glomerular filtration rate
hsCRP	high-sensitivity C-reactive protein
ROC	receiver operating characteristic
AUC	area under the curve
TMth	thigh muscle thickness
COPD	chronic obstructive pulmonary disease
HbA1c	hemoglobin A1c
MVIC	maximum voluntary isometric contraction
ELISA	enzyme-linked immunosorbent assay
ICU	intensive care unit
ACS	acute coronary syndrome
AKI	acute kidney disease
BIA	bioelectric impedance analyzer
HF	heart failure
HT	hypertension
HD	hemodialysis
CKD	chronic kidney disease

References

1. Partridge, J.S.; Harari, D.; Dhesi, J.K. Frailty in the older surgical patient: A review. *Age Ageing* **2012**, *41*, 142–147. [CrossRef] [PubMed]
2. Clegg, A.; Young, J.; Iliffe, S.; Rikkert, M.O.; Rockwood, K. Frailty in elderly people. *Lancet* **2013**, *381*, 752–762. [CrossRef]
3. Makary, M.A.; Segev, D.L.; Pronovost, P.J.; Syin, D.; Bandeen-Roche, K.; Patel, P.; Takenaga, R.; Devgan, L.; Holzmueller, C.G.; Tian, J.; et al. Frailty as a predictor of surgical outcomes in older patients. *J. Am. Coll. Surg.* **2010**, *210*, 901–908. [CrossRef] [PubMed]
4. Shimura, T.; Yamamoto, M.; Kano, S.; Kagase, A.; Kodama, A.; Koyama, Y.; Tsuchikane, E.; Suzuki, T.; Otsuka, T.; Kohsaka, S.; et al. OCEAN-TAVI Investigators. Impact of the Clinical Frailty Scale on Outcomes After Transcatheter Aortic Valve Replacement. *Circulation* **2017**, *135*, 2013–2024. [CrossRef] [PubMed]
5. Afilalo, J.; Alexander, K.P.; Mack, M.J.; Maurer, M.S.; Green, P.; Allen, L.A. Frailty assessment in the cardiovascular care of older adults. *J. Am. Coll. Cardiol.* **2014**, *63*, 747–762. [CrossRef]
6. Rosenberg, I.H. Sarcopenia: Origins and clinical relevance. *J. Nutr.* **1997**, *127* (Suppl. 5), 990S–991S. [CrossRef]

7. Chen, L.K.; Liu, L.K.; Woo, J.; Assantachai, P.; Auyeung, T.W.; Bahyah, K.S.; Chou, M.Y.; Chen, L.Y.; Hsu, P.S.; Krairit, O.; et al. Sarcopenia in Asia: Consensus report of the Asian Working Group for Sarcopenia. *J. Am. Med. Dir. Assoc.* **2014**, *15*, 95–101. [CrossRef]
8. Mimeault, M.; Batra, S.K. Divergent molecular mechanisms underlying the pleiotropic functions of macrophage inhibitory cytokine-1 in cancer. *J. Cell. Physiol.* **2010**, *224*, 626–635. [CrossRef]
9. Shi, Y.; Massagué, J. Mechanisms of TGF-beta signaling from cell membrane to the nucleus. *Cell* **2003**, *113*, 685–700. [CrossRef]
10. Bootcov, M.R.; Bauskin, A.R.; Valenzuela, S.M.; Moore, A.G.; Bansal, M.; He, X.Y.; Zhang, H.P.; Donnellan, M.; Mahler, S.; Pryor, K.; et al. MIC-1, a novel macrophage inhibitory cytokine, is a divergent member of the TGF-beta superfamily. *Proc. Natl. Acad. Sci. USA* **1997**, *94*, 11514–11519. [CrossRef]
11. Dandrea, T.; Hellmold, H.; Jonsson, C.; Zhivotovsky, B.; Hofer, T.; Wärngård, L.; Cotgreave, I. The transcriptosomal response of human A549 lung cells to a hydrogen peroxide-generating system: Relationship to DNA damage, cell cycle arrest, and caspase activation. *Free Radic. Biol. Med.* **2004**, *36*, 881–896. [CrossRef] [PubMed]
12. Kempf, T.; Eden, M.; Strelau, J.; Naguib, M.; Willenbockel, C.; Tongers, J.; Heineke, J.; Kotlarz, D.; Xu, J.; Molkentin, J.D.; et al. The transforming growth factor-beta superfamily member growth-differentiation factor-15 protects the heart from ischemia/reperfusion injury. *Circ. Res.* **2006**, *98*, 351–360. [CrossRef] [PubMed]
13. Lind, L.; Wallentin, L.; Kempf, T.; Tapken, H.; Quint, A.; Lindahl, B.; Olofsson, S.; Venge, P.; Larsson, A.; Hulthe, J.; et al. Growth-differentiation factor-15 is an independent marker of cardiovascular dysfunction and disease in the elderly: Results from the Prospective Investigation of the Vasculature in Uppsala Seniors (PIVUS) Study. *Eur. Heart J.* **2009**, *30*, 2346–2353. [CrossRef] [PubMed]
14. Eggers, K.M.; Kempf, T.; Wallentin, L.; Wollert, K.C.; Lind, L. Change in growth differentiation factor 15 concentrations over time independently predicts mortality in community-dwelling elderly individuals. *Clin. Chem.* **2013**, *59*, 1091–1098. [CrossRef] [PubMed]
15. Wollert, K.C.; Kempf, T.; Wallentin, L. Growth Differentiation Factor 15 as a Biomarker in Cardiovascular Disease. *Clin. Chem.* **2017**, *63*, 140–151. [CrossRef] [PubMed]
16. George, M.; Jena, A.; Srivatsan, V.; Muthukumar, R.; Dhandapani, V.E. GDF 15-A Novel Biomarker in the Offing for Heart Failure. *Curr. Cardiol. Rev.* **2016**, *12*, 37–46. [CrossRef] [PubMed]
17. Preeshagul, I.; Gharbaran, R.; Jeong, K.H.; Abdel-Razek, A.; Lee, L.Y.; Elman, E.; Suh, K.S. Potential biomarkers for predicting outcomes in CABG cardiothoracic surgeries. *J. Cardiothorac. Surg.* **2013**, *8*, 176. [CrossRef]
18. Wollert, K.C.; Kempf, T.; Lagerqvist, B.; Lindahl, B.; Olofsson, S.; Allhoff, T.; Peter, T.; Siegbahn, A.; Venge, P.; Drexler, H.; et al. Growth differentiation factor 15 for risk stratification and selection of an invasive treatment strategy in non ST-elevation acute coronary syndrome. *Circulation* **2007**, *116*, 1540–1548. [CrossRef]
19. Khan, S.Q.; Ng, K.; Dhillon, O.; Kelly, D.; Quinn, P.; Squire, I.B.; Davies, J.E.; Ng, L.L. Growth differentiation factor-15 as a prognostic marker in patients with acute myocardial infarction. *Eur. Heart J.* **2009**, *30*, 1057–1065. [CrossRef]
20. Kempf, T.; von Haehling, S.; Peter, T.; Allhoff, T.; Cicoira, M.; Doehner, W.; Ponikowski, P.; Filippatos, G.S.; Rozentryt, P.; Drexler, H.; et al. Prognostic utility of growth differentiation factor-15 in patients with chronic heart failure. *J. Am. Coll. Cardiol.* **2007**, *50*, 1054–1060. [CrossRef]
21. Breit, S.N.; Carrero, J.J.; Tsai, V.W.; Yagoutifam, N.; Luo, W.; Kuffner, T.; Bauskin, A.R.; Wu, L.; Jiang, L.; Barany, P.; et al. Macrophage inhibitory cytokine-1 (MIC-1/GDF15) and mortality in end-stage renal disease. *Nephrol. Dial. Transplant.* **2012**, *27*, 70–75. [CrossRef] [PubMed]
22. Ho, J.E.; Hwang, S.J.; Wollert, K.C.; Larson, M.G.; Cheng, S.; Kempf, T.; Vasan, R.S.; Januzzi, J.L.; Wang, T.J.; Fox, C.S. Biomarkers of cardiovascular stress and incident chronic kidney disease. *Clin. Chem.* **2013**, *59*, 1613–1620. [CrossRef] [PubMed]
23. Nair, V.; Robinson-Cohen, C.; Smith, M.R.; Bellovich, K.A.; Bhat, Z.Y.; Bobadilla, M.; Brosius, F.; de Boer, I.H.; Essioux, L.; Formentini, I.; et al. Growth Differentiation Factor-15 and Risk of CKD Progression. *J. Am. Soc. Nephrol.* **2017**, *28*, 2233–2240. [CrossRef] [PubMed]
24. Heringlake, M.; Charitos, E.I.; Gatz, N.; Käbler, J.H.; Beilharz, A.; Holz, D.; Schön, J.; Paarmann, H.; Petersen, M.; Hanke, T. Growth differentiation factor 15: A novel risk marker adjunct to the EuroSCORE for risk stratification in cardiac surgery patients. *J. Am. Coll. Cardiol.* **2013**, *66*, 672–681. [CrossRef] [PubMed]

25. Kahli, A.; Guenancia, C.; Zeller, M.; Grosjean, S.; Stamboul, K.; Rochette, L.; Girard, C.; Vergely, C. Growth differentiation factor-15 (GDF-15) levels are associated with cardiac and renal injury in patients undergoing coronary artery bypass grafting with cardiopulmonary bypass. *PLoS ONE* **2014**, *9*, e105759. [CrossRef] [PubMed]
26. Krau, N.C.; Lünstedt, N.S.; Freitag-Wolf, S.; Brehm, D.; Petzina, R.; Lutter, G.; Bramlage, P.; Dempfle, A.; Frey, N.; Frank, D. Elevated growth differentiation factor 15 levels predict outcome in patients undergoing transcatheter aortic valve implantation. *Eur. J. Heart Fail.* **2015**, *17*, 945–955. [CrossRef] [PubMed]
27. Guenancia, C.; Kahli, A.; Laurent, G.; Hachet, O.; Malapert, G.; Grosjean, S.; Girard, C.; Vergely, C.; Bouchot, O. Pre-operative growth differentiation factor 15 as a novel biomarker of acute kidney injury after cardiac bypass surgery. *Int. J. Cardiol.* **2015**, *197*, 66–71. [CrossRef] [PubMed]
28. Yuan, Z.; Li, H.; Qi, Q.; Gong, W.; Qian, C.; Dong, R.; Zang, Y.; Li, J.; Zhou, M.; Cai, J.; et al. Plasma levels of growth differentiation factor-15 are associated with myocardial injury in patients undergoing off-pump coronary artery bypass grafting. *Sci. Rep.* **2016**, *6*, 28221. [CrossRef]
29. Fujita, Y.; Taniguchi, Y.; Shinkai, S.; Tanaka, M.; Ito, M. Secreted growth differentiation factor 15 as a potential biomarker for mitochondrial dysfunctions in aging and age-related disorders. *Geriatr. Gerontol. Int.* **2016**, *16* (Suppl. 1), 17–29. [CrossRef]
30. Patel, M.S.; Lee, J.; Baz, M.; Wells, C.E.; Bloch, S.; Lewis, A.; Donaldson, A.V.; Garfield, B.E.; Hopkinson, N.S.; Natanek, A.; et al. Growth differentiation factor-15 is associated with muscle mass in chronic obstructive pulmonary disease and promotes muscle wasting in vivo. *J. Cachexia Sarcopenia Muscle* **2016**, *7*, 436–448. [CrossRef]
31. Bloch, S.A.; Lee, J.Y.; Wort, S.J.; Polkey, M.I.; Kemp, P.R.; Griffiths, M.J. Sustained elevation of circulating growth and differentiation factor-15 and a dynamic imbalance in mediators of muscle homeostasis are associated with the development of acute muscle wasting following cardiac surgery. *Crit. Care Med.* **2013**, *41*, 982–989. [CrossRef] [PubMed]
32. Bloch, S.A.; Lee, J.Y.; Syburra, T.; Rosendahl, U.; Griffiths, M.J.; Kemp, P.R.; Polkey, M.I. Increased expression of GDF-15 may mediate ICU-acquired weakness by down-regulating muscle microRNAs. *Thorax* **2015**, *70*, 219–228. [CrossRef] [PubMed]
33. Lerner, L.; Hayes, T.G.; Tao, N.; Krieger, B.; Feng, B.; Wu, Z.; Nicoletti, R.; Chiu, M.I.; Gyuris, J.; Garcia, J.M. Plasma growth differentiation factor 15 is associated with weight loss and mortality in cancer patients. *J. Cachexia Sarcopenia Muscle* **2015**, *6*, 317–324. [CrossRef] [PubMed]
34. Yasuda, T.; Nakajima, T.; Sawaguchi, T.; Nozawa, N.; Arakawa, T.; Takahashi, R.; Mizushima, Y.; Katayanagi, S.; Matsumoto, K.; Toyoda, S.; et al. Short Physical Performance Battery for cardiovascular disease inpatients: Implications for critical factors and sarcopenia. *Sci. Rep.* **2017**, *7*, 17425. [CrossRef] [PubMed]
35. Wang, T.J.; Gona, P.; Larson, M.G.; Tofler, G.H.; Levy, D.; Newton-Cheh, C.; Jacques, P.F.; Rifai, N.; Selhub, J.; Robins, S.J.; et al. Multiple biomarkers for the prediction of first major cardiovascular events and death. *N. Engl. J. Med.* **2006**, *355*, 2631–2639. [CrossRef]
36. Sarnak, M.J.; Levey, A.S.; Schoolwerth, A.C.; Coresh, J.; Culleton, B.; Hamm, L.L.; McCullough, P.A.; Kasiske, B.L.; Kelepouris, E.; Klag, M.J.; et al. American Heart Association Councils on Kidney in Cardiovascular Disease, High Blood Pressure Research, Clinical Cardiology, and Epidemiology and Prevention. Kidney disease as a risk factor for development of cardiovascular disease: A statement from the American Heart Association Councils on Kidney in Cardiovascular Disease, High Blood Pressure Research, Clinical Cardiology, and Epidemiology and Prevention. *Circulation* **2003**, *108*, 2154–2169. [PubMed]
37. Wali, R.K.; Henrich, W.L. Chronic kidney disease: A risk factor for cardiovascular disease. *Cardiol. Clin.* **2005**, *23*, 343–362. [CrossRef]
38. Ibáñez, J.; Riera, M.; Saez de Ibarra, J.I.; Carrillo, A.; Fernández, R.; Herrero, J.; Fiol, M.; Bonnin, O. Effect of preoperative mild renal dysfunction on mortality and morbidity following valve cardiac surgery. *Interact. Cardiovasc. Thorac. Surg.* **2007**, *6*, 748–752. [CrossRef] [PubMed]
39. Thourani, V.; Keeling, W.B.; Sarin, E.L.; Guyton, R.A.; Kilgo, P.D.; Dara, A.B.; Puskas, J.D.; Chen, E.P.; Cooper, W.A.; Vega, J.D.; et al. Impact of preoperative renal dysfunction on long-term survival for patients undergoing aortic valve replacement. *Ann. Thorac. Surg.* **2011**, *91*, 1798–1806. [CrossRef]
40. Gibson, P.H.; Croal, B.L.; Cuthbertson, B.H.; Chiwara, M.; Scott, A.E.; Buchan, K.G.; El-Shafei, H.; Gibson, G.; Jeffrey, R.R.; Hillis, G.S. The relationship between renal function and outcome from heart valve surgery. *Am. Heart J.* **2008**, *156*, 893–899. [CrossRef]

41. Bauskin, A.R.; Brown, D.A.; Kuffner, T.; Johnen, H.; Luo, X.W.; Hunter, M.; Breit, S.N. Role of macrophage inhibitory cytokine-1 in tumorigenesis and diagnosis of cancer. *Cancer Res.* **2006**, *66*, 4983–4986. [CrossRef]
42. Krintus, M.; Braga, F.; Kozinski, M.; Borille, S.; Kubica, J.; Sypniewska, G.; Panteghini, M. A study of biological and lifestyle factors, including within-subject variation, affecting concentrations of growth differentiation factor 15 in serum. *Clin. Chem. Lab. Med.* **2019**, *57*, 1035–1043. [CrossRef] [PubMed]
43. Rothenbacher, D.; Dallmeier, D.; Christow, H.; Koenig, W.; Denkinger, M.; Klenk, J.; ActiFE study group. Association of growth differentiation factor 15 with other key biomarkers, functional parameters and mortality in community-dwelling older adults. *Age Ageing* **2019**, *48*, 541–546. [CrossRef] [PubMed]
44. Semba, R.D.; Gonzalez-Freire, M.; Tanaka, T.; Biancotto, A.; Zhang, P.; Shardell, M.; Moaddel, R.; Ferrucci, L.; CHI Consortium. Elevated Plasma Growth and Differentiation Factor-15 is Associated with Slower Gait Speed and Lower Physical Performance in Healthy Community-Dwelling Adults. *J. Gerontol. A Biol. Sci. Med. Sci.* **2019**. [CrossRef]
45. Welsh, J.B.; Sapinoso, L.M.; Kern, S.G.; Brown, D.A.; Liu, T.; Bauskin, A.R.; Ward, R.L.; Hawkins, N.J.; Quinn, D.I.; Russell, P.J.; et al. Large-scale delineation of secreted protein biomarkers overexpressed in cancer tissue and serum. *Proc. Natl. Acad. Sci. USA* **2003**, *100*, 3410–3415. [CrossRef]
46. Johnen, H.; Lin, S.; Kuffner, T.; Brown, D.A.; Tsai, V.W.; Bauskin, A.R.; Wu, L.; Pankhurst, G.; Jiang, L.; Junankar, S.; et al. Tumor-induced anorexia and weight loss are mediated by the TGF-beta superfamily cytokine MIC-1. *Nat. Med.* **2007**, *13*, 1333–1340. [CrossRef] [PubMed]
47. Tsai, V.W.; Macia, L.; Johnen, H.; Kuffner, T.; Manadhar, R.; Jørgensen, S.B.; Lee-Ng, K.K.; Zhang, H.P.; Wu, L.; Marquis, C.P.; et al. TGF-b superfamily cytokine MIC-1/GDF15 is a physiological appetite and body weight regulator. *PLoS ONE* **2013**, *8*, e55174. [CrossRef]
48. Hubbard, R.E.; O'Mahony, M.S.; Savva, G.M.; Calver, B.L.; Woodhouse, K.W. Inflammation and frailty measures in older people. *J. Cell. Mol. Med.* **2009**, *13*, 3103–3109. [CrossRef] [PubMed]
49. Utech, A.E.; Tadros, E.M.; Hayes, T.G.; Garcia, J.M. Predicting survival in cancer patients: The role of cachexia and hormonal, nutritional and inflammatory markers. *J. Cachexia Sarcopenia Muscle* **2012**, *3*, 245–251. [CrossRef]
50. Schaap, L.A.; Pluijm, S.M.; Deeg, D.J.; Harris, T.B.; Kritchevsky, S.B.; Newman, A.B.; Colbert, L.H.; Pahor, M.; Rubin, S.M.; Tylavsky, F.A.; et al. Health ABC Study. Higher inflammatory marker levels in older persons: Associations with 5-year change in muscle mass and muscle strength. *J. Gerontol. A Biol. Sci. Med. Sci.* **2009**, *64*, 1183–1189. [CrossRef] [PubMed]
51. von Haehling, S.; Steinbeck, L.; Doehner, W.; Springer, J.; Anker, S.D. Muscle wasting in heart failure: An overview. *Int. J. Biochem. Cell Biol.* **2013**, *45*, 2257–2265. [CrossRef] [PubMed]
52. Leng, S.X.; Cappola, A.R.; Andersen, R.E.; Blackman, M.R.; Koenig, K.; Blair, M.; Walston, J.D. Serum levels of insulin-like growth factor-I (IGF-I) and dehydroepiandrosterone sulfate (DHEA-S), and their relationships with serum interleukin-6, in the geriatric syndrome of frailty. *Aging Clin. Exp. Res.* **2004**, *16*, 153–157. [CrossRef] [PubMed]
53. Wang, T.; Liu, J.; McDonald, C.; Lupino, K.; Zhai, X.; Wilkins, B.J.; Hakonarson, H.; Pei, L. GDF15 is a heart-derived hormone that regulates body growth. *EMBO. Mol. Med.* **2017**, *9*, 1150–1164. [CrossRef] [PubMed]

Left Ventricular Function and Myocardial Triglyceride Content on 3T Cardiac MR Predict Major Cardiovascular Adverse Events and Readmission in Patients Hospitalized with Acute Heart Failure

Kuang-Fu Chang [1,2,†], Gigin Lin [2,3,4,†], Pei-Ching Huang [2], Yu-Hsiang Juan [2], Chao-Hung Wang [5], Shang-Yueh Tsai [6], Yu-Ching Lin [1], Ming-Ting Wu [7], Pen-An Liao [2], Lan-Yan Yang [8], Min-Hui Liu [5], Yu-Chun Lin [2,3], Jiun-Jie Wang [2,3], Koon-Kwan Ng [1,*] and Shu-Hang Ng [2,*]

1 Department of Radiology, Chang Gung Memorial Hospital, Keelung and Chang Gung University, Keelung 20401, Taiwan; kc1116@cgmh.org.tw (K.-F.C.); yuching1221@cgmh.org.tw (Y.-C.L.)
2 Department of Medical Imaging and Intervention, Chang Gung Memorial Hospital, Linkou and Chang Gung University, Taoyuan 33305, Taiwan; giginlin@cgmh.org.tw (G.L.); spookie@cgmh.org.tw (P.-C.H.); 8801131@cgmh.org.tw (Y.-H.J.); wakefield1006@gmail.com (P.-A.L.); jack805@gmail.com (Y.-C.L.); jiunjie.wang@gmail.com (J.-J.W.)
3 Imaging Core Lab, Institute for Radiological Research, Chang Gung University, Taoyuan 333, Taiwan
4 Clinical Metabolomics Core Lab, Chang Gung Memorial Hospital, Taoyuan 333, Taiwan
5 Department of Cardiology and Heart Failure Center, Chang Gung Memorial Hospital, Keelung 20401, Taiwan; bearty54@gmail.com (C.-H.W.); khfoffice@gmail.com (M.-H.L.)
6 Graduate Institute of Applied Physics, National Chengchi University, Taipei 11605, Taiwan; syytsai@gmail.com
7 Department of Radiology, Kaohsiung Veterans General Hospital, Kaohsiung 81362, Taiwan; wu.mingting@gmail.com
8 Clinical Trial Center, Chang Gung Memorial Hospital at Linkou, Taoyuan 333, Taiwan; lyyang0111@gmail.com
* Correspondence: ngkk@ms14.hinet.net (K.-K.N.); shuhangng@gmail.com (S.-H.N.);

† These authors contributed equally to this work.

Abstract: Background: This prospective study was designed to investigate whether myocardial triglyceride (TG) content from proton magnetic resonance spectroscopy (MRS) and left ventricular (LV) function parameters from cardiovascular magnetic resonance imaging (CMR) can serve as imaging biomarkers in predicting future major cardiovascular adverse events (MACE) and readmission in patients who had been hospitalized for acute heart failure (HF). Methods: Patients who were discharged after hospitalization for acute HF were prospectively enrolled. On a 3.0 T MR scanner, myocardial TG contents were measured using MRS, and LV parameters (function and mass) were evaluated using cine. The occurrence of MACE and the HF-related readmission served as the endpoints. Independent predictors were identified using univariate and multivariable Cox proportional hazard regression analyses. Results: A total of 133 patients (mean age, 52.4 years) were enrolled. The mean duration of follow-up in surviving patients was 775 days. Baseline LV functional parameters—including ejection fraction, LV end-diastolic volume, LV end-diastolic volume index (LVEDVI), and LV end-systolic volume ($p < 0.0001$ for all), and myocardial mass ($p = 0.010$)—were significantly associated with MACE. Multivariable analysis revealed that LVEDVI was the independent predictor for MACE, while myocardial mass was the independent predictor for 3- and 12-month readmission. Myocardial TG content (lipid resonances δ 1.6 ppm) was significantly associated with readmission in patients with ischemic heart disease. Conclusions: LVEDVI and myocardial mass are potential imaging biomarkers that independently predict MACE and readmission, respectively, in patients discharged after hospitalization for acute HF. Myocardial TG predicts readmission in patients with a history of ischemic heart disease.

Keywords: cardiac magnetic resonance imaging; heart failure; left ventricular systolic function; magnetic resonance spectroscopy; myocardial triglyceride content

---

1. Introduction

Heart failure (HF) is a complex clinical syndrome that results from a variety of conditions preventing the left ventricle (LV) from supporting physiological circulation [1]. Patients with HF are at an increased risk of major adverse cardiovascular events (MACE)—including death, myocardial infarction, stroke, and hospitalizations [2,3]—which pose a significant public health burden globally. The 3-month readmission rates of patients with acute HF remains as high as 25–50%, with 5-year survival rates <50% [4]. Optimized risk sFCtratification would help to prioritize the surveillance for those who are prone to experience MACE.

Cardiomyocytes primarily depend on the oxidation of fatty acids as their source of energy [5]. Because the heart does not serve as a storage depot for fat, the concentration of triglycerides (TG) in the myocardium is low under physiological conditions. However, cardiac steatosis may develop as a result of abnormal regulation of fatty acids uptake or alterations in lipid metabolism. TG accumulation in the heart has been recognized as a risk factor for cardiovascular (CV) disease [6–8]. Vilahur et al. have shown that intramyocardial lipids impaired myofibroblast-related collagen synthesis with resultant poor healing of the myocardial scar post-myocardial infarction, while excess cardiac lipids exacerbated apoptosis and led to extensive myocardial infarcts [9]. Proton magnetic resonance spectroscopy (^{1}H-MRS) has been used to obtain in vivo quantitative measures of myocardial TG content in patients with CV disorders [10–12]. We have previously used 3.0 T CMR to analyze the association between myocardial unsaturated fatty acids (UFA) content and left ventricular (LV) function in patients who had been hospitalized for acute HF [13]. Furthermore, cardiac magnetic resonance imaging (CMR) is well established as the gold standard in the assessment of cardiac structure and function, with incremental diagnostic and prognostic information in HF [14–16]. We, therefore, hypothesize that the quantitative information about myocardial TG content from ^{1}H-MRS and LV function parameters from CMR may help predict the occurrence of future MACE and readmission in patients who have been hospitalized for acute HF.

This prospective study was designed to investigate whether myocardial TG content from ^{1}H-MRS (primary aim) and LV function parameters from CMR (secondary aim) can serve as imaging biomarkers in predicting future MACE and readmission in patients who have been hospitalized for acute HF.

2. Methods

2.1. Ethics Approval and Consent to Participate

Ethical approval was granted by the Institutional Review Board of the Keelung Chang Gung Memorial Hospital (IRB 102-2772A3). The study is reported in accordance with the STROBE (STrengthening the Reporting of OBservational studies in Epidemiology) statement and has been registered at ClinicalTrials.gov (Identifier: NCT02378402) on 21 February 2015. All patients provided their written informed consent.

2.2. Study Design and Patient Population

Between March 2014 and June 2016, we prospectively screened 200 patients and enrolled a total of 147 patients who were hospitalized with acute HF at a tertiary referral hospital with a dedicated HF center (IRB 102-2772A3, ClinicalTrial.gov: NCT02378402). Patients were scanned whose medical condition had become stable after treatment, specifically when they (1) had an oral medication regimen stable for at least 24 h; (2) had no intravenous vasodilator or inotropic agents for at least 24 h; and (3) were ambulatory before discharge to assess functional capacity. Patients aged between 20 and 70 years with acute HF, with initial HF stage C, classified according to the American College of Cardiology (ACC) and the American Heart Association (AHA) HF classification system [4], were eligible. Patients who were unwilling to participate or presenting with general contraindications to CMR (e.g., claustrophobia, metal-containing implants, cardiac pacemakers, or unable to comply with the examiners) were excluded. Additional exclusion criteria were as follows: Positive history of open cardiac surgery; pregnancy or breastfeeding; and inability to adhere to treatment and/or follow-up. All of the medical records underwent a central review by a multidisciplinary team to confirm that the identified patients were suitable for inclusion. The following variables were collected at baseline: Demographic data (age, sex, height, and weight), cardiovascular risk factors (smoking, hypertension, diabetes), previous history of cardiovascular disease (angina, myocardial infarction, dilated cardiomyopathy, myocarditis), and medication use. Serum lipid levels (total cholesterol, very-low-density lipoprotein cholesterol, low-density lipoprotein cholesterol, high-density lipoprotein cholesterol, and TG) were measured 1 month before CMR imaging. Patients with a previous history of angina or myocardial infarction were defined as an ischemic group, while the others as non-ischemic group. Previously, 48 of the 133 patients have been reported in a cross-sectional interim report to study the association of LV function and myocardial TG on CMR [13]. In this study, we further evaluated their predictive value in a longitudinal observational study. The patient flow diagram is present in Figure 1.

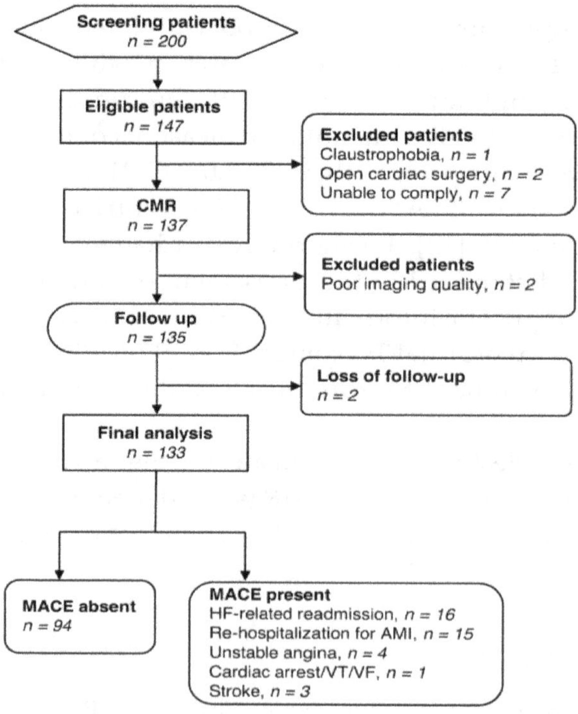

Figure 1. Flow diagram of the study cohort. Note.—AMI, acute myocardial infarction; CMR, cardiac magnetic resonance; HF, heart failure; MACE, major cardiovascular event; VT, ventricular tachycardia; VF, ventricular fibrillation.

2.3. *H-MRS*

Clinical MRS was acquired before contrast administration using the same settings and anatomical localizations as previously reported [13]. In brief, respiratory-triggered cardiac-gated point-resolved spectroscopy (PRESS) [17] was implemented to acquire localized ^{1}H MRS voxels to a $2 \times 2 \times 1$ cm^3 spectroscopic volume within the interventricular septum during the end-systolic phase. The MRS acquisition parameters were as follows: Nominal TR (repetition time)/TE (echo time), 550 ms/33 ms;

64 averages; window size, 1024 points; bandwidth, 2000 Hz [18–21]. Spectra with and without water suppression were used to obtain water and myocardial TG signals, respectively [22].

2.4. CMR Imaging

Patients were required to fast overnight before undergoing CMR examinations on a 3.0-Tesla Siemens Skyra MR scanner (Siemens, Erlangen, Germany). No pre-medications were used. The scanner was equipped with an 18-channel phased-array receiver body coil and operated on a VD13 platform. Steady-state free precession (SSFP) cine imaging was used to produce images with both short-axis (contiguous 8 mm slice thickness) and standard long-axis views (2-, 3- and 4-chamber views). Late gadolinium enhancement (LGE) at 10 min after gadolinium injection in the short-axis (9 to 13 images covering the entire LV), 2-chamber, and 4-chamber planes. The following settings were employed: Echo time, 1.2 ms; repetition time, 3.4 ms; field of view, 34−40 cm; matrix, 256 × 256.

2.5. Image Analysis

Left ventricular ejection fraction (LVEF) was measured on short-axis cine LV images with post-processing software (VB17, Argus Viewer and Function, Siemens, Erlangen, Germany) on a separate workstation. LV endocardial and epicardial borders were manually drawn at end-diastole and end-systole on short-axis cine images and LVEF and end-diastolic LV mass from each slice were measured accordingly. Papillary muscles were not included in the LV mass. Left ventricular end-diastolic volume (LVEDV) and end-systolic volume (LVESV) were calculated using the same methodology. The left ventricular end-diastolic volume index (LVEDVI) was determined by dividing the LVEDV by the body surface area (BSA). The LV global function index (LVGFI) was calculated with the following formula:

$$\text{LVGFI} = [\text{LVESV}/(\text{LVEDV}+\text{LVESV})/2 + (\text{LV mass}/1.05)] \times 100 \tag{1}$$

LCModel 6.2 software package (http://s-provencher.com/pages/lcmodel.shtml) was used for the quantification of TG by fitting the time-domain ^{1}H-MRS spectra (Figure 2). Multiple resonance peaks of fat including methyl ($–(CH_2)_n–CH_3$) peak δ 0.9 ppm, methylene ($–(CH_2)_n–$) peaked at 1.3 ppm, beta-carboxyl ($–CO\text{-}CH_2\text{-}CH_2–$) at 1.6 ppm, alpha-allylic ($–CH_2–CH=CH–CH_2–$) peaked at 2.02 ppm (denote by Lip2.1), alpha-carboxyl ($–CO\text{-}CH_2\text{-}CH_2–$) peaked at 2.24 ppm (denote by Lip2.3), diacyl ($–CH=CH–CH_2–CH=CH–$) peaked at 2.75 ppm (denote by Lip2.8), olefinic ($–CH=CH–$) at 5.29 ppm (denote by Lip5.3) were fitted. Water-suppressed spectra were used to quantify the total myocardial TG resonance and its—including FA (lipid resonances δ 0.9, 1.3 and 1.6 ppm) and UFA (lipid resonance δ 2.02 ppm, 2.24 ppm, 2.75 ppm, and 5.29 ppm), i.e., the ratio of the metabolite resonance area to the unsuppressed water resonance area. Water resonance (~δ 4.7 ppm) without water suppression was also determined for normalization. Cramer-Rao lower bound (CRLB) of TG provided by the LCModel was served as a goodness-of-fit, and used for the evaluation of the spectra quality.

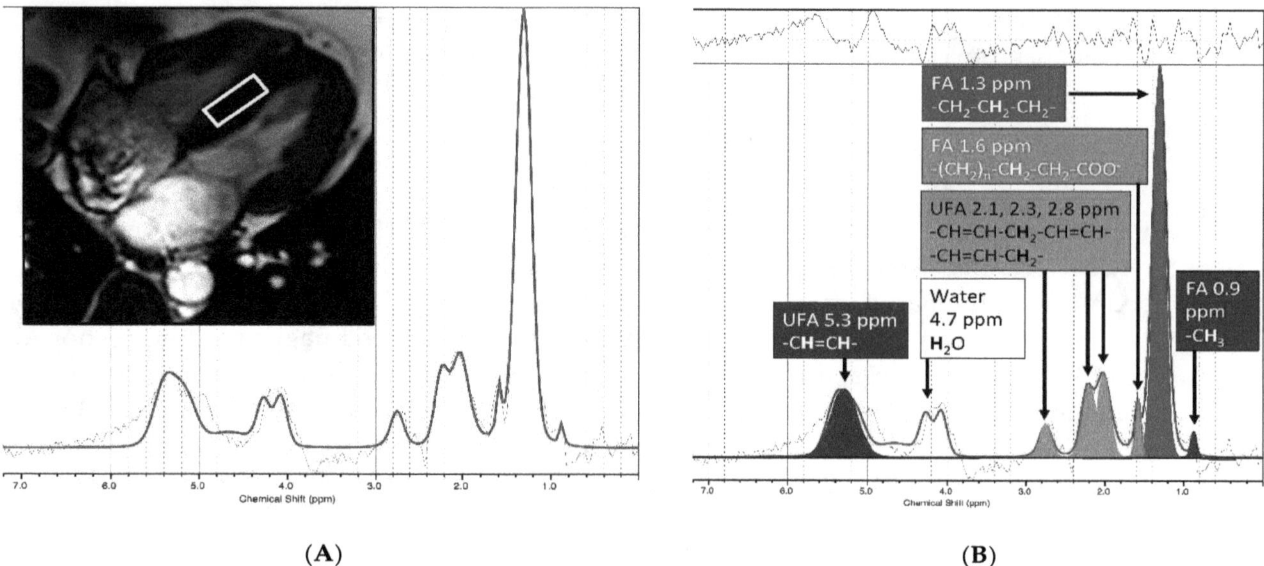

Figure 2. Example myocardial CMR spectroscopy. (**A**) A 2 × 2 × 1 cm^3 spectroscopic volume (white box) was acquired from the interventricular septum during the systolic phase to generate an input spectrum. (**B**) ^{1}H-CMR spectra were fitted and analyzed using the LCModel 6.2 software package (right). We quantified the components of myocardial triglyceride resonances, i.e., fatty acids (FA, lipid resonances δ 0.9, 1.3, and 1.6 ppm) and unsaturated fatty acids (UFA, lipid resonance δ 2.1 and 2.3, 2.8, 5.3 ppm).

2.6. *Treatment and Definition of the Study Outcomes*

Patients were clinically followed on a monthly basis by a dedicated HF team, who were aware of conventional CMR but blinded to the MRS results. MACE is a composite of clinical events without standard definition, because individual outcomes used to make this composite endpoint vary by study [2,3,23]. According to our study endpoints, we used the term MACE to comprise the composite of the events including HF worsening, HF-related readmissions, cardiac catheterization, unstable angina, stroke, cardiac arrest/ventricular tachycardia (VT)/ventricular fibrillation (VF), and cardiac death. However, the HF related-readmission rates were not included in MACE and, thus, were separately considered. The appropriate length of the 2-year follow-up was determined based on our previous heart failure cohort study [24].

2.7. *Data Analysis*

Univariate and stepwise multivariable regression analyses (Wald statistics) were used to assess CMR parameters. A complete-case analysis was implemented (missing data were not excluded). Survival curves were plotted with the Kaplan-Meier method (log-rank test). Two-group comparisons of continuous and categorical variables were performed with the Student's *t*-test (two-group comparisons) and chi-square test, respectively. Continuous variables were determined by the recursive partitioning method to obtain the optimal cut-off values. Independent predictors of MACE and readmission rates were identified using univariate and multivariable Cox proportional hazard regression analyses. A Bonferroni posthoc correction was conducted to reduce Type I Error by dividing the original α-value by the number of analyses on the dependent variable. Data correlation was evaluated based on the Spearman rank test. Data analyses were performed using the following software: SPSS (version 11; SPSS Inc., Chicago, IL, USA), MedCalc (version 9.2.0.0; MedCalc Software, Mariakerke, Belgium), and R (version 3.5.3, R Foundation for Statistical Computing, Vienna, Austria, www.r-project.org).

3. Results

3.1. Patient Characteristics

A total of 133 consecutive patients (mean age, 52.4 years) entered the final analysis, with the mean follow-up time for surviving patients being 775 days. Table S1 details the baseline LV functional parameters. The baseline LVEF of this patient population was 52.2 (52.2 ± 21.7%). There were more patients with preserved EF ≥55% (n = 71) than reduced EF <55% (n = 62). MACE was observed in 39 cases (29.3%). The MACE with their distribution being as follows: HF-related readmission (n = 16; ischemic/non-ischemic 6/10), re-hospitalization for acute myocardial infarction (n = 15; 15/0), unstable angina (n = 4; 4/0), cardiac arrest (n = 1; 1/0), and stroke (n = 3; 0/3). There were no cases of cardiac death. The baseline clinical characteristics of the study participants are summarized in Table 1. Patients who experienced MACE did not differ from those who did not in terms of baseline clinical characteristics. As far as HF-related events are concerned, 6 patients (4.5%) were readmitted within 3 months and 18 patients (13.5%) within 12 months. Only one patient (0.8%) was readmitted within 30 days. Ischemic heart disease was identified in 50 patients, with the involvement of the left main (n = 2), left anterior descending (n = 36), left circumflex (n = 26), and right coronary artery (n = 23), verified by the presence of a myocardial scar on LGE. The remaining 83 patients had no history of ischemic heart disease and had no myocardial scar on LGE.

Table 1. Baseline characteristics of the study patients (n = 133).

Variable	MACE (n = 39)	Non-MACE (n = 94)	p Value
Clinical profile			
Male sex (%)	74.2%	57.5%	0.088
Age (years)	52.3 ± 10.0	52.7 ± 10.3	0.846
Height (m)	1.7 ± 0.1	1.7 ± 0.1	0.656
Weight (kg)	70.5 ± 13.8	69.6 ± 15.9	0.751
BMI (kg/m^2)	25.7 ± 3.9	25.6 ± 5.3	0.953
Heart rate	73.8 ± 14.2	71.3 ± 13.2	0.350
SBP (mmHg)	125.3 ± 19.5	131.9 ± 21.1	0.087
DBP (mmHg)	73.0 ± 11.7	76.4 ± 10.2	0.116
Smoking	53.8%	42.5%	0.316
Comorbidities			
Hypertension	47.3%	45.0%	0.956
DM	23.7%	20.0%	0.813
Angina	36.6%	32.5%	0.802
MI	36.6%	32.5%	0.802
DCM	16.1%	10.0%	0.512
Myocarditis	2.2%	5.0%	0.742
CAD	35.5%	32.5%	0.894
Medications			
DM drugs	16.1%	20.0%	0.771
Anti-platelets	39.8%	37.5%	0.957
Statins	23.7%	17.5%	0.576
Thrombolytic agents	6.5%	0.0%	0.235
Antiarrhythmic drugs	14.0%	10.0%	0.729
Diuretics	39.8%	30.0%	0.381
Calcium channel blockers	10.8%	7.5%	0.794
Beta blockers	68.8%	62.5%	0.611
ACEI/ARB	68.8%	57.5%	0.289
Vasodilators	16.1%	5.0%	0.139
Iron supplements	5.4%	2.5%	0.781

Table 1. *Cont.*

Variable	MACE (n = 39)	Non-MACE (n = 94)	p Value
Laboratory data			
AST (U/L)	31.4 ± 28.5	27.9 ± 24.3	0.556
ALT (U/L)	28.1 ± 16.5	39.8 ± 49.3	0.187
HDL (mg/dL)	43.5 ± 12.4	43.5 ± 12.1	0.988
VLDL (mg/dL)	30.3 ± 15.7	28.6 ± 13.0	0.598
LDL (mg/dL)	106.2 ± 53.2	109.7 ± 38.4	0.737
Total cholesterol/HDL	5.1 ± 5.3	4.4 ± 1.1	0.449
LDL/HDL	2.8 ± 1.2	2.7 ± 1.0	0.663
Total cholesterol (mg/dL)	189.3 ± 49.4	185.2 ± 35.7	0.672
Triglyceride (mg/dL)	165.5 ± 129.1	151.2 ± 86.2	0.564
Non-HDL (mg/dL)	145.8 ± 45.0	141.7 ± 35.4	0.662
Glucose (mg/dL)	113.2 ± 31.2	123.5 ± 51.2	0.210
HbA1c (mg/dL)	6.2 ± 1.2	6.4 ± 1.6	0.421
TIBC (ug/dL)	377.9 ± 85.8	346.7 ± 52.2	0.413
Troponin (ng/mL)	2.0 ± 8.9	0.3 ± 0.7	0.428
BNP (pg/mL)	342.9 ± 583.0	450.4 ± 569.7	0.470
Neutrophil count (%)	62.7 ± 12.6	57.5 ± 12.4	0.078
Hemoglobin (g/dL)	14.4 ± 3.5	13.5 ± 1.5	0.129
MCV (fl)	87.7 ± 6.7	86.4 ± 8.0	0.322
MCH (pg)	29.6 ± 2.7	29.0 ± 3.1	0.240
MCHC (%)	33.7 ± 1.0	41.0 ± 47.5	0.337

Note—Categorical data are expressed as numbers (%), whereas continuous variables are given as means ± standard deviations unless otherwise specified. Abbreviations: BMI, body mass index; CAD, coronary artery disease; SBP, systolic blood pressure; DBP, diastolic blood pressure; MACE, major adverse cardiac events; DM, diabetes mellitus; MI, myocardial infarction; DCM, dilated cardiomyopathy; ACEI, angiotensin-converting enzyme inhibitors; ARB, angiotensin receptor blockers; AST, aspartate aminotransferase; ALT, alanine transaminase; HDL, high-density lipoprotein; VLDL, very-low-density lipoprotein; LDL, low-density lipoprotein; TIBC, total iron-binding capacity; BNP, B-type natriuretic peptide; MCV, mean corpuscular volume; MCH, mean corpuscular hemoglobin; MCHC, mean corpuscular hemoglobin concentration.

3.2. Associations between CMR, and ^{1}H-MRS Parameters with MACE and HF-Related Readmission

All of the CMR parameters (EF, LVEDV, LVEDVI, LVESV, LV mean cavity volume, LV global volume, and LVGFI) were reciprocally correlated with one another ($p < 0.0001$). The results of univariate Cox regression analysis for MACE and HF-related readmission are shown in Tables 2 and 3. After allowance for potential confounders in multivariable analysis, LVEDVI was identified as an independent predictor for MACE, whereas myocardial mass independently predicted 3- and 12-month readmission rates. Kaplan-Meier survival analysis (Figure 3) demonstrated that patients with low LVEDVI (≤90.2 mL/m^2) had a lower probability for MACE than those with high LVEDVI (>90.2 mL/m^2, log-rank test, $p < 0.0001$).

Table 2. Univariate and stepwise multivariable Cox regression analysis of CMR and ^{1}H-MRS factors associated with major adverse cardiovascular events.

CMR& MRS Parameters	Overall (n = 133)				Ischemia (n = 50)				Non-Ischemia (n = 83)			
	Univariate		Stepwise Multivariable		Univariate		Stepwise Multivariable		Univariate		Stepwise Multivariable	
Variable	HR	p Value	HR	p Value	HR	p Value	HR	p Value	HR	p Value	HR	p Value
EF (%)	0.97	<0.001			0.99	0.456			0.95	0.001		
LV EDV (mL)	1.01	<0.001			1.00	0.099			1.01	<0.001		
LV EDVI (mL/m^2)	1.01	<0.001	1.01	<0.001 *	1.01	0.041			1.02	<0.001		
LV ESV (mL)	1.01	<0.001			1.00	0.189			1.01	<0.001		
Cardiac output (L/min)	1.08	0.463			1.25	0.067	1.32	0.044	0.95	0.768		
Myocardial mass (g)	1.01	0.001			1.01	0.144			1.01	<0.001	1.32	0.044
LV stroke volume (mL)	1.00	0.635			1.01	0.341			1.01	0.836		
LV mean cavity volume (mL)	1.01	<0.001			1.00	0.132			1.01	<0.001		
LV myocardial volume (mL)	1.01	0.001			1.01	0.144			1.01	<0.001		
LV global volume (mL)	1.00	<0.001			1.00	0.103			1.00	<0.001		
LVGFI (%)	0.97	0.001			0.99	0.562			0.95	<0.001		
FA 0.9 ppm	1.00	0.508			1.00	0.573			1.00	0.671		
FA 1.3 ppm	1.00	0.599			1.00	0.697			1.00	0.764		
FA 1.6 ppm	1.00	0.967			1.00	0.472			1.00	0.706		
UFA 2.1 ppm	1.00	0.557			1.00	0.938			1.00	0.779		
UFA 2.3 ppm	1.00	0.796			1.00	0.876			0.94	0.604		
UFA 2.8 ppm	1.00	0.796			1.00	0.753			0.18	0.772		
FA (09,13,16)	1.00	0.617			1.00	0.701			1.00	0.748		
UFA (21,23,28,53)	1.00	0.881			1.00	0.640			1.00	0.722		
TG (FA+UFA)	1.00	0.592			1.00	0.643			1.00	0.740		
FA/TG	1.68	0.219			1.89	0.292			1.60	0.605		
UFA/TG	0.60	0.219			0.53	0.292			0.62	0.605		
FA/UFA	1.00	0.089			1.01	0.023	1.01	0.022	0.98	0.426		

Note.—Abbreviations: HR, hazard ratio; CI, confidence interval; BMI, body mass index; SBP, systolic blood pressure; DBP, diastolic blood pressure; EF, ejection fraction; LV, left ventricular; EDV, end-diastolic volume; EDVI, end-diastolic volume index; ESV, end-systolic volume; FA, fatty acid; LVGFI, left ventricular global volume index; TG, triglycerides; UFA, unsaturated fatty acids. * significant after Bonferroni correction.

Table 3. Univariate and stepwise multivariable Cox regression analysis of CMR and ^{1}H-MRS factors associated with heart failure-related readmission.

CMR& MRS Parameters	Overall (n = 133)				Ischemia (n = 50)				Non-Ischemia (n = 83)			
	Univariate		Stepwise Multivariable		Univariate		Stepwise Multivariable		Univariate		Stepwise Multivariable	
Variable	HR	p Value	HR	p Value	HR	p Value	HR	p Value	HR	p Value	HR	p Value
EF (%)	0.96	<0.001			0.97	0.184			0.94	0.001		
LV EDV (mL)	1.01	<0.001			1.01	0.152			1.01	<0.001		
LV EDVI (mL/m^2)	1.02	<0.001	1.02	<0.001 *	1.02	0.106			1.02	0.001	1.01	<0.001 *
LV ESV (mL)	1.01	<0.001			1.01	0.119			1.01	<0.001		
Cardiac output (L/min)	0.85	0.348			0.92	0.781			0.81	0.326		
Myocardial mass (g)	1.01	<0.001			1.01	0.177	1.02	0.001 *	1.01	0.001		
LV stroke volume (mL)	0.99	0.447			0.99	0.699			0.99	0.408		
LV mean cavity volume (mL)	1.01	<0.001			1.01	0.130			1.01	<0.001		
LV myocardial volume (mL)	1.01	<0.001			1.01	0.177			1.01	0.001		
LV global volume (mL)	1.01	<0.001	1.01	<0.001 *	1.01	0.107			1.01	<.001	1.01	0.002 *
LVGFI (%)	0.94	<0.001			0.95	0.148			0.94	<0.001		
FA 0.9 ppm	0.70	0.523			0.86	0.708			0.00	0.555		
FA 1.3 ppm	1.00	0.746			0.96	0.832			1.00	0.769		
FA 1.6 ppm	0.68	0.635				0.006		0.003 *	0.22	0.735		
UFA 2.1 ppm	0.34	0.629			0.50	0.723			0.16	0.766		
UFA 2.3 ppm	0.65	0.718			0.82	0.737			0.24	0.770		
UFA 2.8 ppm	0.04	0.619			0.71	0.780				0.487		
FA (09,13,16)	0.99	0.589			0.96	0.0718			1.00	0.795		
UFA (21,23,28,53)	0.93	0.581			0.77	0.708			0.96	0.635		
TG (FA+UFA)	0.99	0.589			0.99	0.851			0.99	0.680		
FA/TG	2.72	0.183			56.41	0.095			1.21	0.818		
UFA/TG	0.37	0.183			0.02	0.095			0.83	0.818		
FA/UFA	1.01	0.396			1.01	0.318			1.00	0.858		

Note.—Abbreviations: HR, hazard ratio; CI, confidence interval; BMI, body mass index; SBP, systolic blood pressure; DBP, diastolic blood pressure; EF, ejection fraction; LV, left ventricular; EDV, end-diastolic volume; EDVI, end-diastolic volume index; ESV, end-systolic volume; FA, fatty acid; LVGFI, left ventricular global volume index; TG, triglycerides; UFA, unsaturated fatty acids. * significant after Bonferroni correction.

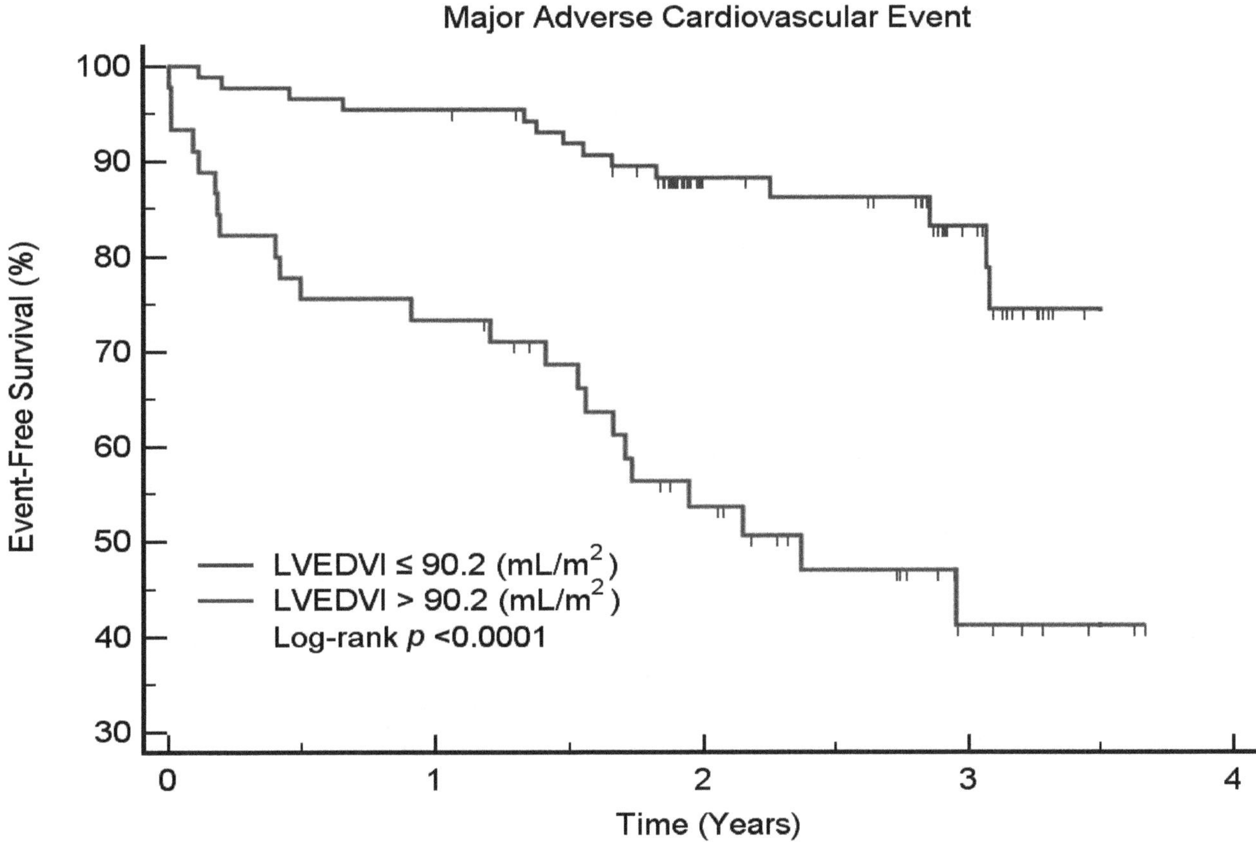

Figure 3. Kaplan-Meier curves for MACE-free survival in patients stratified according to the left ventricular end-diastolic volume index (LVEDVI) on CMR. Note—Kaplan-Meier survival analysis demonstrated that all patients with low LVEDVI (≤90.2 mL/m^2) had a lower probability for MACE than those with high LVEDVI (>90.2 mL/m^2, log-rank test, $p < 0.0001$). MACE, major cardiovascular event.

We found that baseline myocardial TG content—FA/UFA ratio—was significantly associated with the MACE, whilst the level of lipid resonances δ 1.6 ppm was significantly associated with HF-related readmission for those patients with ischemic heart disease. Kaplan-Meier survival analysis (Figure 4) demonstrated that ischemic patients with a low level of lipid resonance δ 1.6 ppm (≤0.99) had a lower probability for HF-related readmission than those with a high lipid resonance δ 1.6 ppm (>0.99, log-rank test, $p < 0.0001$). In non-ischemic patients, Kaplan-Meier survival analysis (Figure 5) demonstrated that patients with low LV global volume (≤231 mL) had a lower probability for HF-related readmission than those with high LV global volume (>231 mL, log-rank test, $p < 0.0001$). Myocardial TG content was not associated with MACE or HF-related readmission in non-ischemic patients. The levels of lipid resonances δ 1.6 ppm inversely correlated with the myocardial mass ($r = -0.290$, $p = 0.009$) and LV global volume ($r = -0.282$, $p = 0.011$) in non-ischemic patients. No correlations between the myocardial TG content and CMR functional parameters were found in the ischemic patient group.

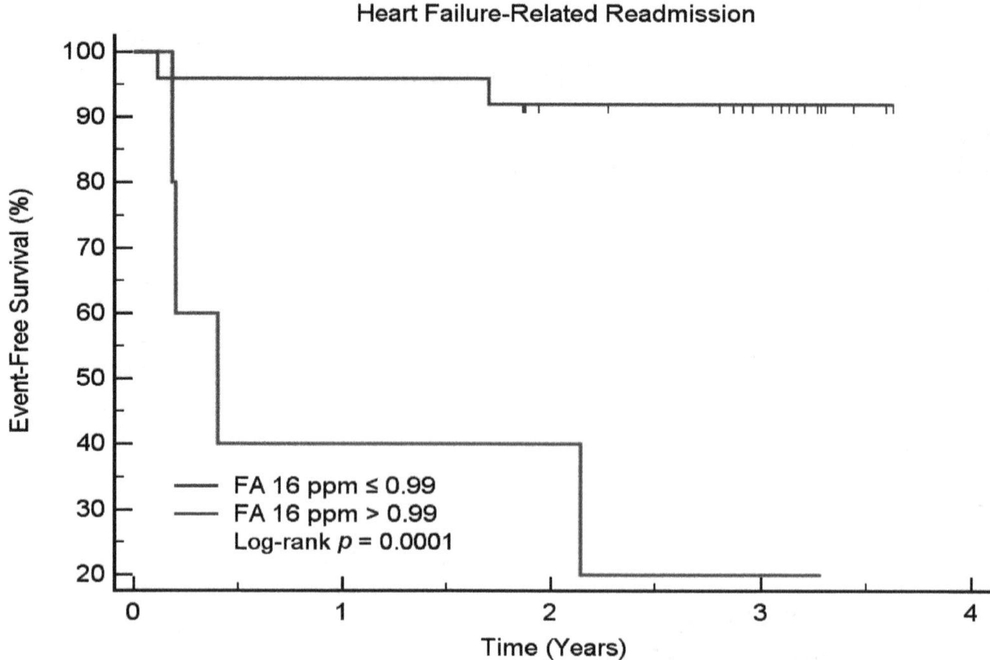

Figure 4. Kaplan-Meier curves for readmission-free survival in ischemic patients stratified according to the level of lipid resonances δ 1.6 ppm on ^{1}H-MRS. Note—Kaplan-Meier survival analysis demonstrated that ischemic patients with low levels of lipid resonances δ 1.6 ppm (≤0.99) had a lower probability for heart failure-related readmission than those with high levels of lipid resonances δ 1.6 ppm (>0.99, log-rank test, $p < 0.0001$). Note.—Abbreviations: FA, fatty acid.

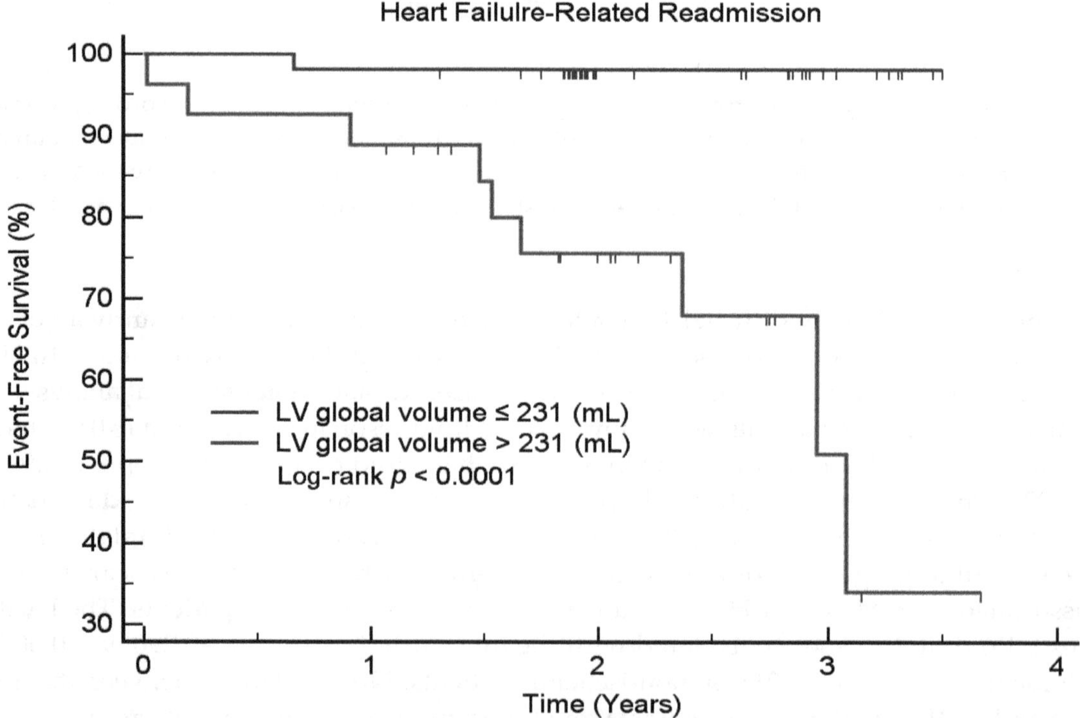

Figure 5. Kaplan-Meier curves for readmission-free survival in non-ischemic patients stratified according to LV (left ventricular) global volume on CMR. Note—Kaplan-Meier survival analysis showed that non-ischemic patients with low LV global volume (≤231 mL) had a lower probability for heart failure-related readmission than those with high LV global volume (>231 mL, log-rank test, $p < 0.0001$).

4. Discussion

This study was designed to simultaneously assess the prognostic significance of myocardial TG content (assessed by ^{1}H-MRS) and LV function parameters (measured on CMR) in the prediction of MACE and readmission in patients hospitalized for acute HF. Our main results can be summarized as follows. First, an increased LVEDVI was identified as an independent predictor of reduced MACE-free survival. Second, myocardial mass was independently associated with 3- and 12-month readmission rates. Finally, we found myocardial TG content—FA/UFA ratio—was significantly associated with MACE, whilst the level of lipid resonances δ 1.6 ppm was significantly associated with HF-related readmission for patients with ischemic heart disease. Taken together, these data indicate that assessment of LV function on CMR may improve the risk stratification of patients who have been hospitalized for acute HF. ^{1}H-MRS assessment might be reserved for patients with a history of ischemic heart disease.

In patients with HF, diastolic wall strain has been reported as an independent predictor of MACE [25], and the global circumferential strain may improve the prognostic stratification [26]. However, both diastolic wall strain and global circumferential strain require expertise for post-processing from cine CMR, and were not performed in the present study. In contrast, LVEDVI (defined as the volume of blood in the LV at end load filling indexed for body surface area) is easier to integrate in the clinical routine. Mewton et al. [27] have reported that LVGFI—a CMR parameter that integrates LV structure with global function—has a strong predictive value of MACE in a multiethnic population of men and women without a history of CVD at baseline. However, in the current study, LVGFI was a significant prognostic predictor in univariate but not in multivariable analysis. It is possible that the weaker predictor value of LVGFI—as compared with LVEDVI—observed in our study could reflect compensatory modifications in LV mass and volumes aimed at preserving systolic function during HF. Because HF is a complex clinical syndrome that results from a variety of conditions preventing the LV from supporting the physiological circulation. Our study explored the possibility of linking the dysregulation of myocardial TG with the future MACE, based on evidence showing the associations of myocardial TG and CV disease [6–8], plus the potential of quantitative readout of MRS in differentiating various lipid species in the myocardium [10]. Using this technique, we have previously shown that patients hospitalized for acute HF are characterized by increased myocardial UFA content [13]. The predictive value of myocardial TG contents—FA/UFA ratio and levels of lipid resonances δ 1.6 ppm, were further validated in the current case-control study. Indeed, increased myocardial TG content is a prerequisite of cardiac steatosis, which may ultimately result in lipotoxicity and heart dysfunction [6–8,10]. In line with our results, Wei et al. [28] demonstrated that myocardial steatosis is mechanistically linked to diastolic dysfunction in women with coronary microvascular dysfunction. The early alterations of myocardial TG measured by using ^{1}H-MRS might be supplementary to the diastolic dysfunction to improve the stratification for patients with ischemic heart disease.

Readmissions are frequent in patients with acute HF and served as a secondary outcome measure in the current study. A previous report demonstrated that diabetes mellitus, hyperlipidemia, CAD, length of stay at the index admission, and prescription of beta-blockers were significant predictors of readmission rates [29]. The 30-day, 3-month, and 12-month readmission rates observed in our study were 0.8%, 4.5%, 13.5%, respectively, being markedly lower than those observed in Western countries [30,31]. Interestingly, we identified myocardial mass measured on CMR as an independent predictor of readmission rates. The present study supports the concept that LV mass measured by CMR is a viable predictor of adverse cardiovascular events [27], either from the MESA (Multi-Ethnic Study of Atherosclerosis) study [32] or the Cardiovascular Health Study [33]. Further independent studies in larger sample sizes are needed to confirm this pilot observation.

Our data should be interpreted in the context of some limitations. First, the single-center of our study may bring into question its generalizability, as the study population was highly selected for those with medical conditions becoming stable and ready to discharge. The number of HF-related readmissions might be too small for meaningful multivariable analyses. However, it is noteworthy that patients were recruited regardless of the underlying cause of HF. The data should be interpreted carefully because pathophysiologically diverse endpoints were included in this study. Second, the resonance δ 1.6 ppm sometimes overlaps with the main CH_2 resonance δ 1.3 ppm. The sum of the signal intensities δ 0.9, 1.3 and 1.6 ppm would have been more reliably extracted from an in vivo cardiac ^{1}H-MRS. Nonetheless, the quantitative analysis was carried out using well-established LC Model software to enhance the generalizability of the current study. Third, longitudinal 3-T CMR and ^{1}H-MRS examinations were not performed and changes in LVEDVI and/or myocardial TG content were not investigated over time. A validation cohort for our findings would help to elucidate the clinical value of such imaging biomarkers, however, it was outside of the pre-specified analysis for this study.

5. Conclusions

Our results indicate that LVEDVI and myocardial mass are potential imaging biomarkers that independently predict MACE and readmission, respectively, in patients discharged after hospitalization for acute HF. Myocardial TG predicts readmission in patients with a history of ischemic heart disease. Further studies are needed to determine whether LVEDVI and myocardial mass, as well as myocardial TG, may serve as therapeutic targets to improve prognoses in targeted patient populations.

Author Contributions: K.-F.C., K.-K.N., C.-H.W., J.-J.W., S.-H.N., and G.L. drafted the manuscript. C.-H.W., M.-H.L., M.-T.W., J.-J.W., S.-H.N., and G.L. designed the study. K.-F.C., P.-A.L., P.-C.H., K.-K.N., Y.-H.J., Y.-C.L. (Yu-Ching Lin), Y.-C.L. (Yu-Chun Lin), J.-J.W., S.-H.N., and G.L. analyzed the data, prepared the Tables and Figures. S.-Y.T. and G.L. carried out the analysis of magnetic resonance spectroscopy data. L.-Y.Y. and G.L. performed the statistical analysis. All authors have read and agreed to the published version of the manuscript.

Acknowledgments: We appreciate statistician Lan-Yan Yang and Hsin-Ying Lu for their assistance in data analysis.

References

1. Ponikowski, P.; Voors, A.A.; Anker, S.D.; Bueno, H.; Cleland, J.G.F.; Coats, A.J.S.; Falk, V.; Gonzalez-Juanatey, J.R.; Harjola, V.P.; Jankowska, E.A.; et al. 2016 ESC Guidelines for the diagnosis and treatment of acute and chronic heart failure: The Task Force for the diagnosis and treatment of acute and chronic heart failure of the European Society of Cardiology (ESC) Developed with the special contribution of the Heart Failure Association (HFA) of the ESC. *Eur. Heart J.* **2016**, *37*, 2129–2200. [PubMed]
2. Tsutsui, H.; Tsuchihashi, M.; Takeshita, A. Mortality and readmission of hospitalized patients with congestive heart failure and preserved versus depressed systolic function. *Am. J. Cardiol.* **2001**, *88*, 530–533. [CrossRef]
3. Yancy, C.W.; Jessup, M.; Bozkurt, B.; Butler, J.; Casey, D.E., Jr.; Drazner, M.H.; Fonarow, G.C.; Geraci, S.A.; Horwich, T.; Januzzi, J.L.; et al. 2013 ACCF/AHA guideline for the management of heart failure: Executive summary: A report of the American College of Cardiology Foundation/American Heart Association Task Force on practice guidelines. *Circulation* **2013**, *128*, 1810–1852. [CrossRef] [PubMed]
4. Hunt, S.A.; Abraham, W.T.; Chin, M.H.; Feldman, A.M.; Francis, G.S.; Ganiats, T.G.; Jessup, M.; Konstam, M.A.; Mancini, D.M.; Michl, K.; et al. ACC/AHA 2005 Guideline Update for the Diagnosis and Management of Chronic Heart Failure in the Adult: A report of the American College of Cardiology/American Heart Association Task Force on Practice Guidelines (Writing Committee to Update the 2001 Guidelines for the Evaluation and Management of Heart Failure): Developed in collaboration with the American College of Chest Physicians and the International Society for Heart and Lung Transplantation: Endorsed by the Heart Rhythm Society. *Circulation* **2005**, *112*, e154–e235. [PubMed]

5. Taegtmeyer, H.; McNulty, P.; Young, M.E. Adaptation and maladaptation of the heart in diabetes: Part I: General concepts. *Circulation* **2002**, *105*, 1727–1733. [CrossRef]
6. Wright, J.J.; Kim, J.; Buchanan, J.; Boudina, S.; Sena, S.; Bakirtzi, K.; Ilkun, O.; Theobald, H.A.; Cooksey, R.C.; Kandror, K.V.; et al. Mechanisms for increased myocardial fatty acid utilization following short-term high-fat feeding. *Cardiovasc. Res.* **2009**, *82*, 351–360. [CrossRef]
7. Turkbey, E.B.; McClelland, R.L.; Kronmal, R.A.; Burke, G.L.; Bild, D.E.; Tracy, R.P.; Arai, A.E.; Lima, J.A.; Bluemke, D.A. The impact of obesity on the left ventricle: The Multi-Ethnic Study of Atherosclerosis (MESA). *JACC Cardiovasc. Imaging* **2010**, *3*, 266–274. [CrossRef]
8. Wende, A.R.; Abel, E.D. Lipotoxicity in the heart. *Biochim. Biophys. Acta* **2010**, *1801*, 311–319. [CrossRef]
9. Vilahur, G.; Casani, L.; Juan-Babot, O.; Guerra, J.M.; Badimon, L. Infiltrated cardiac lipids impair myofibroblast-induced healing of the myocardial scar post-myocardial infarction. *Atherosclerosis* **2012**, *224*, 368–376. [CrossRef]
10. Faller, K.M.; Lygate, C.A.; Neubauer, S.; Schneider, J.E. (1) H-MR spectroscopy for analysis of cardiac lipid and creatine metabolism. *Heart Fail. Rev.* **2013**, *18*, 657–668. [CrossRef]
11. Bizino, M.B.; Hammer, S.; Lamb, H.J. Metabolic imaging of the human heart: Clinical application of magnetic resonance spectroscopy. *Heart* **2014**, *100*, 881–890. [CrossRef] [PubMed]
12. Mahmod, M.; Bull, S.; Suttie, J.J.; Pal, N.; Holloway, C.; Dass, S.; Myerson, S.G.; Schneider, J.E.; De Silva, R.; Petrou, M.; et al. Myocardial steatosis and left ventricular contractile dysfunction in patients with severe aortic stenosis. *Circ. Cardiovasc. Imaging* **2013**, *6*, 808–816. [CrossRef] [PubMed]
13. Liao, P.A.; Lin, G.; Tsai, S.Y.; Wang, C.H.; Juan, Y.H.; Lin, Y.C.; Wu, M.T.; Yang, L.Y.; Liu, M.H.; Chang, T.C.; et al. Myocardial triglyceride content at 3 T cardiovascular magnetic resonance and left ventricular systolic function: A cross-sectional study in patients hospitalized with acute heart failure. *J. Cardiovasc. Magn. Reson.* **2016**, *18*, 9. [CrossRef] [PubMed]
14. Aljizeeri, A.; Sulaiman, A.; Alhulaimi, N.; Alsaileek, A.; Al-Mallah, M.H. Cardiac magnetic resonance imaging in heart failure: Where the alphabet begins! *Heart Fail. Rev.* **2017**, *22*, 385–399. [CrossRef] [PubMed]
15. Todiere, G.; Marzilli, M. Role of cardiac imaging in heart failure. *Minerva Cardioangiol.* **2012**, *60*, 347–362. [PubMed]
16. Partington, S.L.; Cheng, S.; Lima, J.A. Cardiac magnetic resonance imaging for stage B heart failure. *Heart Fail. Clin.* **2012**, *8*, 179–190. [CrossRef]
17. Bottomley, P.A. Spatial localization in NMR spectroscopy in vivo. *Ann. N. Y. Acad. Sci.* **1987**, *508*, 333–348. [CrossRef]
18. Liu, C.Y.; Bluemke, D.A.; Gerstenblith, G.; Zimmerman, S.L.; Li, J.; Zhu, H.; Lai, S.; Lai, H. Myocardial steatosis and its association with obesity and regional ventricular dysfunction: Evaluated by magnetic resonance tagging and 1H spectroscopy in healthy African Americans. *Int. J. Cardiol.* **2014**, *172*, 381–387. [CrossRef]
19. Reingold, J.S.; McGavock, J.M.; Kaka, S.; Tillery, T.; Victor, R.G.; Szczepaniak, L.S. Determination of triglyceride in the human myocardium by magnetic resonance spectroscopy: Reproducibility and sensitivity of the method. *Am. J. Physiol. Endocrinol. Metab.* **2005**, *289*, E935–E939. [CrossRef]
20. van der Meer, R.W.; Doornbos, J.; Kozerke, S.; Schar, M.; Bax, J.J.; Hammer, S.; Smit, J.W.; Romijn, J.A.; Diamant, M.; Rijzewijk, L.J.; et al. Metabolic imaging of myocardial triglyceride content: Reproducibility of 1H MR spectroscopy with respiratory navigator gating in volunteers. *Radiology* **2007**, *245*, 251–257. [CrossRef]
21. O'Connor, R.D.; Xu, J.; Ewald, G.A.; Ackerman, J.J.; Peterson, L.R.; Gropler, R.J.; Bashir, A. Intramyocardial triglyceride quantification by magnetic resonance spectroscopy: In vivo and ex vivo correlation in human subjects. *Magn. Reson. Med.* **2011**, *65*, 1234–1238. [CrossRef] [PubMed]
22. Weiss, K.; Summermatter, S.; Stoeck, C.T.; Kozerke, S. Compensation of signal loss due to cardiac motion in point-resolved spectroscopy of the heart. *Magn. Reson. Med.* **2014**, *72*, 1201–1207. [CrossRef] [PubMed]
23. Kip, K.E.; Hollabaugh, K.; Marroquin, O.C.; Williams, D.O. The problem with composite end points in cardiovascular studies: The story of major adverse cardiac events and percutaneous coronary intervention. *J. Am. Coll. Cardiol.* **2008**, *51*, 701–707. [CrossRef]
24. Cheng, M.L.; Wang, C.H.; Shiao, M.S.; Liu, M.H.; Huang, Y.Y.; Huang, C.Y.; Mao, C.T.; Lin, J.F.; Ho, H.Y.; Yang, N.I. Metabolic disturbances identified in plasma are associated with outcomes in patients with heart failure: Diagnostic and prognostic value of metabolomics. *J. Am. Coll. Cardiol.* **2015**, *65*, 1509–1520. [CrossRef] [PubMed]

25. Minamisawa, M.; Miura, T.; Motoki, H.; Ueki, Y.; Shimizu, K.; Shoin, W.; Harada, M.; Mochidome, T.; Yoshie, K.; Oguchi, Y.; et al. Prognostic Impact of Diastolic Wall Strain in Patients at Risk for Heart Failure. *Int. Heart J.* **2017**, *58*, 250–256. [CrossRef] [PubMed]
26. Mordi, I.; Bezerra, H.; Carrick, D.; Tzemos, N. The Combined Incremental Prognostic Value of LVEF, Late Gadolinium Enhancement, and Global Circumferential Strain Assessed by CMR. JACC. *Cardiovasc. Imaging* **2015**, *8*, 540–549.
27. Mewton, N.; Opdahl, A.; Choi, E.Y.; Almeida, A.L.; Kawel, N.; Wu, C.O.; Burke, G.L.; Liu, S.; Liu, K.; Bluemke, D.A.; et al. Left ventricular global function index by magnetic resonance imaging—A novel marker for assessment of cardiac performance for the prediction of cardiovascular events: The multi-ethnic study of atherosclerosis. *Hypertension* **2013**, *61*, 770–778. [CrossRef]
28. Wei, J.; Nelson, M.D.; Szczepaniak, E.W.; Smith, L.; Mehta, P.K.; Thomson, L.E.; Berman, D.S.; Li, D.; Bairey Merz, C.N.; Szczepaniak, L.S. Myocardial steatosis as a possible mechanistic link between diastolic dysfunction and coronary microvascular dysfunction in women. *Am. J. Physiol. Heart Circ. Physiol.* **2016**, *310*, H14–H19. [CrossRef]
29. Deeka, H.; Skouri, H.; Noureddine, S. Readmission rates and related factors in heart failure patients: A study in Lebanon. *Collegian* **2016**, *23*, 61–68. [CrossRef]
30. Butler, J.; Kalogeropoulos, A. Worsening heart failure hospitalization epidemic we do not know how to prevent and we do not know how to treat! *J. Am. Coll. Cardiol.* **2008**, *52*, 435–437. [CrossRef]
31. Desai, A.S.; Stevenson, L.W. Rehospitalization for heart failure: Predict or prevent? *Circulation* **2012**, *126*, 501–506. [CrossRef] [PubMed]
32. Bluemke, D.A.; Kronmal, R.A.; Lima, J.A.; Liu, K.; Olson, J.; Burke, G.L.; Folsom, A.R. The relationship of left ventricular mass and geometry to incident cardiovascular events: The MESA (Multi-Ethnic Study of Atherosclerosis) study. *J. Am. Coll. Cardiol.* **2008**, *52*, 2148–2155. [CrossRef] [PubMed]
33. de Simone, G.; Gottdiener, J.S.; Chinali, M.; Maurer, M.S. Left ventricular mass predicts heart failure not related to previous myocardial infarction: The Cardiovascular Health Study. *Eur. Heart J.* **2008**, *29*, 741–747. [CrossRef] [PubMed]

5

Biophysical and Lipidomic Biomarkers of Cardiac Remodeling Post-Myocardial Infarction in Humans

Valerie Samouillan [1], Ignacio Miguel Martinez de Lejarza Samper [2,3], Aleyda Benitez Amaro [4,5], David Vilades [2,3], Jany Dandurand [1], Josefina Casas [6,7], Esther Jorge [2,3], David de Gonzalo Calvo [4,5], Alberto Gallardo [8], Enrique Lerma [8], Jose Maria Guerra [2,3], Francesc Carreras [2,3], Ruben Leta [2,3] and Vicenta Llorente Cortes [3,4,5,*]

1 CIRIMAT, Université de Toulouse, Université Paul Sabatier, Equipe PHYPOL, 31062 Toulouse, France; valerie.samouillan@univ-tlse3.fr (V.S.); jany.lods@univ-tlse3.fr (J.D.)
2 Department of Cardiology, Hospital de la Santa Creu i Sant Pau, Biomedical Research Institute Sant Pau (IIB Sant Pau), Universitat Autonoma de Barcelona, 08193 Barcelona, Spain; IMartinezL@santpau.cat (I.M.M.d.L.S.); DVilades@santpau.cat (D.V.); EJorge@santpau.cat (E.J.); JGuerra@santpau.cat (J.M.G.); FCarreras@santpau.cat (F.C.); RLeta@santpau.cat (R.L.)
3 CIBERCV, Institute of Health Carlos III, 28029 Madrid, Spain
4 Institute of Biomedical Research of Barcelona (IIBB), Spanish National Research Council (CSIC), 08036 Barcelona, Spain; ABenitez@santpau.cat (A.B.A.); david.degonzalo@gmail.com (D.d.G.C.)
5 Group of Lipids and Cardiovascular Pathology, Biomedical Research Institute Sant Pau (IIB Sant Pau), Hospital de la Santa Creu i Sant Pau, 08041 Barcelona, Spain
6 Research Unit on BioActive Molecules (RUBAM), Department of Biological Chemistry, Institute for Advanced Chemistry of Catalonia (IQAC-CSIC), 08034 Barcelona, Spain; fina.casas@iqac.csic.es
7 CIBEREHD Institute of Health Carlos III, 28029 Madrid, Spain
8 Department of Pathology, Hospital de la Santa Creu i Sant Pau, 08041 Barcelona, Spain; AGallardo@santpau.cat (A.G.); ELerma@santpau.cat (E.L.)
* Correspondence: cllorente@santpau.cat or vicenta.llorente@iibb.csic.es

Abstract: Few studies have analyzed the potential of biophysical parameters as markers of cardiac remodeling post-myocardial infarction (MI), particularly in human hearts. Fourier transform infrared spectroscopy (FTIR) illustrates the overall changes in proteins, nucleic acids and lipids in a single signature. The aim of this work was to define the FTIR and lipidomic pattern for human left ventricular remodeling post-MI. A total of nine explanted hearts from ischemic cardiomyopathy patients were collected. Samples from the right ventricle (RV), left ventricle (LV) and infarcted left ventricle (LV INF) were subjected to biophysical (FTIR and differential scanning calorimetry, DSC) and lipidomic (liquid chromatography–high-resolution mass spectrometry, LC–HRMS) studies. FTIR evidenced deep alterations in the myofibers, extracellular matrix proteins, and the hydric response of the LV INF compared to the RV or LV from the same subject. The lipid and esterified lipid FTIR bands were enhanced in LV INF, and both lipid indicators were tightly and positively correlated with remodeling markers such as collagen, lactate, polysaccharides, and glycogen in these samples. Lipidomic analysis revealed an increase in several species of sphingomyelin (SM), hexosylceramide (HexCer), and cholesteryl esters combined with a decrease in glycerophospholipids in the infarcted tissue. Our results validate FTIR indicators and several species of lipids as useful markers of left ventricular remodeling post-MI in humans.

Keywords: biophysical markers; cardiac remodeling post-MI; lipidomics; Fourier transform infrared spectroscopy; heart failure

1. Introduction

Ischemic heart disease is the primary cause of death in Western countries, and myocardial infarction occupies about 50% of deaths in this group. Despite the important improvements in the management of myocardial infarction, adverse left ventricular remodeling, which occurs in up to 30% of cases following ST-segment elevation myocardial infarction (STEMI), is strongly associated with poor patient outcomes. Chronic left ventricular remodeling (LVR) is, apart from infarct size and infarct wound healing, the primary determinant of heart failure post-myocardial infarction (MI) [1,2]. Adverse LVR after MI involves crucial changes in the composition and organization of the extracellular matrix (ECM) [3].

The location, size and shape of MI is commonly determined by imaging techniques at the clinical level or by histopathology at the experimental level. Detailed information about the chemical composition and physical structure of infarct zones post-MI remains limited. Previous studies from our group have shown that Fourier transform infrared (FTIR) spectroscopy has the potential to highlight the main alterations that occur in cardiac remodeling in a post-MI mice model [4], as well as in a pig model of tachycardia-induced dilated cardiomyopathy [5]. The FTIR spectra of freeze-dried mice's left ventricles showed amides I and II to be the major absorptions bands. Collagen possesses a specific band at 1338 cm^{-1} [6] that can be used to compile a collagen/protein indicator. Finally, the sub-resolution of the FTIR spectra determined by Fourier self-deconvolution (FSD) and the second derivative method in the amide I/II zone is useful for determining the secondary structures of proteins [7]. In a mice model, we showed that an increase in the collagen indicator in the infarcted tissue is associated with the predominance of the triple helical conformation of proteins, evidencing a deep remodeling of this zone.

In addition to structural remodeling, infarcted tissue undergoes what is called "metabolic remodeling", which includes a set of metabolic changes that occur in the cardiac tissue exposed to ischemia. These metabolic changes include partial insulin resistance, associated with reduced fatty acid oxidation and impaired mitochondrial biogenesis [8,9], downregulation of metabolic genes [10], and upregulation of lipoprotein receptors that contribute to increasing the intracellular lipids in cardiomyocytes [11–14]. A high prevalence of myocardial lipids has been found in areas of chronic MI in humans [15]. Patients with cardiac lipid deposition had larger infarctions, as well as decreased wall thickening and impaired endocardial wall motion. The hydrolysis of lipid species such as phospholipids in the membrane of cardiomyocytes during ischemic processes is intimately linked to the pathogenesis of myocardial infarction [16,17]. Clinical studies have identified new circulating metabolites that are derived from phospholipidic metabolism in serum and are useful as potential new biomarkers in cardiac remodeling post-MI [18–22]. To the best of our knowledge, only one lipidomic study has been performed in cardiac infarcted tissues, and was developed using pigs [13].

The objective of the current investigation was to identify conformational, biophysical, and lipidomic alterations that are useful as biomarkers of cardiac adverse remodeling in human infarcted hearts.

2. Materials and Methods

2.1. Collection of Human Samples

A total of 9 explanted human hearts from ischemic cardiomyopathy patients were collected and immediately processed. These hearts were from patients undergoing cardiac transplantation in the Department of Cardiology. The myocardial samples from the explanted hearts were collected in the Department of Pathology (both departments from Santa Creu I Sant Pau Hospital, Barcelona). Clinical data, electrocardiograms, Doppler echocardiography, hemodynamic studies, and coronary angiography were available for all patients. All patients were functionally classified according to the New York Heart Association (NYHA) criteria and received medical treatment according to the guidelines of the European Society of Cardiology [23] using diuretics 89%, angiotensin-converting enzyme inhibitors 86%, β-blockers 48%, aldosterone antagonists 71%, digoxin 49% and statins 82% (Table 1).

Table 1. Clinical and echocardiographic characteristics from whom explanted ischemic hearts were obtained.

	ICM (n = 9)
Age (years)	57.67 ± 12.02
Gender male (%)	78
Prior Hypertension (%)	44
Diabetes mellitus (%)	11
Dislipemia (%)	75
Perfusion abnormalities * (%)	72
Echo-Doppler study	
Ejection fraction (%)	29.88 ± 8.90
Intraventricular septum in diastole (mm)	11.63 ± 4.63
Left ventricular posterior wall in diastole (mm)	9.53 ± 0.75
Left ventricular end-diastolic diameter (mm)	60.38 ± 14.15
Left ventricular end-systolic diameter (mm)	56.25 ± 2.79
Treatment (%)	
Diuretics	89
Angiotensin-converting enzyme inhibitors	86
β-blockers	48
Aldosteron antagonists	71
Digoxin	49
Statins	82

ICM, ischemic cardiomyopathy; * the patients with perfusion abnormalities were considered those subjected to coronary interventions (i.e. by-pass, angioplasty, stents and others).

Hearts were weighed and measured, and samples from the right ventricle (RV) (n = 9), left ventricle (LV) (n = 9), and infarcted left ventricle (LV INF) (n = 9) were excised and frozen at −80 °C for immunohistochemical, biophysical and lipidomic studies. The project was approved by the local Ethics Committee of Hospital de la Santa Creu i Sant Pau, Barcelona, Spain, and was conducted in accordance with the guidelines of the Declaration of Helsinki. All patients gave written informed consent that was obtained according to our institutional guidelines.

2.2. *Tissue Homogenization and Preparation of the Samples for the Different Studies*

One portion of collected tissue was embedded in optimal cutting temperature compound (OCT) and used for immunohistochemical studies. Other portion was frozen under N_2, pulverized using a mortar and a pestle in liquid nitrogen and used for the biophysical studies. A 5 mg aliquot was freeze dried and used for vibrational characterization and a 25 mg aliquot was used for differential scanning calorimetry (DSC). Another aliquot of pulverized tissue (500 µg) was dissolved in a lysis buffer (Tris-HCl 1 M, KCl 1 M, and protease inhibitors 1 µg/mL) and used for the lipidomic studies.

2.3. *Immunohistochemical Analysis*

Myocardial collagen was immunohistochemically assessed by Sirius Red Staining as previously described [24].

2.4. *Vibrational Characterization*

The Fourier transform infrared spectroscopy/attenuated total reflectance (FTIR/ATR) spectra of the freeze-dried tissues were acquired using a Nicolet 5700 FTIR instrument (Thermo Fisher Scientific, Waltham, MA, USA) equipped with an ATR device with a KBr beam splitter and an MCT/B detector. The ATR accessory used was a Smart Orbit with a type IIA diamond crystal (refractive index 2.4, Thermo Fisher Scientific, Waltham, MA, USA). Samples were directly deposited on the entire active surface of the crystal and gently compressed using a Teflon tip to ensure good contact. For each sample, 80 interferograms were recorded in the 4000–450 cm^{-1} region, co-added and Fourier-transformed to generate an average spectrum of the segmented heart part with a nominal resolution of 1 cm^{-1} using Omnic 8.0 (Thermo Fisher Scientific, Waltham, MA, USA). The single-beam background spectrum was collected from the clean diamond crystal before each experiment, and this background was subtracted from the spectra.

To circumvent the attenuation of penetration depth in the samples at large wave numbers in the ATR mode, spectra were subjected to advanced ATR correction. Then, the spectra were baseline corrected and normalized using the maximum of the amide II peak. These spectra were subsequently used to calculate the integrated band intensities and their ratios. For semi-quantitative comparison between groups, the areas of the different absorption bands were computed from the individual spectrum of each tissue, and the appropriate ratio of areas was used according to the literature data in trans-reflectance or ATR mode [25,26]. Second derivatives were used to enhance the chemical information present in the overlapping infrared absorption bands of the spectra. All spectra processing was performed using Omnic 8.0. The spectra presented for each group were calculated by averaging the spectra of all samples within each group.

2.5. *Differential Scanning Calorimetry*

Calorimetric analyses were performed using a DSC Pyris calorimeter (Perkin Elmer, Waltham, MA). The calorimeter was calibrated using Hg and In resulting in a temperature accuracy of 0.1 °C and an enthalpy accuracy of 0.2 J/g. Fresh samples, 5–10 mg in weight, were set into hermetic aluminum pans and equilibrated at the initial temperature for 5 min before cooling to −100 °C at 10 °C/min. Then, the thermograms were recorded during heating at 10 °C/min until reaching 90 °C. After the DSC measurements were performed, the pans were reweighed to check that they had been correctly sealed.

2.6. *Lipidomic Analysis of the Heart*

Phospholipids (PLs) and sphingolipids (SLs extracts) were prepared and analyzed using the following protocols previously described [27,28], with minor modifications.

2.6.1. Phospholipids and Neutral Lipids

A 750 μL methanol–chloroform (1:2, *v*/*v*) solution containing standards was transferred to borosilicate glass test tubes with Teflon caps, and 0.25 mL methanol and 0.5 mL chloroform were subsequently added. This mixture was fortified with the internal standards of lipids (200 pmol each). The following standards were added to myocardial samples: 16:0 D31_18:1 phosphocholine, 16:0 D31_18:1 phosphoethanolamine, 16:0 D31-18:1 phosphoserine, 17:0 lyso-phosphocholine, 17:1 lyso-phosphoethanolamine, 17:1 lyso-phosphoserine, 17:0/17:0/17:0 triacylglycerol, and C17:0 cholesteryl ester; 0.2 nmol of each standard (from Avanti Polar Lipids). The samples were vortexed and sonicated until they appeared dispersed and were then incubated at 48 °C overnight. The solvent was removed using a Speed Vac Savant SPD131DDA (Thermo Scientific). Lipids were solubilized in 0.5 mL of methanol and transferred to 1.5 mL Eppendorf tubes and evaporated again. The samples were resuspended in 150 μL of methanol. The tubes were centrifuged at 13,000× *g* for 3 min, and 130 μL of the supernatants was transferred to ultra-performance liquid chromatography (UPLC) vials for injection and analysis.

2.6.2. Sphingolipids

A 750 μL methanol–chloroform (2:1, *v*/*v*) solution containing internal standards (N-dodecanoylsphingosine, N-dodecanoylglucosylsphingosine, N-dodecanoylsphingosylphosphorylcholine, and C17-sphinganine, 0.2 nmol each, from Avanti Polar Lipids) was added to the myocardial samples. The samples were extracted at 48 °C overnight and cooled. Then, 75 μL of 1 M KOH in methanol was added to saponify phospholipids and prevent their possible interference in the detection of sphingolipids, and the mixture was incubated for 2 h at 37 °C. Following the addition of 75 μL of 1 M acetic acid, the samples were evaporated to dryness, and stored at −20 °C until analysis. Before analysis, 150 μL of methanol was added to the samples. Then, the samples were centrifuged at 13,000× *g* for 5 min, and 130 μL of the supernatant was transferred to a new vial and injected.

2.6.3. UPLC Coupled to HRMS Analysis

Ultra Performance Liquid chromatography (UPLC) coupled to high-resolution mass spectrometry (HRMS) analysis was performed using an Acquity ultra-high-performance liquid chromatography (UHPLC) system (Waters, USA) connected to a Time of Flight (LCT Premier XE) Detector. The full-scan spectra from 50 to 1800 Da were acquired, and individual spectra were summed to produce data points each being 0.2 s. Mass accuracy at a resolving power of 10,000 and reproducibility were maintained using an independent reference spray via LockSpray interference.

Lipid extracts were injected onto an Acquity UPLC BEH C8 column (1.7 μm particle size, 100 mm × 2.1 mm, Waters Ireland) at a flow rate of 0.3 mL/min and a column temperature of 30 °C. The mobile phases were water with 2 mM of ammonium formate and 0.2% of formic acid (A) and methanol with 2 mM of ammonium formate and 0.2% of formic acid (B).The UPLC conditions were programmed as follows: 0.0 min_80% B; 3 min_90% B (linear gradient); 6 min_90% B (isocratic); 15 min_99% B (linear gradient); 18 min_99% B (isocratic); 20 min_80% B (linear gradient); 22 min_80% B (isocratic).

Positive identification of compounds was based on the accurate mass measurement and its LC retention time, compared with that of a standard (<2%). Selected ions for SLs and glycerophospholipids correspond to $[M + H]^+$, whereas ammonia adduct were used for neutral lipids (Table S1). The ceramide (Cer) standards used were N-palmitoyl-sphingosine, N-stearoyl-sphingosine, N-lignoceroyl-sphingosine and N-nervonoyl-sphingosine. The sphingomyelin (SM) standards used were N-palmitoylsphingosyl phosphorylcholine, egg SMs (predominant C16:0SM) and brain SMs (C18:0SM, C24:0SM and C24:1SM in known percentages). The glucosylceramide standard used was N-palmitoylglucosylsphingosine. The lactosylceramide standard used was N-palmitoyl-lactosylsphingosine. The diacylphospholipid standards used were 1,2-dipalmitoyl -snglycero- 3-phosphocholine, 1-palmitoyl-2-oleoyl-sn-glycero- 3-phosphocholine, 1-palmitoyl-2-oleoyl -sn-glycero-3-phosphoethanolamine and 1-palmitoyl-2-oleoyl-sn-glycero- 3-phospho-L-serine. The lysophospholipid standards used were 1-stearoyl-2-hydroxy-sn-glycero-3-phosphocholine, 1-oleoyl-2-hydroxy-sn-glycero-3-phosphoethanolamine and 1-oleoyl-2-hydroxy-sn-glycero-3-phospho -L-serine. The triacylglycerol standard used was 1,2,3-tri-(9Z-octadecenoyl)-glycerol. The cholesteryl ester standard used was cholesteryl cis-9-octadecenoate. When authentic standards were not available, identification was achieved based on their accurate mass measurement, elemental composition, calculated mass, error, double-bond equivalents and retention times. Quantification was carried out using the extracted ion chromatogram of each compound, obtained with a mass chromatogram absolute window value of 0.05 Da. As an example, representative ion chromatograms for sphingolipids (Figure S1), glycerophospholipids (Figures S2 and S3) and neutral lipids (Figure S4) of the right, left and infarcted left ventricle from the same patient are shown. The linear dynamic range was determined by injecting mixtures of internal and natural standards indicated above. If values were above the linear dynamic range, samples were diluted and analyzed again. Since standards for all identified lipids were not available, the amounts of lipids are given as pmol equivalents relative to each specific standard (Table S1).

Sphingolipids (Cer: ceramide; SM: sphingomyelin; CDH: Ceramide dihexoside; HexCer: hexosylceramides), glycerophospholipids (PC: phosphatidylcholine; LPC: lysophosphatidylcholine; PE: phosphatidylethanolamine; LPE: lysophosphatidylethanolamine; PS: phosphatidylserine; LPS: lysophosphatidylserine, PG: phosphatidylglycerol), and neutral lipids (TAG: triacylglycerol; CE: cholesteryl esters; free cholesterol: FC) were detected. All glycerophospholipid and neutral lipid species were annotated using the "lipid subclass" and "C followed by the total fatty acid (FA) chain length:total number of unsaturated bonds" (e.g., PC (32:2)).

2.7. Statistical Analysis

Variables were compared two by two among the 3 groups (RV, LV and LV INF) using Student's *t*-test or a Mann–Whitney U test for paired samples (myocardial samples were from the same patient), respectively, depending on whether the variables were normal. Normality was tested with a Shapiro–Wilk and Lilliefors test. p values were adjusted with Bonferroni's correction, we performed 3 comparisons for each variable.

The correlations between variables were studied in each group using Pearson's correlation. p values were adjusted with Bonferroni's correction because we tested the correlation among all lipidomic and biophysical variables. $p < 0.05$ was considered statistically significant.

Lipidomic variables whose differences were significant in some of the study groups were represented in a heatmap. Each variable was represented as a logarithm of the quotient of the group mean and the mean value in all groups.

Statistical power was calculated afterwards as few lipidomic studies in human hearts have been performed until now and it was difficult to estimate the effect size in some lipidomic variables. Assuming the differences obtained in the significant variables as the real effect size, we obtained a range of values of statistical power between 0.64 and 0.98 in differential analysis and a range between 0.79 and 1 in correlation analysis.

All data analyses were performed using R 4.0.2 software [29].

3. Results

3.1. Identification of the Main FTIR Bands in the Human Heart

To compare the spectral signature of the human heart with previous data collected from animal hearts [4,5], the average FTIR spectra of mice, pig, and human right ventricles were superimposed (Figure 1). Table S2 summarizes the different FTIR absorption bands detected in human compared to pig and mice right ventricles, as well as their assignments, according to previously published data in transmission or ATR mode [5,6,30–37]. The major absorption bands in these spectra were the amide A, the amide I, and the amide II, which are mainly associated with proteins in freeze-dried tissues. Since Amide A is located in the large wave number zone where FTIR-ATR is not the more appropriate mode, the intensity of this mode has not been used for further semi-quantitative analysis. The primary ventricular proteins are cardiomyocyte myofibrillar (myosin, α-actin) and sarcoplasmic proteins and the structural proteins of the extracellular matrix (ECM), i.e., fibrillar collagens I and III. Among these different vibrations, the 1338 cm^{-1} band (wagging of the proline side chain) [6,25,36] corresponds to a specific signature of the structural proteins of the ECM since it is the only one that does not overlap with absorption or other components, e.g., DNA, lipids, or proteoglycans. As shown in Figure 1, the spectral signatures of the structural proteins of the ECM and the myofibers from mice, pigs and humans are very similar.

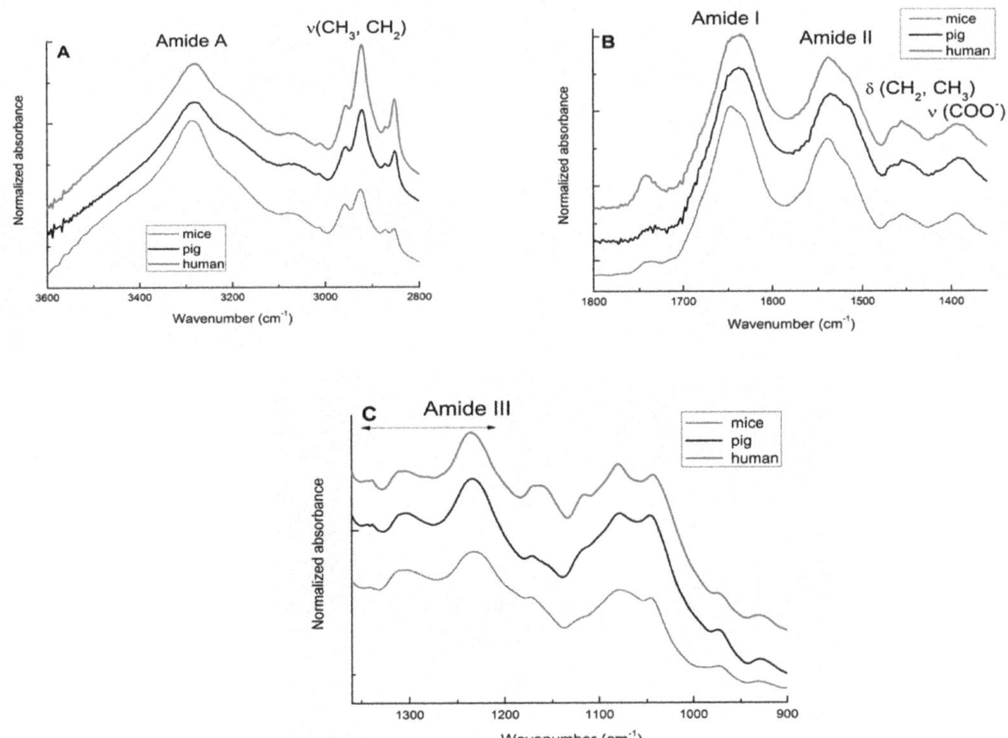

Figure 1. Averaged Fourier transform infrared spectroscopy (FTIR) spectra of the right ventricles from the mice, pig, and human samples. Line graphs showing the 3600–2800 cm^{-1} (**A**), 1800–1350 cm^{-1} (**B**), and 1350–900 cm^{-1} (**C**) spectral regions of mice, pig, and human right ventricles.

The complex FTIR spectra of the ventricles also include lipids with their classic markers at 2800–3000 cm^{-1} (especially the CH_2 stretching of long hydrocarbon chains) (Figure 1A) and at 1475–1450 cm^{-1} (CH_2 scissoring and CH3 bending) (Figure 1B). These lipids are mainly phospholipids of the plasmatic membranes, confirmed by the presence of the C=O stretching of ester groups, the CO-O-C and $PO_2{}^-$ stretching bands, triglycerides, cholesteryl esters, free cholesterol and free fatty acids (C=O stretching at 1712 cm^{-1} and COO^- stretching at 1392 cm^{-1}). Unsaturated lipids are specifically marked by the 3013 cm^{-1} band.

Where the band position of the lipids is quasi-identical among the three species, the lipid vibrational response is more intense in human ventricles (for both the ν(CH2) and ν(C=O) bands) than in pig and mice ventricles.

Finally, as shown in Figure 1C, other ventricular components contributed to this complex vibrational response including DNA, specifically at 974 cm^{-1} [37]; proteoglycans (contributing to the 1079 cm^{-1} band and the overlapping 1226 cm^{-1} band); glycogen; and other polysaccharides (1200–1000 cm^{-1}). The composite (1240–1100 cm^{-1}) zone is subjected to fine differences due to disparities in the nature or proportion of these components among the three compared species.

3.2. Characterization of the Human Heart Lipidome

UPLC–HRMS analysis electrospray ionization mass spectrometry revealed 44 species of sphingolipids, 60 species of glycerophospholipids, and 60 species of neutral lipids in the human heart. The relative amount of each lipid in the whole family was expressed as the percentage of each lipid area compared to the total number of lipids of the same family in the right and left ventricles (Figures S5–S7).

The relative abundance of the species present for each particular lipid among the family of sphingolipids in the human heart is also shown (Figure S5A–E). The most abundant sphingolipid in the human heart is sphingomyelin d18:1 (SM, 88.53%), particularly the species with long fatty acid chains (from 14 to 18 C) (Figure S5A). Minor species include ceramide d18:1 (Cer, 6.94%) (Figure S5B), followed by dihydrosphingomyelin d18:0 (dhSM, 3.56%) (Figure S5C), hexosylceramide (d18:1) (HexCer, 0.58%) (Figure S5D) and ceramide dihexoside (18:1) (CDH, 0.39%) (Figure S5E). CDH (d18:14:0) was significantly higher in LV than in RV (p = 0.045) (Figure S5E).

The most abundant glycerophospholipids in human cardiac tissue are phosphatidylcholine (PC, 75.24%), mainly species with long fatty acid (FA) chains (from 32 to 38 C) (Figure S6A); followed by phosphatidylserine (PS, 8.43%) (Figure S6B); lyso-phosphatidylcholine (LPC, 6.62%) (Figure S6C), phosphatidylethanolamine (PE, 4.96%) (Figure S6D), lyso-phosphatidylethanolamine (LPE, 2.88%) (Figure S6E), lyso- phosphatidylserine (LPS, 1.12%) (Figure S6F) and phosphatidylglycerol (PG, 0.76%) (Figure S6G).

Finally, as shown in Figure S7, the neutral lipids in the human hearts contain a high percentage of triglycerides (TAG, 97.06%) (Figure S7A). Several TAG species with longer unsaturated chains of fatty acids (FAs), decreased in the LV compared to the RV. These TAG species were C53:2 ($p = 0.041$), C54:1 ($p = 0.036$), and C54:2 ($p = 0.033$). The decrease in TAG in human LV compared to RV was previously reported in a porcine model [5] and likely reflects a higher effort and more energetic consumption of LV. Most of the cholesterol was found in the form of free cholesterol (FC, 2.03%) (Figure S7B), with a minor proportion found as cholesteryl esters (CE, 0.90%) (Figure S7C). There were no statistically significant differences in FC or CE between RV and LV.

3.3. Identification of the Alterations of the FTIR Bands Related to Myofibers and Structural Extracellular Matrix Proteins in Human LV INF compared to LV and RV

Table S3 shows a comparison of the IR bands between RVs, LVs and LV INFs of the human hearts compiled from IR spectra. Specific assignments of these bands were performed according to the literature [5,6,30–37]. Most of the IR bands previously described in murine and porcine cardiac control tissues are also present in the RV, LV, and LV INF of human hearts.

In agreement with the deep remodeling of infarcted tissue assessed by immunohistochemistry (Figure 2A), FTIR analyses revealed the profound alteration of the IR band pattern at 1300–860 cm^{-1} in the LV INF compared to the LV or RV samples (Figure 2B). A distinct feature of the collagen-specific absorption band at 1338 cm^{-1} was found in the human LV INF sample but not in the RV or LV samples. The indicator collagen/amide II (1338 cm^{-1}/1540 cm^{-1}), which reflects the content of structural proteins related to the total proteins, was significantly increased in LV INF compared to LV ($p = 0.023$) and RV ($p = 0.023$) (Figure 2C). The second derivative FTIR spectra (which allows increased resolution) showed the exclusive presence of certain IR bands in LV INF at 1140 and 1095 cm^{-1} (Figure 2D, asterisks) in the ν(C-O-C)/ν(C-OH) absorption zone, indicating deep alterations in oligosaccharides and also in glycolipids, phospholipids, and nucleic acids in the infarcted area. In addition, intense absorptions at 1120 cm^{-1} (characteristic of ν(C-O) in lactate, polysaccharides, and glycogen), 1236 cm^{-1} (amide III), and 1160 cm^{-1} (hydroxyproline residues, collagen specific) were detected in human LV INF compared to LV and RV (Figure 2B,D, arrows). The increase of 1236 and 1160 cm^{-1} band absorptions could be due to augmented collagen deposition in the infarcted zone, while that of 1120 cm^{-1} is associated with elevated levels of lactate and/or polysaccharides in this zone ($p = 0.047$) (Figure 2E).

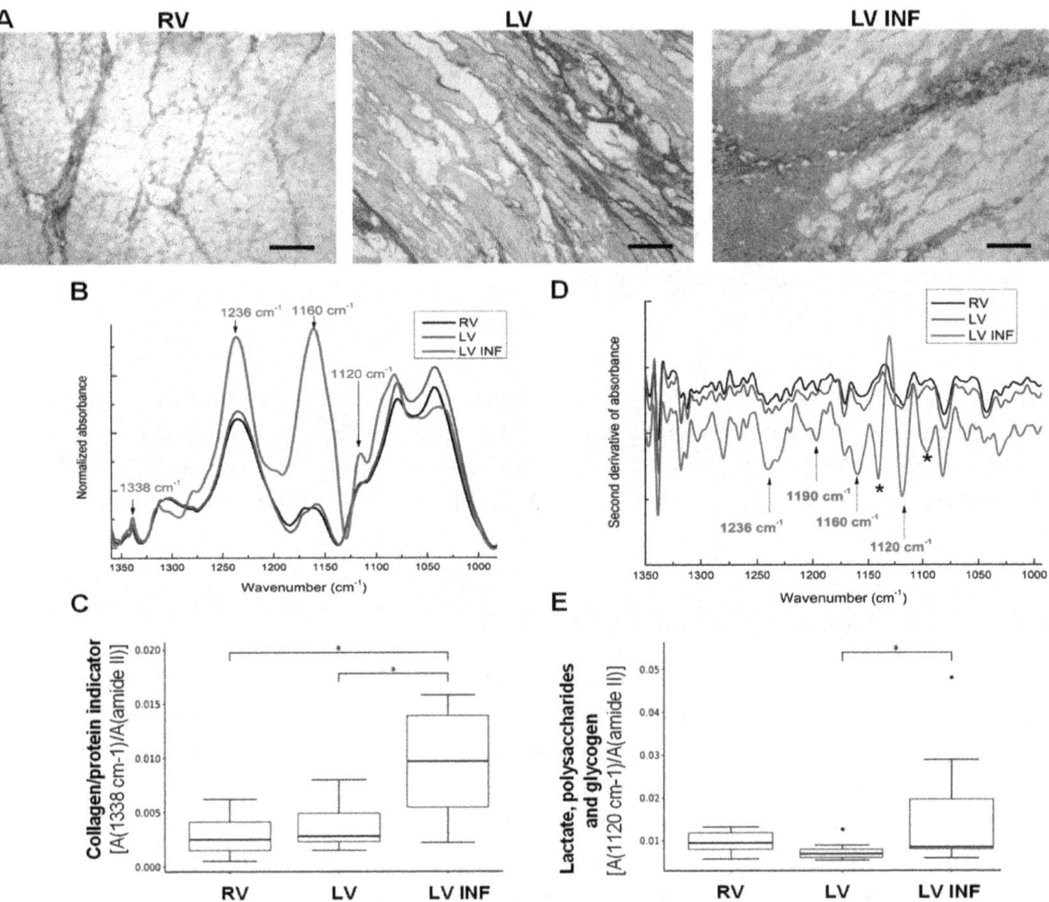

Figure 2. Immunohistochemical and FTIR analyses of fibrosis in human ventricle samples. Sirius Red Staining was used to distinguish the collagen (in red) in the right ventricle (RV), left ventricle (LV) and infarcted left ventricle (LV INF) samples. Scale Bar: 20 μm (**A**). Line graphs showing the 1350–1000 cm^{-1} averaged FTIR spectra of RV, LV, and LV INF (**B**). Boxplot analysis of the FTIR collagen/protein indicator (1338 cm^{-1}/amide II) in the three groups (**C**). Line graphs showing the average second derivative spectra in the 1370–1000 cm^{-1} region (**D**). Arrows indicate the bands altered in the LV INF samples. Asterisks indicate the occurrence of new absorption bands in the LV INF samples. Boxplots showing lactate, polysaccharide, and glycogen/protein indicator (1220 cm^{-1}/amide II) in the three groups (n = 9/group) (**E**). * $p < 0.05$. RV: right ventricle, LV: left ventricle, LV INF: infarcted left ventricle.

3.4. Identification of the Alterations in the FTIR Bands Corresponding to DNA Response in Human LV INF Compared to LV and RV

As reported in Figure 3A, FTIR spectra corresponding to 1000–850 cm^{-1} where the DNA/RNA response prevails, showed differences between the three myocardial samples, which were quantified by the nucleic acid/protein indicator (band area ratio 974 cm^{-1}/1540 cm^{-1}, Figure 3B). There was a significant decrease in the DNA/protein ratio from the right to left ischemic ventricles, reaching significance in LV INF vs. LV (p = 0.0056) and RV (p = 0.0061) (Figure 3B).

This evolution is consistent with previous FTIR imaging results on infarcted myocardium, indicating that nucleic acids are widespread in a normal myocardium but destroyed in an infarcted myocardium [38]. All changes revealed the profound remodeling of the ECM in human infarcted tissue.

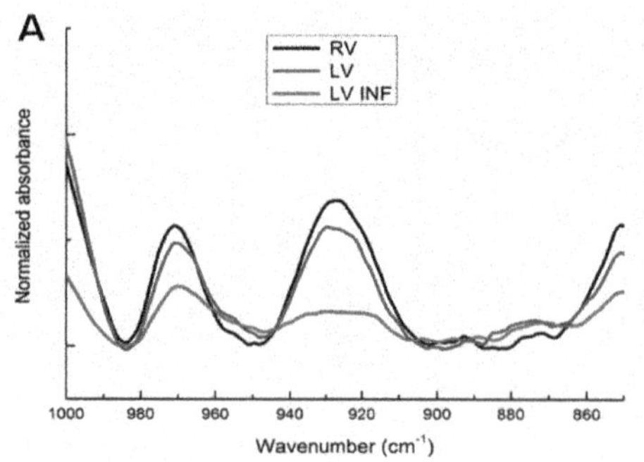

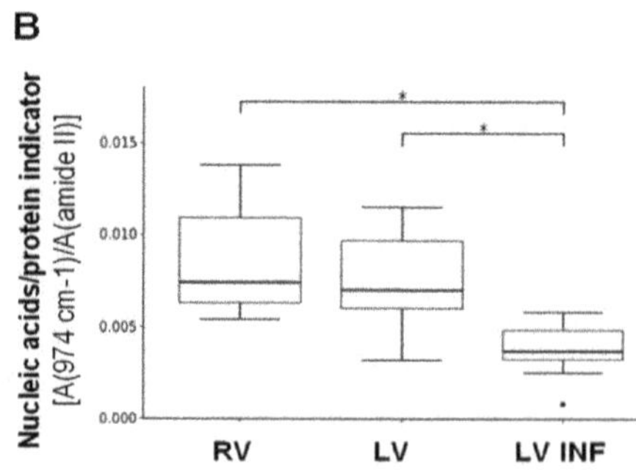

Figure 3. FTIR analysis of the nucleic acids in the human ventricle samples. Line graphs showing the 1000–850 cm^{-1} average FTIR spectra corresponding to the signal of nucleic acids in the RV, LV, and LV INF samples (**A**). Boxplot analysis of nucleic acid/protein FITR indicator (974 cm^{-1}/amide II) (**B**) in the three groups (n = 9/group). * $p < 0.05$. RV: right ventricle, LV: left ventricle, LV INF: infarcted left ventricle.

3.5. Study of the Hydric Response of Human RV, LV and LV INF

Representative DSC thermograms (normalized to the initial mass) of fresh human ventricles corresponding to cooling from 20 to −100 °C and successive heating from −100 to 25 °C are reported in Figure S8A. The cooling thermograms are characterized by an intense exothermic peak corresponding to the crystallization of free water (namely, water not bound to hydrophilic components and able to form ice). The onset temperature of the peak (Ton) is attributed to the transition temperature of this thermal event. The heating thermograms are characterized by an endothermic peak corresponding to the melting of previously frozen water. Weak and multiple thermal events are detectable in the (50–85 °C) zone and attributed to the denaturation of cardiac muscle proteins, including myosin, sarcoplasmic proteins, collagen and actin as already observed in a previous study [4]. There is a significant decrease in the temperature of water crystallization Tc for LV INF compared to LV ($p = 0.044$) (Figure S8B). A similar trend is observed for the ice melting recorded in the heating scans. The increase in aqueous salt concentrations could explain such a depression of the melting/crystallization temperature. However, the typical signature of aqueous salts, namely the eutectic phase transition at lower temperature, was not detected in the DSC thermograms of myocardial samples. Since water crystallization and ice melting are related to the pore size in porous [39] and biological materials [40], the differences between the infarcted and non-infarcted zones can be interpreted as changes in the architecture associated with a decrease of the pore's nominal radius. Cardiac remodeling, including the replacement of myofibers by collagen fibers marking a difference in the tissue architecture (pore size), could explain this peculiar thermal behavior.

3.6. Study of the Associations between FITR Variables in Human RV, LV and LV INF

The FTIR spectra show that the CH_2 bands (2921 cm^{-1} and 2850 cm^{-1}) in the (CH_2, CH_3) stretching zone (3000–2800 cm^{-1}) are mainly associated with the lipid signature (Figure 4A) and the C=O stretching zones of the ester carbonyl groups of phospholipids, triglycerides, and cholesteryl esters (Figure 4B). There was an intensification of the lipid bands in the left infarcted ventricles, and a close correlation (R = 1, $p = 8.7 \times 10^{-8}$) between the total lipid (2921–2850 cm^{-1}/1540 cm^{-1}) and the esterified lipid (1745 cm^{-1}/1540 cm^{-1}) indicators (Figure 4C) in this zone. There were no correlations statistically significant between total and esterified lipids in RV or LV (R = 0.93, $p = 1$; R = 0.89, $p = 1$, respectively), suggesting that most of the lipids are esterified in the infarcted LV, but not in the RV or LV.

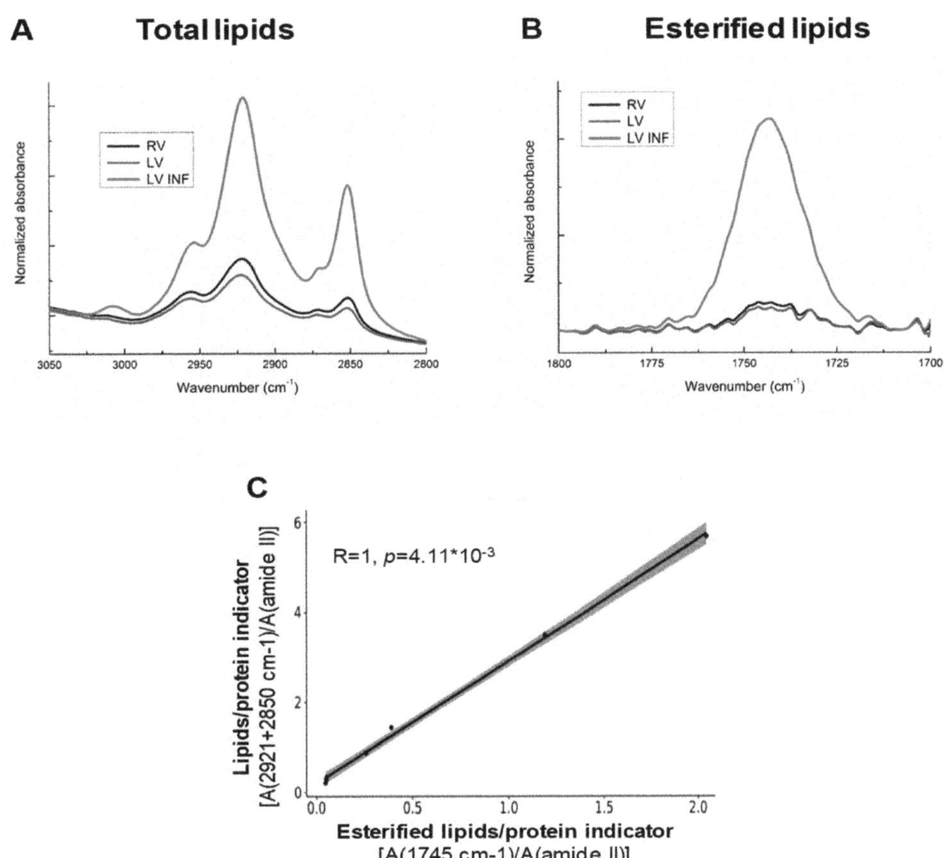

Figure 4. FTIR analysis of the total and esterified lipids in the human ventricle samples. Line graphs showing the 3050–2800 cm^{-1} (**A**) and 1800–1700 cm^{-1} (**B**) average FTIR spectra corresponding to the signals of the total and esterified lipids, respectively, in right ventricle (RV), left ventricle (LV), and infarcted left ventricle (LV INF). (**C**) Correlation analysis between the FTIR indicators of the total and esterified lipids in LV INF. The correlation was studied with Pearson's correlation, and the *p*-values were adjusted with Bonferroni's correction. RV: right ventricle, LV: left ventricle, LV INF: infarcted left ventricle.

3.7. Identification of the Alterations in Sphingolipids, Glycerophospholipids and Neutral Lipids in Human LV INF Compared to LV and RV

Lipidomic studies reflected deep lipid remodeling in the infarcted tissue. As visualized in the heatmap of Figure 5, cholesteryl ester and several sphingolipid species were significantly increased in LV INF compared to RV or LV, while most of the glycerophospholipid species were significantly decreased in the infarcted cardiac tissue. As shown in Table 2, SM 18:1 (14:0 and 14:1) and 16:1, dhSM 18:0 (16:0 and 18:0), and HexCer 18:1 species (16:0, 22:0, 24:0, 24:1) were significantly increased, while Cer 18:1 (18:0, 20:0, 20:1, 22:1 and 24:1) species were significantly decreased in the LV infarcted tissue (Table 2). There were no significant differences in CDH or the rest of the sphingolipid species between LV INF and LV or RV (Table S4). Like Cer, the main glycerophospholipids, including PE (34:2, 36:4), LPE (18:2), PC (32:2, 34:1, 34:2, 34:3, 34:4, 36:2, 36:3, 36:5), and PG (34:1, 34:2), were significantly decreased in human infarcted tissue (Table 3). There were no significant differences in the PS, LPS, or LPC and the rest of glycerophospholipid species between LV INF and LV or RV (Table S5). Finally, among the neutral lipids, only cholesteryl esters were found to be significantly increased in the infarcted tissue (18:3) (Table 4). There were no differences in the highly abundant TAG species or minor FC species between LV INF and LV or RV (Table S6).

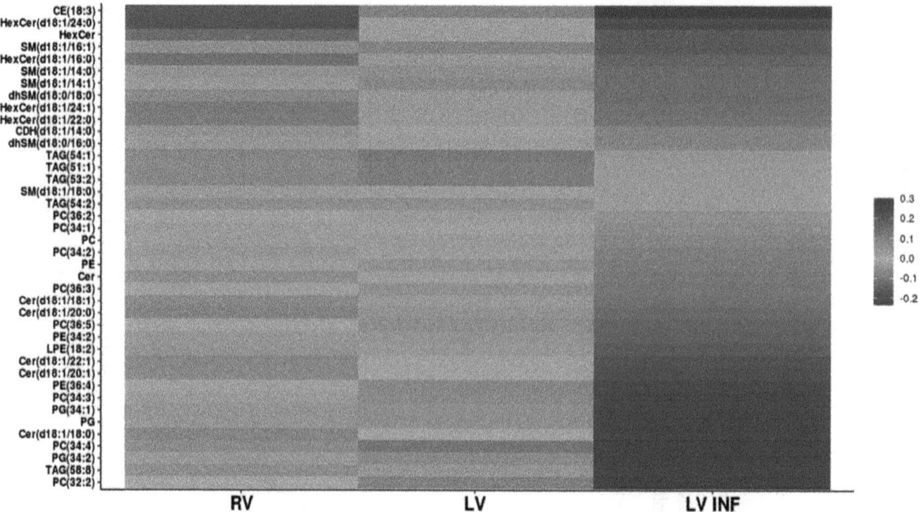

Figure 5. Lipidomic analysis of the human right ventricle, left ventricle and infarcted left ventricle. Heatmap of the nine human heart samples (in columns) based in the quantification of 40 differential lipid species (in rows) that exhibited statistically significant differences among right ventricle (RV), left ventricle (LV), and infarcted left ventricle (LV INF) samples. The heatmap colors represent a decimal logarithm of the quotient of the group mean and the mean value in all groups for each variable. Blue cells indicate values below the mean value of the variables in all groups, while red cells indicate values above the mean value of the variables in all groups. CE: cholesteryl esters, HexCer: hexosylceramide, SM: sphingomyelin, dhSM: dihydrosphingomyelin, CDH: ceramide dihexoside, TAG: triacylglycerols, PC: phosphatidylcholine, PE: phosphatidylethanolamine, LPE: lysophosphatidylethanolamine, Cer: ceramide, PG: phosphatidylglycerol. RV: right ventricle, LV: left ventricle, LV INF: infarcted left ventricle.

Table 2. Sphingolipid species with differential concentrations in the infarcted left ventricle compared to left ventricle or right ventricle from human explanted ischemic hearts.

Variable	RV	LV	LV INF	*p* vs. LV	*p* vs. RV
SM(d18:1/14:0)	308.5 ± 77.4	309.5 ± 95.9	430.5 ± 95.3	0.024	0.055
SM(d18:1/14:1)	3 ± 1.2	2.8 ± 1	3.9 ± 1.4	0.029	0.096
SM(d18:1/16:1)	164 ± 39.5	160.1 ± 56.8	258.8 ± 105.8	0.029	0.041
SM(d18:1/18:0)	1199.2 ± 156.3	1138.7 ± 128.5	1086.2 ± 142.7	0.485	0.038
Total Cer	753 ± 261.6	592.7 ± 240.1	549.5 ± 179.1	0.932	0.044
Cer(d18:1/18:0)	30.4 ± 13.5	22.9 ± 14.5	15 ± 4.9	0.115	0.029
Cer(d18:1/18:1)	7.2 ± 2.3	5.2 ± 2	4.6 ± 1.1	0.456	0.006
Cer(d18:1/20:0)	14.5 ± 3.6	11.1 ± 4	9.6 ± 2.8	0.457	0.01
Cer(d18:1/20:1)	4.4 ± 0.8	3.4 ± 1.3	2.6 ± 0.6	0.13	0.006
Cer(d18:1/22:1)	28.7 ± 22.9	20.2 ± 16.1	17.5 ± 20.1	0.804	0.018
dhSM(d18:0/16:0)	179.4 ± 41.3	207.5 ± 91.7	226.4 ± 65	0.931	0.029
dhSM(d18:1/18:0)	46.3 ± 13.4	49.5 ± 23.3	64.5 ± 16.3	0.174	0.041
Total HexCer	48.1 ± 26.6	63.9 ± 31.2	91.3 ± 36.6	0.114	0.006
HexCer(d18:1/16:0)	2.3 ± 1.5	3.2 ± 1.7	4.4 ± 3.1	0.474	0.023
HexCer(d18:1/22:0)	10.9 ± 5.8	16.1 ± 13.2	16 ± 5.6	1	0.012
HexCer(d18:1/24:0)	19.6 ± 10.4	25.3 ± 13.6	44.3 ± 25.1	0.127	0.018
HexCer(d18:1/24:1)	15.5 ± 10.5	20 ± 5.6	26.7 ± 13.5	0.102	0.006

Data are expressed as mean ± SD, $n = 9$ (RV, LV and LV INF). SM: sphingomyelin, Cer: Ceramide, dhSM: dihydrosphingomyelin, HexCer: Hexosylceramide, SD: standard deviation, RV: right ventricle, LV: left ventricle, LV INF: infarcted left ventricle.

Table 3. Glycerophospholipid species with differential concentrations in the infarcted left ventricle compared to left ventricle or right ventricle from human explanted ischemic hearts.

Variable	RV	LV	LV INF	*p* vs. LV	*p* vs. RV
Total PC	54,624.9 ± 11408.6	56,737 ± 5670.8	48,392.9 ± 4893.7	0.012	0.335
PC(32:2)	342.5 ± 146.2	389.6 ± 115.9	221.1 ± 103.4	0.029	0.102
PC(34:1)	14,602.8 ± 2506.6	15,143.9 ± 1769.8	13,505.1 ± 1492.7	0.029	0.556
PC(34:2)	13,397 ± 2572.8	13,827.1 ± 1685	11,574.9 ± 1501.8	0.006	0.232
PC(34:3)	120.7 ± 54.3	133.2 ± 46.3	71.9 ± 21.8	0.012	0.049
PC(34:4)	100.7 ± 52.6	133.8 ± 67.5	64.7 ± 34.1	0.041	0.077
PC(36:2)	4753.8 ± 1047.4	4902.2 ± 444.3	4439.5 ± 328.1	0.025	0.698
PC(36:3)	3650 ± 1035	3884.2 ± 936.2	2866.5 ± 856.6	0.003	0.122
PC(36:5)	391.6 ± 437.5	376.8 ± 327.3	236.4 ± 269.4	0.041	0.069
Total PE	3502.5 ± 1052.4	3840.7 ± 914.1	2986.4 ± 769	0.004	0.285
PE(34:2)	203.1 ± 65.5	205.2 ± 47	144.1 ± 37.9	0.008	0.028
PE(36:4)	1014.5 ± 300.8	1309.3 ± 502.6	629.4 ± 269.1	0.011	0.036
LPE(18:2)	144.7 ± 60.3	142.7 ± 43.4	95 ± 30.3	0.006	0.052
Total PG	538.9 ± 135.4	581.8 ± 188.7	329.2 ± 152.5	0.045	0.041
PG(34:1)	483 ± 121.9	523 ± 176.8	300.9 ± 139.4	0.052	0.042
PG(34:2)	55.9 ± 20.6	58.8 ± 19.1	28.3 ± 14.9	0.028	0.047

Data are expressed as mean ± SD, $n = 9$ (RV, LV and LV INF). PC: phosphatidylcholine, PE:phosphatidylethanolamine, LPE: lysophosphatidylethanolamine, PG: phosphatidylglycerol, SD: standard deviation, RV: right ventricle, LV: left ventricle, LV INF: infarcted left ventricle.

Table 4. Neutral lipid species with differential concentrations in the infarcted left ventricle compared to left ventricle or right ventricle from human explanted ischemic hearts.

Variable	RV	LV	LV INF	*p* vs. LV	*p* vs. RV
TAG(58:8)	2856 ± 1534.1	3364.8 ± 3160.3	1978.9 ± 1520.3	0.018	0.075
CE(18:3)	269.5 ± 248.3	352.3 ± 319.7	575.9 ± 583.5	0.239	0.018

Data are expressed as mean ± SD, $n = 9$ (RV, LV and LV INF). TAG: triacylglycerols, CE: cholesteryl esters, SD: standard deviation, RV: right ventricle, LV: left ventricle, LV INF: infarcted left ventricle.

3.8. Study of the Association between FTIR and Lipidomic Variables in RV, LV and LV INF

As shown in Figure 6, biophysical studies revealed that ECM remodeling was closely associated with lipid indicators, such as total lipids (2921–2850 cm^{-1}) ($R = 1$, $p = 1.6 \times 10^{-8}$) (Figure 6A) and esterified lipids (1745 cm^{-1}/amide II) ($R = 0.99$, $p = 9.3 \times 10^{-7}$) (Figure 6B) specifically in LV INF. In addition, other extracellular matrix markers such as lactate, polysaccharides, and glycogen, were also closely associated with total lipids ($R = 1$, $p = 3.6 \times 10^{-11}$) (Figure 6C) and esterified lipids ($R = 0.99$, $p = 9.1 \times 10^{-7}$) (Figure 6D) in the cardiac infarcted tissue. There was no significant correlation between lipid and ECM remodeling FITR indicators in human RV ($R = 0.54$, $p = 1$) or LV ($R = 0.68$, $p = 1$).

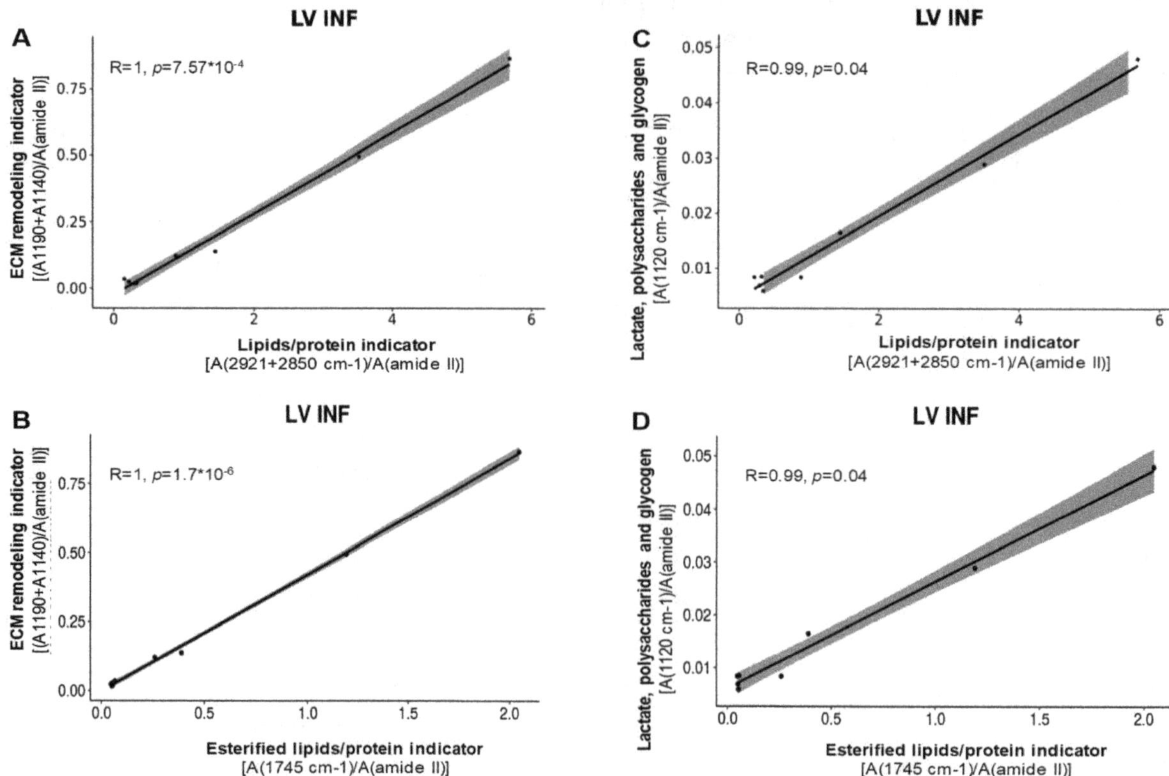

Figure 6. Correlation analysis of FTIR indicators of cardiac remodeling and lipids in the human heart. Correlation between the extracellular matrix (ECM) remodeling indicator and both total lipids (**A**) and esterified lipids (**B**), as well as between lactate, polysaccharide, and glycogen and both total lipids (**C**) and esterified lipids (**D**), in human infarcted left ventricle. The correlation was studied with Pearson's correlation, and p values were adjusted with Bonferroni's correction. LV INF: infarcted left ventricle.

4. Discussion

In this work, we used the FTIR spectrum to illustrate the overall variety of changes in proteins, nucleic acids, and lipids that occur in human cardiac infarcted tissue. FTIR spectroscopy is very sensitive to variations in cell metabolism, making it highly suitable for defining the structure in the infarcted areas where the tissue has undergone strong cardiometabolic alterations primarily associated with the process of ischemia [41].

The spectral signatures of the structural proteins of ECM and the myofibers in the human heart are similar to those previously reported in murine [4] and porcine hearts [5]. One of the most significant alterations observed in the FTIR spectra of human LV INF vs. LV or RV was a strong increase in the 1338 cm^{-1} band, which has been shown to be specific to collagen [6,25,36]. The utility of this particular FTIR band to monitor the evolution of cardiac pathology and therapeutics was previously validated in a rat MI model [6]. Another FTIR band that is deeply altered in the context of MI is the 974 cm^{-1} band assigned to nucleic acids that, as expected, suffered a strong decline in LV INF compared to LV and RV. These changes reflected a profound remodeling of the LV INF accompanying cardiomyocyte death in the context of myocardial infarction and highlighted the potential of infrared markers to trace the incidence of ischemia in cardiac remodeling.

The spectral signatures of lipids are also quasi-identical in the human heart to those in previous murine [4] and pig [5] hearts. The vibrational response of the lipids is much more intense (for both the ν(CH2) and ν(C=O) bands, corresponding to the total lipids and ester carbonyl groups of PL and neutral lipids) in human than in murine or porcine ventricles. Lipidomic analysis of the human heart revealed that the main lipids present are SM (d18:1) (88% of the total sphingolipids), PC (75% of the total glycerophospholipids) and TAGs (97% of the total neutral lipids). There are few detailed lipidomic studies of ventricles and almost none on humans, likely due to the difficulty of obtaining human heart samples. We found several species belonging to the sphingolipid, glycerophospholipid, and neutral lipid families that were altered in LV INF but not in RV and LV. Most of the glycerophospholipids decreased, while most of the sphingolipids and, specific species of cholesteryl esters increased in the infarcted human cardiac tissue.

Between sphingolipids, the levels of several species of SM, dhSM, and HexCer were increased in LV INF compared to LV or RV. The increase in the SM content of infarcted tissue found in the present work seems to be coherent with the decreased sphingomyelinase (SMase) activity previously described [42]. The increase in SM that we found in humans differs from the results showing lower SM levels in the infarcted brains of in vivo models of ischemic stroke [43]. The cleavage of SM by acid or neutral SMase results in the liberation of ceramide, a sphingolipid that acts as an intracellular messenger regulating the activity of kinases, phosphatases, and transcription factors. Ceramides were reported to be upregulated in the ischemic zones of the heart in several in vivo models of ischemia/reperfusion [13,44,45]. This increase in ceramides after ischemia reperfusion appears to be transient and linked with reperfusion injury, as shown in a model of ischemic-reperfused myocardium in rats [42]. It has also been shown that the post-MI increase in cardiac ceramide is not caused by increased SMase activity but instead by decreased ceramidase activity. In addition, it has been recently demonstrated that a transient increase in acid ceramidase is sufficient to induce cardioprotection post-MI [46]. Ceramide is utilized for the synthesis of other bioactive sphingolipids, including sphingosine-1-phosphate, sphingosine, and the glycosphingolipids lactosylceramide and hexosylceramide (HexCer). Here, several species of HexCer were found accumulated in human infarcted hearts. Previous studies have reported the accumulation of HexCer in several organs from in vivo models of aging [47,48]. Clinically, increased circulating levels of both SM and Cer have been correlated with an increased risk of coronary artery disease [49,50].

Between glycerophospholipids, we found that the levels of the main PL, phosphatidylcholine (PC), and other less abundant PLs, such as phosphatidylethanolamine (PE) and phosphatidylglycerol (PG), were significantly decreased in LV INF compared to LV. These results are in agreement with previous studies performed in in vivo MI models [16,17] showing a strong PL decay caused by ischemia-induced phospholipolysis of the cardiomyocyte membranes. Increased phospholipolysis can be caused, among other factors, by the upregulatory effect of hypoxia on phospholipase activity [51,52]. Unbalanced levels of anionic phospholipids such as PG seem to have harmful consequences for mitochondrial morphology and function. PG plays a pivotal role in the formation of cardiolipin, which is essential in the control of mitochondrial inflammation and oxidative stress [53,54], and respiratory activity [54]. In this study, we found a significant loss of PG that could, indeed, contribute to a serious decrease in mitochondrial oxidative metabolism in infarcted tissue. The strong decrease in mitochondrial respiratory activity combined with acute phospholipolysis, which actively generates fatty acids [16,17], could be a determinant for increased FA esterification. An additional source of esterified lipids in the infarcted tissue is circulating lipoproteins. Several groups, including ours, have reported the upregulatory effect of hypoxia/ischemia on lipoprotein receptors such as Very low-density lipoprotein receptor VLDLR and Low-density lipoprotein receptor related-protein 1 LRP1, which bind and internalize lipoproteins such as Very low-density lipoprotein (VLDL) and Low-density lipoprotein (LDL) (lipoproteins highly enriched in cholesteryl esters) [11–13,55,56]. Here, the close correlation between esterified lipids and remodeling in the human infarcted tissue pointed to FTIR lipid indicators as potential biomarkers of remodeling, at least in the context of ischemia. Previous studies from our group demonstrated that the levels of intracellular esterified lipids in cardiomyocytes determine the structural and physical characteristics of secreted tropoelastin through an increase in cathepsin S mature protein levels [57]. The intracellular esterified lipids stored in lipid droplets are the subject of an intense debate over their potential beneficial/harmful effects on cell functionality [58]. The differential implications of triglyceride and cholesteryl ester proportions in these lipid droplets are also under discussion [59].

5. Conclusions

As a general conclusion, FTIR studies showed that human cardiac infarcted tissue suffers deep alterations in proteins, nucleic acids, and—especially—lipids. Liquid chromatography coupled to high-resolution mass spectrometry (LC–HRMS) revealed the strong lipid remodeling that results in reduced levels of PC, PE, LPE and PG and increased levels of SM, HexCer and cholesteryl esters in human cardiac infarcted tissue. We found a strong and positive association between esterified lipids and adverse cardiac remodeling in the context of human cardiac remodeling post-MI. The specific conclusions are that (i) there are deep alterations of the FTIR bands related to myofibers and structural extracellular matrix proteins in human LV INF compared to LV and RV, (ii) there are strong differences in the FTIR spectra corresponding to DNA responses in human LV INF compared to RV and LV, (iii) there is a differential hydric response of human LV INF compared to RV and LV, (iv) FTIR combined with lipidomic studies showed a strong intensification of lipids, particularly esterified lipids concomitantly with deep phospholipid remodeling in human infarcted hearts, and (v) esterified lipids are closely related with adverse cardiac remodeling in human infarcted heart. Thus, we have shown that FTIR lipid indicators are potential biomarkers of cardiac remodeling and validated certain lipid species as crucial in human pathological ventricular remodeling post-MI.

Limitations of This Study: The main limitation of this study is the low number of patients included due to the difficulty of (i) obtaining samples from ischemic cardiomyopathy patients and (ii) performing biophysical and lipidomic studies on an elevated number of series. However, great differences in some variables were found between ventricle samples, as well as strong correlations between variables. There was also a high correlation between ECM remodeling indicators and the total and esterified lipids in LV INF. Furthermore, we have obtained relatively high values of statistical power (between 0.64–0.98), despite the low number of samples, due to the big differences in some variables between the ventricles. Regardless, more studies are needed to confirm our results and provide higher statistical power. We also consider, as limitation of this study, the impossibility to characterize the infarcted right ventricle due to the low prevalence and diagnose of this entity. Finally, we could not assess the levels of cardiolipin, a crucial lipid in cardiovascular disease, due to the technical unavailability to perform this analysis.

Supplementary Materials

Figure S1: Representative ion chromatograms of ceramides and sphingomyelins detected in the right, left and infarcted left ventricle of the same patient; Figure S2: Representative ion chromatograms of phosphatidylcholines (PCs) and phosphatidylethanolamines (PEs) detected in the right, left and infarcted left ventricle of the same patient; Figure S3: Representative ion chromatograms of phosphatidylserines (PSs) and lysophospholipids (PEs) detected in the right, left and infarcted left ventricle of the same patient; Figure S4: Representative ion chromatograms of neutral lipids detected in the right, left and infarcted left ventricle of the same patient; Figure S5: Levels of sphingolipids species in right and left ventricles from human explanted ischemic hearts; Figure S6: Levels of glycerolipids species in right and left ventricles from human explanted ischemic hearts; Figure S7: Levels of neutral lipid species in right and left ventricles from human explanted ischemic hearts; Figure S8: Hydric response of the right, left and left infarcted ventricles from human explanted ischemic hearts; Table S1: Lipids identified in the myocardial samples; Table S2: FTIR band position and assignment in human, pig and mice right ventricle samples; Table S3: FTIR band position and assignment in right, left and left infarcted ventricles from human explanted ischemic hearts; Table S4: Levels of sphingolipids species (pmol equiv/mg prot) in right, left and left infarcted ventricles from human ischemic hearts; Table S5: Levels of glycerophospholipid species (pmol equiv/mg prot) in right, left and left infarcted ventricles from human ischemic hearts; Table S6: Levels of neutral lipid species (pmol equiv/mg prot) in right, left and left infarcted ventricles from human ischemic hearts.

Author Contributions: Conceptualization, D.V., J.D., J.C., D.d.G.C., E.L., J.M.G., F.C., R.L., V.L.C.; Data curation, I.M.M.d.L.S., A.B.A.; Formal analysis, V.S., I.M.M.d.L.S., J.D., J.C., E.J., V.L.C.; Funding acquisition, V.L.C. and J.M.G.; Investigation, V.S., A.B.A., D.V., J.D., J.C., E.J., A.G., J.M.G., F.C., R.L.,V.L.C.; Methodology, V.S., I.M.M.d.L.S., A.B.A., J.D., J.C., D.d.G.C., A.G., E.L., V.L.C.; Project administration, V.S., A.B.A., F.C., V.L.C.; Resources, A.G., E.L., J.M.G., R.L., V.L.C.; Software, I.M.M.d.L.S.; Supervision, V.S., J.D., F.C., R.L., V.L.C.; Validation, I.M.M.d.L.S., D.V., D.d.G.C.; Writing—original draft, V.S., V.L.C. All authors have read and agreed to the published version of the manuscript.

References

1. Pfeffer, M.A.; Braunwald, E. Ventricular remodeling after myocardial infarction. Experimental observations and clinical implications. *Circulation* **1990**, *81*, 1161–1172. [CrossRef] [PubMed]
2. Opie, L.H.; Commerford, P.J.; Gersh, B.J.; Pfeffer, M.A. Controversies in ventricular remodelling. *Lancet* **2006**, *367*, 356–367. [CrossRef]
3. Jugdutt, B.I. Ventricular remodeling after infarction and the extracellular collagen matrix: When is enough enough? *Circulation* **2003**, *108*, 1395–1403. [CrossRef] [PubMed]
4. Samouillan, V.; Revuelta-López, E.; Soler-Botija, C.; Dandurand, J.; Benitez-Amaro, A.; Nasarre, L.; de Gonzalo-Calvo, D.; Bayes-Genis, A.; Lacabanne, C.; Llorente-Cortés, V. Conformational and thermal characterization of left ventricle remodeling post-myocardial infarction. *Biochim. Biophys. Acta-Mol. Basis Dis.* **2017**, *1863*, 1500–1509. [CrossRef] [PubMed]
5. Benitez-Amaro, A.; Samouillan, V.; Jorge, E.; Dandurand, J.; Nasarre, L.; de Gonzalo-Calvo, D.; Bornachea, O.; Amoros-Figueras, G.; Lacabanne, C.; Vilades, D.; et al. Identification of new biophysical markers for pathological ventricular remodelling in tachycardia-induced dilated cardiomyopathy. *J. Cell. Mol. Med.* **2018**, *22*, 4197–4208. [CrossRef] [PubMed]
6. Cheheltani, R.; Rosano, J.M.; Wang, B.; Sabri, A.K.; Pleshko, N.; Kiani, M.F. Fourier transform infrared spectroscopic imaging of cardiac tissue to detect collagen deposition after myocardial infarction. *J. Biomed. Opt.* **2012**, *17*, 56014. [CrossRef]
7. Kong, J.; Yu, S. Fourier Transform Infrared Spectroscopic Analysis of Protein Secondary Structures Protein FTIR Data Analysis and Band Assign- ment. *Acta Biochim. Biophys. Sin.* **2007**, *39*, 549–559. [CrossRef]
8. Amorim, P.A.; Nguyen, T.D.; Shingu, Y.; Schwarzer, M.; Mohr, F.W.; Schrepper, A.; Doenst, T. Myocardial infarction in rats causes partial impairment in insulin response associated with reduced fatty acid oxidation and mitochondrial gene expression. *J. Thorac. Cardiovasc. Surg.* **2010**, *140*, 1160–1167. [CrossRef]
9. Heather, L.C.; Clarke, K. Metabolism, hypoxia and the diabetic heart. *J. Mol. Cell. Cardiol.* **2011**, *50*, 598–605. [CrossRef]
10. Rosenblatt-Velin, N.; Montessuit, C.; Papageorgiou, I.; Terrand, J.; Lerch, R. Postinfarction heart failure in rats is associated with upregulation of GLUT-1 and downregulation of genes of fatty acid metabolism. *Cardiovasc. Res.* **2001**, *52*, 407–416. [CrossRef]
11. Cal, R.; Castellano, J.; Revuelta-López, E.; Aledo, R.; Barriga, M.; Farré, J.; Vilahur, G.; Nasarre, L.; Hove-Madsen, L.; Badimon, L.; et al. Low-density lipoprotein receptor-related protein 1 mediates hypoxia-induced very low density lipoprotein-cholesteryl ester uptake and accumulation in cardiomyocytes. *Cardiovasc. Res.* **2012**, *94*, 469–479. [CrossRef]
12. Cal, R.; Juan-Babot, O.; Brossa, V.; Roura, S.; Gálvez-Montón, C.; Portoles, M.; Rivera, M.; Cinca, J.; Badimon, L.; Llorente-Cortés, V. Low density lipoprotein receptor-related protein 1 expression correlates with cholesteryl ester accumulation in the myocardium of ischemic cardiomyopathy patients. *J. Transl. Med.* **2012**, *10*, 160. [CrossRef]
13. Drevinge, C.; Karlsson, L.O.; Ståhlman, M.; Larsson, T.; Perman Sundelin, J.; Grip, L.; Andersson, L.; Borén, J.; Levin, M.C. Cholesteryl Esters Accumulate in the Heart in a Porcine Model of Ischemia and Reperfusion. *PLoS ONE* **2013**, *8*, e61942. [CrossRef]
14. De Lima, A.D.; Guido, M.C.; Tavares, E.R.; Carvalho, P.O.; Marques, A.F.; de Melo, M.D.T.; Salemi, V.M.C.; Kalil-Filho, R.; Maranhão, R.C. The Expression of Lipoprotein Receptors Is Increased in the Infarcted Area After Myocardial Infarction Induced in Rats With Cardiac Dysfunction. *Lipids* **2018**, *53*, 177–187. [CrossRef]
15. Goldfarb, J.W.; Roth, M.; Han, J. Myocardial fat deposition after left ventricular myocardial infarction: Assessment by using MR water-fat separation imaging. *Radiology* **2009**, *253*, 65–73. [CrossRef] [PubMed]
16. Turer, A.T. Using metabolomics to assess myocardial metabolism and energetics in heart failure. *J. Mol. Cell. Cardiol.* **2013**, *55*, 12–18. [CrossRef]
17. Nam, M.; Jung, Y.; Ryu, D.H.; Hwang, G.S. A metabolomics-driven approach reveals metabolic responses and mechanisms in the rat heart following myocardial infarction. *Int. J. Cardiol.* **2017**, *227*, 239–246. [CrossRef]
18. Feng, L.; Yang, J.; Liu, W.; Wang, Q.; Wang, H.; Shi, L.; Fu, L.; Xu, Q.; Wang, B.; Li, T. Lipid biomarkers in acute myocardial infarction before and after percutaneous coronary intervention by lipidomics analysis. *Med. Sci. Monit.* **2018**, *24*, 4175–4182. [CrossRef]

19. Mundra, P.A.; Barlow, C.K.; Nestel, P.J.; Barnes, E.H.; Kirby, A.; Thompson, P.; Sullivan, D.R.; Alshehry, Z.H.; Mellett, N.A.; Huynh, K.; et al. Large-scale plasma lipidomic profiling identifies lipids that predict cardiovascular events in secondary prevention. *JCI Insight* **2018**, *3*. [CrossRef]
20. Floegel, A.; Kühn, T.; Sookthai, D.; Johnson, T.; Prehn, C.; Rolle-Kampczyk, U.; Otto, W.; Weikert, C.; Illig, T.; von Bergen, M.; et al. Serum metabolites and risk of myocardial infarction and ischemic stroke: A targeted metabolomic approach in two German prospective cohorts. *Eur. J. Epidemiol.* **2018**, *33*, 55–66. [CrossRef]
21. Lewis, G.D.; Asnani, A.; Gerszten, R.E. Application of Metabolomics to Cardiovascular Biomarker and Pathway Discovery. *J. Am. Coll. Cardiol.* **2008**, *52*, 117–123. [CrossRef] [PubMed]
22. Dang, V.T.; Huang, A.; Werstuck, G.H. Untargeted Metabolomics in the Discovery of Novel Biomarkers and Therapeutic Targets for Atherosclerotic Cardiovascular Diseases. *Cardiovasc. Hematol. Disord. Targets* **2018**, *18*, 166–175. [CrossRef] [PubMed]
23. Swedberg, K.; Cleland, J.; Dargie, H.; Drexler, H.; Follath, F.; Komajda, M.; Tavazzi, L.; Smiseth, O.A.; Gavazzi, A.; Haverich, A.; et al. Guidelines for the diagnosis and treatment of chronic heart failure: Executive summary (update 2005). *Eur. Heart J.* **2005**, *26*, 1115–1140. [CrossRef]
24. Kiernan, J.A. *Histological and Histochemical Methods: Theory and Practice*, 3rd ed.; Butterworth Heinemann: Oxford, UK, 1999; Volume 12, p. 679.
25. Staniszewska, E.; Malek, K.; Baranska, M. Rapid approach to analyze biochemical variation in rat organs by ATR FTIR spectroscopy. *Spectrochim. Acta. A Mol. Biomol. Spectrosc.* **2014**, *118*, 981–986. [CrossRef]
26. Wang, Q.; Sanad, W.; Miller, L.M.; Voigt, A.; Klingel, K.; Kandolf, R.; Stangl, K.; Baumann, G. Infrared imaging of compositional changes in inflammatory cardiomyopathy. *Vib. Spectrosc.* **2005**, *38*, 217–222. [CrossRef]
27. Simbari, F.; McCaskill, J.; Coakley, G.; Millar, M.; Maizels, R.M.; Fabriás, G.; Casas, J.; Buck, A.H. Plasmalogen enrichment in exosomes secreted by a nematode parasite versus those derived from its mouse host: Implications for exosome stability and biology. *J. Extracell. Vesicles* **2016**, *5*, 30741. [CrossRef]
28. Weber, M.; Mera, P.; Casas, J.; Salvador, J.; Rodríguez, A.; Alonso, S.; Sebastián, D.; Soler-Vázquez, M.C.; Montironi, C.; Recalde, S.; et al. Liver CPT1A gene therapy reduces diet-induced hepatic steatosis in mice and highlights potential lipid biomarkers for human NAFLD. *FASEB J.* **2020**, *34*, 11816–11837. [CrossRef]
29. R Core Team. R: A Language and Environment for Statistical Computing 2020. R Foundation for Statistical Computing: Vienna, Austria. Available online: https://www.R-project.org/ (accessed on 21 October 2020).
30. Bozkurt, O.; Severcan, M.; Severcan, F. Diabetes induces compositional, structural and functional alterations on rat skeletal soleus muscle revealed by FTIR spectroscopy: A comparative study with EDL muscle. *Analyst* **2010**, *135*, 3110. [CrossRef]
31. Gough, K.M.; Zelinski, D.; Wiens, R.; Rak, M.; Dixon, I.M.C. Fourier transform infrared evaluation of microscopic scarring in the cardiomyopathic heart: Effect of chronic AT1 suppression. *Anal. Biochem.* **2003**, *316*, 232–242. [CrossRef]
32. Jerônimo, D.P.; de Souza, R.A.; da Silva, F.F.; Camargo, G.L.; Miranda, H.L.; Xavier, M.; Sakane, K.K.; Ribeiro, W. Detection of creatine in rat muscle by FTIR spectroscopy. *Ann. Biomed. Eng.* **2012**, *40*, 2069–2077. [CrossRef]
33. Kirschner, C.; Ofstad, R.; Skarpeid, H.-J.; Høst, V.; Kohler, A. Monitoring of denaturation processes in aged beef loin by Fourier transform infrared microspectroscopy. *J. Agric. Food Chem.* **2004**, *52*, 3920–3929. [CrossRef]
34. Petibois, C.; Gouspillou, G.; Wehbe, K.; Delage, J.-P.; Déléris, G. Analysis of type I and IV collagens by FT-IR spectroscopy and imaging for a molecular investigation of skeletal muscle connective tissue. *Anal. Bioanal. Chem.* **2006**, *386*, 1961–1966. [CrossRef]
35. Zohdi, V.; Wood, B.R.; Pearson, J.T.; Bambery, K.R.; Black, M.J. Evidence of altered biochemical composition in the hearts of adult intrauterine growth-restricted rats. *Eur. J. Nutr.* **2013**, *52*, 749–758. [CrossRef]
36. Belbachir, K.; Noreen, R.; Gouspillou, G.; Petibois, C. Collagen types analysis and differentiation by FTIR spectroscopy. *Anal. Bioanal. Chem.* **2009**, *395*, 829–837. [CrossRef]
37. Wood, B.R. The importance of hydration and DNA conformation in interpreting infrared spectra of cells and tissues. *Chem. Soc. Rev.* **2016**, *45*, 1980–1998. [CrossRef]
38. Yang, T.T.; Weng, S.F.; Zheng, N.; Pan, Q.H.; Cao, H.L.; Liu, L.; Zhang, H.D.; Mu, D.W. Histopathology mapping of biochemical changes in myocardial infarction by Fourier transform infrared spectral imaging. *Forensic Sci. Int.* **2011**, *207*, e34–e39. [CrossRef] [PubMed]

39. Landry, M.R. Thermoporometry by differential scanning calorimetry: Experimental considerations and applications. *Thermochim. Acta* **2005**, *433*, 27–50. [CrossRef]
40. Fathima, N.N.; Kumar, M.P.; Rao, J.R.; Nair, B.U. A DSC investigation on the changes in pore structure of skin during leather processing. *Thermochim. Acta* **2010**, *501*, 98–102. [CrossRef]
41. Mignolet, A.; Derenne, A.; Smolina, M.; Wood, B.R.; Goormaghtigh, E. FTIR spectral signature of anticancer drugs. Can drug mode of action be identified? *Biochim. Biophys. Acta-Proteins Proteom.* **2016**, *1864*, 85–101. [CrossRef] [PubMed]
42. Zhang, D.X.; Fryer, R.M.; Hsu, A.K.; Zou, A.P.; Gross, G.J.; Campbell, W.B.; Li, P.L. Production and metabolism of ceramide in normal and ischemic-reperfused myocardium of rats. *Basic Res. Cardiol.* **2001**, *96*, 267–274. [CrossRef]
43. Wang, H.-Y.J.; Liu, C.B.; Wu, H.-W.; Kuo, S., Jr. Direct profiling of phospholipids and lysophospholipids in rat brain sections after ischemic stroke. *Rapid Commun. Mass Spectrom.* **2010**, *24*, 2057–2064. [CrossRef]
44. Beresewicz, A.; Dobrzyn, A.; Gorski, J. Accumulation of specific ceramides in ischemic/reperfused rat heart; effect of ischemic preconditioning. *J. Physiol. Pharmacol.* **2002**, *53*, 371–382.
45. Bielawska, A.E.; Shapiro, J.P.; Jiang, L.; Melkonyan, H.S.; Piot, C.; Wolfe, C.L.; Tomei, L.D.; Hannun, Y.A.; Umansky, S.R. Ceramide is involved in triggering of cardiomyocyte apoptosis induced by ischemia and reperfusion. *Am. J. Pathol.* **1997**, *151*, 1257–1263. [PubMed]
46. Hadas, Y.; Vincek, A.S.; Youssef, E.; Żak, M.M.; Chepurko, E.; Sultana, N.; Sharkar, M.T.K.; Guo, N.; Komargodski, R.; Kurian, A.A.; et al. Altering sphingolipid metabolism attenuates cell death and inflammatory response after myocardial infarction. *Circulation* **2020**, *141*, 916–930. [CrossRef] [PubMed]
47. Hernández-Corbacho, M.J.; Jenkins, R.W.; Clarke, C.J.; Hannun, Y.A.; Obeid, L.M.; Snider, A.J.; Siskind, L.J. Accumulation of long-chain glycosphingolipids during aging is prevented by caloric restriction. *PLoS ONE* **2011**, *6*, e20411. [CrossRef]
48. Trayssac, M.; Hannun, Y.A.; Obeid, L.M. Role of sphingolipids in senescence: Implication in aging and age-related diseases. *J. Clin. Investig.* **2018**, *128*, 2702–2712. [CrossRef]
49. Laaksonen, R.; Ekroos, K.; Sysi-Aho, M.; Hilvo, M.; Vihervaara, T.; Kauhanen, D.; Suoniemi, M.; Hurme, R.; März, W.; Scharnagl, H.; et al. Plasma ceramides predict cardiovascular death in patients with stable coronary artery disease and acute coronary syndromes beyond LDL-cholesterol. *Eur. Heart J.* **2016**, *37*, 1967–1976. [CrossRef]
50. Wang, D.D.; Toledo, E.; Hruby, A.; Rosner, B.A.; Willett, W.C.; Sun, Q.; Razquin, C.; Zheng, Y.; Ruiz-Canela, M.; Guasch-Ferré, M.; et al. Plasma ceramides, mediterranean diet, and incident cardiovascular disease in the PREDIMED trial (prevención con dieta mediterránea). *Circulation* **2017**, *135*, 2028–2040. [CrossRef]
51. Hazen, S.L.; Ford, D.A.; Gross, R.W. Activation of a membrane-associated phospholipase A2 during rabbit myocardial ischemia which is highly selective for plasmalogen substrate. *J. Biol. Chem.* **1991**, *266*, 5629–5633.
52. Ford, D.A.; Hazen, S.L.; Saffitz, J.E.; Gross, R.W. The rapid and reversible activation of a calcium-independent plasmalogen-selective phospholipase A2 during myocardial ischemia. *J. Clin. Investig.* **1991**, *88*, 331–335. [CrossRef]
53. Chen, W.W.; Chao, Y.J.; Chang, W.H.; Chan, J.F.; Hsu, Y.H.H. Phosphatidylglycerol Incorporates into Cardiolipin to Improve Mitochondrial Activity and Inhibits Inflammation. *Sci. Rep.* **2018**, *8*. [CrossRef]
54. Pokorná, L.; Čermáková, P.; Horváth, A.; Baile, M.G.; Claypool, S.M.; Griač, P.; Malínský, J.; Balážová, M. Specific degradation of phosphatidylglycerol is necessary for proper mitochondrial morphology and function. *Biochim. Biophys. Acta* **2016**, *1857*, 34–45. [CrossRef]
55. Castellano, J.; Aledo, R.; Sendra, J.; Costales, P.; Juan-Babot, O.; Badimon, L.; Llorente-Cortés, V. Hypoxia stimulates low-density lipoprotein receptor-related protein-1 expression through hypoxia-inducible factor-1α in human vascular smooth muscle cells. *Arterioscler. Thromb. Vasc. Biol.* **2011**, *31*, 1411–1420. [CrossRef]
56. Castellano, J.; Farré, J.; Fernandes, J.; Bayes-Genis, A.; Cinca, J.; Badimon, L.; Hove-Madsen, L.; Llorente-Cortés, V. Hypoxia exacerbates Ca(2+)-handling disturbances induced by very low density lipoproteins (VLDL) in neonatal rat cardiomyocytes. *J. Mol. Cell. Cardiol.* **2011**, *50*, 894–902. [CrossRef]
57. Samouillan, V.; Revuelta-López, E.; Dandurand, J.; Nasarre, L.; Badimon, L.; Lacabanne, C.; Llorente-Cortés, V. Cardiomyocyte intracellular cholesteryl ester accumulation promotes tropoelastin physical alteration and degradation: Role of LRP1 and cathepsin S. *Int. J. Biochem. Cell Biol.* **2014**, *55*, 209–219. [CrossRef]
58. Goldberg, I.J.; Reue, K.; Abumrad, N.A.; Bickel, P.E.; Cohen, S.; Fisher, E.A.; Galis, Z.S.; Granneman, J.G.; Lewandowski, E.D.; Murphy, R.; et al. Deciphering the role of lipid droplets in cardiovascular disease. *Circulation* **2018**, *138*, 305–315. [CrossRef]

6

Tissue-Specific miRNAs Regulate the Development of Thoracic Aortic Aneurysm: The Emerging Role of KLF4 Network

Stasė Gasiulė [1,†], Vaidotas Stankevičius [1,*,†], Vaiva Patamsytė [2], Raimundas Ražanskas [1], Giedrius Žukovas [3], Žana Kapustina [4], Diana Žaliaduonytė [5], Rimantas Benetis [2], Vaiva Lesauskaitė [2] and Giedrius Vilkaitis [1,*]

1 Institute of Biotechnology, Vilnius University, LT-10257 Vilnius, Lithuania; stase.gasiule@bti.vu.lt (S.G.); raimundas.razanskas@bti.vu.lt (R.R.)
2 Institute of Cardiology, Lithuanian University of Health Sciences, LT-50103 Kaunas, Lithuania; vaiva.patamsyte@lsmuni.lt (V.P.); rimantas.benetis@kaunoklinikos.lt (R.B.); vaiva.lesauskaite@lsmuni.lt (V.L.)
3 Department of Cardiac, Thoracic and Vascular Surgery, Lithuanian University of Health Sciences, LT-50103 Kaunas, Lithuania; giedrews@yahoo.com
4 Thermo Fisher Scientific Baltics, LT-02241 Vilnius, Lithuania; zana.kapustina@thermofisher.com
5 Department of Cardiology, Lithuanian University of Health Sciences, LT-50161 Kaunas, Lithuania; diana.zaliaduonyte@kaunoklinikos.lt
* Correspondence: vaidotas.stankevicius@gmc.vu.lt (V.S.); giedrius@ibt.lt (G.V.)
† These authors contributed equally to this manuscript.

Abstract: MicroRNAs (miRNAs) are critical regulators of the functional pathways involved in the pathogenesis of cardiovascular diseases. Understanding of the disease-associated alterations in tissue and plasma will elucidate the roles of miRNA in modulation of gene expression throughout development of sporadic non-syndromic ascending thoracic aortic aneurysm (TAA). This will allow one to propose relevant biomarkers for diagnosis or new therapeutic targets for the treatment. The high-throughput sequencing revealed 20 and 17 TAA-specific miRNAs in tissue and plasma samples, respectively. qRT-PCR analysis in extended cohort revealed sex-related differences in miR-10a-5p, miR-126-3p, miR-155-5p and miR-148a-3p expression, which were the most significantly dysregulated in TAA tissues of male patients. Unexpectedly, the set of aneurysm-related miRNAs in TAA plasma did not resemble the tissue signature suggesting more complex organism response to the disease. Three of TAA-specific plasma miRNAs were found to be restored to normal level after aortic surgery, further signifying their relationship to the pathology. The panel of two plasma miRNAs, miR-122-3p, and miR-483-3p, could serve as a potential biomarker set (AUC = 0.84) for the ascending TAA. The miRNA-target enrichment analysis exposed TGF-β signaling pathway as sturdily affected by abnormally expressed miRNAs in the TAA tissue. Nearly half of TAA-specific miRNAs potentially regulate a key component in TGF-β signaling: TGF-β receptors, SMADs and KLF4. Indeed, using immunohistochemistry analysis we detected increased KLF4 expression in 27% of TAA cells compared to 10% of non-TAA cells. In addition, qRT-PCR demonstrated a significant upregulation of ALK1 mRNA expression in TAA tissues. Overall, these observations indicate that the alterations in miRNA expression are sex-dependent and play an essential role in TAA via TGF-β signaling.

Keywords: aortic disease; aneurysm; miRNA; TGF-β pathway; KLF4; synthetic phenotype

1. Introduction

Thoracic aortic aneurysms (TAAs) are usually silent and therefore deadly if not detected and repaired on time [1]. Most of them are affecting the root or ascending aorta [2]. TAA is categorized as syndromic (Marfan, Loyes-Dietz, Ehlers-Danlos, etc.), familial non-syndromic and sporadic [3]. The incidence of TAA is permanently increasing and remains much higher in males than females [4]. Similar trends are observed in hospital admissions for TAA [5]. The aortic diseases are more common in males but the outcome is worse in female patients, although reasons for sex differences are unknown [6]. Therefore, further investigation of molecular mechanisms for these differences are required as well [7]. Vascular smooth muscle cells (VSMC) have been shown to possess a natural plasticity to switch between contractile and synthetic phenotypes in order to repair small vascular injuries [8]. For the last few decades, VSMC dedifferentiation has been recognized as one of the key processes involved in arterial maintenance and development of vascular diseases [9]. This led to the identification of various regulators of VSMC phenotype including a transcription activator myocardin (*MyoCD*) [10], transcription factor Krüppel-like factor 4 (*KLF4*) [11], and components of a transforming growth factor beta (*TGF-β*) signalling pathway [12]. During the formation of TAA, VSMCs are thought to lose their contractile ability and start secretion of various extracellular matrix proteins and their inhibitors, but the mechanism of this phenotypic shift remains unknown.

Recent studies have focused on the emerging epigenetic regulation of gene expression and the short non-coding microRNAs (miRNAs) involved in post-transcriptional regulation of a target messenger RNA (mRNA) [13]. MiRNAs have been implicated in the pathogenesis of various cardiovascular diseases [14] and show the potential to be utilised as biomarkers in diagnosis, prognosis, and selection of treatment [15]. Over the last decade a variety of miRNAs have been identified in the regulation of VSMC phenotype [16–18] some of which have been associated with the formation of TAA [19,20]. The majority of miRNAs association studies were done using PCR or microarray techniques [21] and only a fraction of miRNAs have been validated in plasma samples [22]. However, to date, the global high-throughput miRNA sequencing data of TAA tissue is still missing. Furthermore, most of miRNA-related mechanistic insights of TAA development are made using cell cultures or knock-out animal models which only mildly represents human disease and could further lead to misinterpretation of biological processes occurring in human tissue *in vivo* [23].

A multidimensional approach is needed in order to uncover the complex mechanisms occurring in the human aortic wall during the formation of TAA and to evaluate the possibility of using circulating miRNAs as biomarkers for the development of the disease. In the present study, we aimed to profile miRNA changes in TAA tissue and blood plasma samples and to assess their role in the pathogenesis of the disease as well as to evaluate their potential to be used as biomarkers. Using high-throughput miRNA sequencing we identified 20 and 17 differentially expressed miRNAs in TAA tissue and TAA plasma samples compared to non-TAA specimens, respectively. Deregulation of selected miRNAs in TAA samples were further confirmed by qRT-PCR analysis, thus verifying reliability of miRNA-Seq results. A subsequent pathway enrichment analysis of miRNA target genes revealed significant relationship between nearly half of dysregulated miRNAs and TGF-β signalling pathway. Finally, we for the first time showed accumulation of KLF4, a master regulator of VSMC differentiation state, in TAA tissue obtained from patients. Altogether our results define potential candidates for TAA diagnostic biomarkers and provide new insights in regulatory miRNA-related mechanisms of TAA development.

2. Materials and Methods

2.1. Patient Samples

All experimental procedures using human tissue and plasma samples conform to the principles outlined in the Declaration of Helsinki and were approved by Kaunas Regional Biomedical Research Ethics Committee (Nr. P2-BE-2-12/2012).

The study included 40 patients with sporadic non-syndromic ascending thoracic aorta aneurysm (TAA group). Exclusion criteria were severe atherosclerosis showing calcified or ulcerating plaques of the ascending aorta, aortitis, phenotypic characteristics of the known genetic disorders such as Marfan, Ehlers Danlos and other syndromes. The diagnosis was confirmed by two-dimensional thoracic aorta echocardiography according to the 2014 ESC guidelines on the diagnosis and treatment of aortic diseases. Echocardiography was performed at the Department of Cardiology, Lithuanian University of Health Sciences (LUHS). TAA group included patients (n = 23) who underwent aortic reconstruction surgery at the Department of Cardiac, Thoracic and Vascular Surgery, LUHS and non-operated patients (n = 17) with ascending aorta aneurysm.

Study subjects without TAA (non-TAA group) included i) heart transplantation donors (n = 6), ii) patients who underwent isolated coronary artery bypass graft surgery (CABG) (n = 72) and iii) healthy volunteers (n = 10). All healthy volunteers were screened using two-dimensional transthoracic echocardiography to ensure the ascending aorta was not dilated. Detailed preparation of patients' tissue and plasma samples can be found in the Supplementary Methods.

2.2. Study Design

Study subjects (n = 32) selected for miRNA expression profiling in aortic tissue consisted of surgical TAA patients (n = 8), donors (n = 4) as well as CABG patients (n = 2). miRNA expression profiling in plasma was done in samples from surgical TAA patients (n = 7) before and 3 months after the aortic surgery (denoted as operated, n = 4), respectively. Seven volunteers without health complaints (n= 7) were used as non-TAA controls. Clinical and demographic characteristics of the groups are summarized in Table 1.

Table 1. Demographic and clinical characteristics of control and thoracic aortic aneurysm (TAA) patients selected for profiling of microRNA (miRNA) expression.

	Tissue		Plasma		
Variables	non-TAA (n = 6)	TAA (n = 8)	non-TAA (n = 7)	TAA (n = 7)	Operated (n = 4)
Age, years ± SD	47 ± 5	62 ± 10	54 ± 12	63 ± 11	64 ± 12
Sex, male (%)	4 (67 %)	6 (75 %)	4 (57 %)	5 (71 %)	3 (75 %)
Ascending aortic diameter, mm	36 ± 0.7 *	50 ± 3	35 ± 3	53 ± 5	52 ± 4
Aortic valve stenosis (%)	0 (0 %)	3 (38 %)	1 (14 %)	2 (29 %)	1 (25 %)
Bicuspid aortic valve (%)	0 (0 %)	5 (63 %)	0 (0 %)	4 (57 %)	2 (50 %)
Aortic valve insufficiency (%)	0 (0 %)	5 (63 %)	1 (14 %)	3 (43 %)	1 (25 %)
Hypertension (%)	2 (100 %) *	7 (88 %)	4 (57 %)	6 (86 %)	4 (100 %)
Smokers (%)	2 (100 %) *	1 (13 %)	1 (14 %)	1 (14 %)	0 (0 %)
Diabetes (%)	0 (0 %)	1 (13 %)	0 (0%)	3 (43 %)	1 (25 %)

Notes: * Data is missing from four aorta donors. Operated denotes patient samples collected after aortic surgery.

Validation group for miRNA expression in aortic tissue consisted of TAA surgical patients (n = 17), donors and CABG patients (n = 35). For the miRNA validation in plasma samples, we were able to collect larger TAA group (n = 28) and non-TAA group (n = 34) which consisted of healthy volunteers and CABG patients. Clinical and demographic characteristics of each validation group are presented in Supplementary Table S1. A significant difference in ascending aortic diameter ($p < 0.001$) was observed between TAA patients and non-TAA in both miRNA profiling groups supporting the selection criteria. Patients with bicuspid aortic valve were predominant in both TAA groups ($p < 0.001$) compared with non-TAA group.

Total RNA isolation, cDNA library sequencing, and miRNA-Seq differential and functional analysis are described in detail in Supplementary Methods. miRNA-Seq data are available at GEO database using accession number GSE122266. Validation of miRNA-Seq data was performed as described previously [24] and detailed qRT-PCR and immunohistochemistry analysis are depicted in Supplementary Methods.

3. Results

3.1. Differential miRNA Expression Analysis in TAA Tissue and Blood Plasma Samples

In order to determine miRNAs which expression levels are potentially deregulated in aorta tissue and blood plasma during the formation of TAA, in the present study we evaluated miRNA expression profiles in a learning set of patient tissue and plasma samples ($n = 32$) using Illumina high-throughput miRNA sequencing platform (Table 1; Figure 1A). The overview of miRNA-Seq experimental design and data quality is depicted in Supplementary Results. miRNA-Seq data analysis revealed a total of 20 differentially expressed miRNAs (selection criteria were fold change ≥ 1.5, p value < 0.05 and base mean higher than 10) in TAA tissue samples compared to non-TAA group (Table 2), among which the majority (15 of 20 miRNAs) were upregulated (Table 3). A detailed differential miRNA-Seq data evaluation of each sample assessed in the present study is depicted in Supplementary File 1 and Supplementary File 2. A heat map of expression signature for these dysregulated miRNAs in all 14 samples clearly clustered aorta tissues according to the presence or absence of aneurysm (Figure 1B).

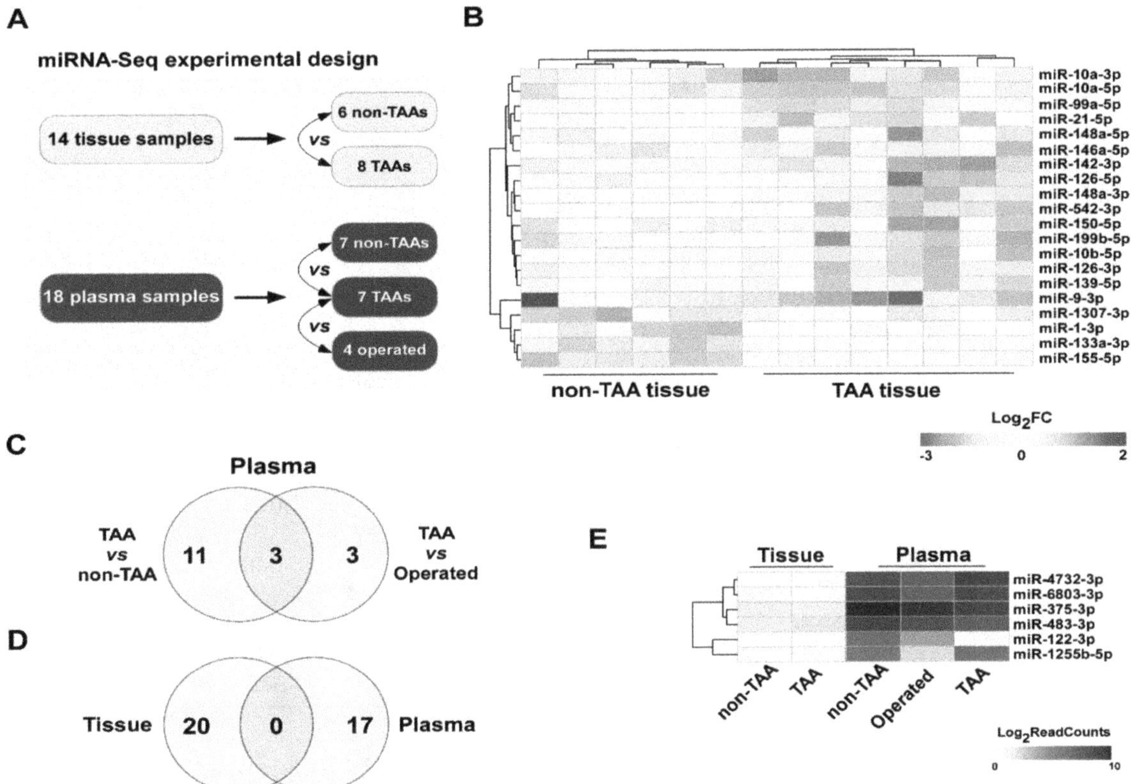

Figure 1. Differential miRNA expression analysis in TAA tissue and plasma samples using high-throughput RNA sequencing. (**A**) Schematic diagram of miRNA-Seq experiment. (**B**) Heat map showing a total of 20 miRNAs differentially expressed (fold change, FC > 1.5, $p < 0.05$, normalized read count average, RC > 10) in TAA tissue samples ($n = 8$) compared to normal aorta tissue ($n = 6$). Red color indicates upregulated log-transformed expression level ratios of corresponding miRNAs, blue – downregulated; (**C**) Venn's diagram showing the number of differentially expressed miRNAs (FC > 1.5, $p \leq 0.05$ and RC > 20) in TAA plasma samples ($n = 7$) compared to non-aneurysmal group ($n = 7$) and plasma samples obtained 3 months after aortic reconstructive surgery ($n = 4$); (**D**) Venn's diagram demonstrating the number of differentially expressed miRNAs in TAA tissue and plasma samples; (**E**) Heat map demonstrating the expression of six miRNAs, which were significantly deregulated in TAA plasma samples, but were almost absent in TAA tissue samples. Color intensity indicates log-transformed normalized read counts of corresponding miRNA.

Table 2. A number of miRNAs differentially expressed (fold change > 1.5) in TAA tissue and blood plasma samples compared to non-TAA controls.

Groups	Number of miRNAs	Upregulated	Downregulated
Tissue			
TAA vs. non-TAA	20	15	5
Plasma			
TAA vs. non-TAA	14	3	11
TAA v.s Op	6	4	2
TAA vs. non-TAA + Op	10	2	8

Notes: TAA—Thoracic Ascending Aneurysm; Op—Operated.

Table 3. List of differentially expressed miRNAs (selection criteria were fold change > 1.5, p value < 0.05 and base mean higher than 10) in TAA aortic tissue samples compared to miRNA expression levels in non-TAA controls.

No.	miRNAs	Fold Change	p Value
	Upregulated		
1	hsa-miR-10a-3p	2.69	2.05E–06
2	hsa-miR-10a-5p	2.45	8.63E–07
3	hsa-miR-150-5p	2.21	2.05E–05
4	hsa-miR-199b-5p	2.12	1.19E–04
5	hsa-miR-126-5p	1.89	7.95E–04
6	hsa-miR-126-3p	1,88	2.10E–05
7	hsa-miR-139-5p	1.74	7.22E–04
8	hsa-miR-148a-3p	1.71	3.44E–05
9	hsa-miR-10b-5p	1.70	7.78E–04
10	hsa-miR-148a-5p	1.70	0.0112
11	hsa-miR-99a-5p	1.68	1.76E–05
12	hsa-miR-21-5p	1.67	1.10E–03
13	hsa-miR-146a-5p	1.67	0.002
14	hsa-miR-142-3p	1.66	0.020
15	hsa-miR-542-3p	1.64	0.009
	Downregulated		
16	hsa-miR-1-3p	−1.59	0.001
17	hsa-miR-133a-3p	−1.64	2.96E–07
18	hsa-miR-1307-3p	−1.68	0.011
19	hsa-miR-9-3p	−1.79	0.021
20	hsa-miR-155-5p	−1.88	7.34E−08

Using the same workflow of miRNA-Seq analysis, we found 14 differentially expressed miRNAs in TAA patient plasma samples compared to non-TAA group. Out of these, 3 were upregulated and 11 were downregulated (Tables 2 and 4). Next, to determine alterations after the removal of aneurysm, we compared the miRNA expression levels between TAA plasma samples collected before and 3 months after aortic surgery. This analysis led to the detection of six differentially expressed miRNAs (Table 4; Supplementary Figure S1). Remarkably, the expression of three of TAA-specific plasma miRNAs, miR-1255b-5p, miR-122-3p and miR-23b-5p, returned to near non-TAA levels after the operation. Finally, to identify the most significantly dysregulated miRNAs in TAA plasma samples, we pooled data from both non-aneurysmal (non-TAA and TAA samples collected after the surgery) cohorts and compared to TAA group. The differential analysis determined ten differentially expressed miRNAs revealing the greatest fold change for miR-122-3p. Thus, the overall evaluation of miRNA expression changes in plasma samples discovered a total of 17 differentially expressed miRNAs in TAA samples compared to non-TAA samples, samples collected after aortic surgery or both groups of samples (Figure 1C).

Table 4. List of differentially expressed miRNAs (fold change > 1.5, p value ≤ 0.05-fold and base mean ≥ 20) in TAA patient blood plasma samples compared to miRNA expression levels in non-TAA controls.

Group	No.	miRNA	Regulation	Fold Change	p Value
TAA vs. non-TAA	1	hsa-miR-146b-3p	up	9.11	0.044
	2	hsa-miR-1255b-5p	up	8.87	0.015
	3	hsa-miR-889-3p	up	7.95	0.047
	4	hsa-miR-375-3p	down	–2.38	0.036
	5	hsa–miR-30a-5p	down	–2.54	0.033
	6	hsa-miR-483-3p	down	–2.68	0.015
	7	hsa-miR-23b-3p	down	–2.79	0.017
	8	hsa-miR-140-3p	down	–4.01	0.010
	9	hsa-miR-100-5p	down	–9.17	0.003
	10	hsa-miR-145-5p	down	–17.36	1.44E–04
	11	hsa-miR-143-3p	down	–17.74	3.27E–05
	12	hsa–miR-23b-5p	down	–24.93	0.013
	13	hsa-miR-122-3p	down	–69.32	3.31E–04
	14	hsa-miR-34a-5p	down	–71.95	4.01E–05
TAA vs. Operated	1	hsa-miR-1255b-5p	up	9.7203	0.045
	2	hsa-miR-4732-3p	up	3.9801	0.050
	3	hsa-miR-6803-3p	up	3.4495	0.011
	4	hsa-miR-22-3p	up	2.5198	0.029
	5	hsa-miR-122-3p	down	–18.4085	0.024
	6	hsa-miR-23b-5p	down	–44.7992	0.001
TAA vs. non-TAA & Operated	1	hsa-miR-1255b-5p	up	11.68	0.004
	2	hsa-miR-22-3p	up	1.73	0.034
	3	hsa-miR-375-3p	down	–2.12	0.049
	4	hsa-miR-483-3p	down	–2.29	0.035
	5	hsa-miR-23b-3p	down	–2.36	0.024
	6	hsa-miR-143-3p	down	–3.83	0.012
	7	hsa-miR-145-5p	down	–4.83	0.019
	8	hsa-miR-23b-5p	down	–29.67	0.003
	9	hsa-miR-34a-5p	down	–48.62	6.26E–05
	10	hsa-miR-122-3p	down	–53.67	2.31E–04

Surprisingly, a pattern of aneurysm-related alterations in plasma's miRNA profiles showed no resemblance to the tissue set. Indeed, none of the differentially expressed miRNAs overlapped in Venn's diagram (Figure 1D). Moreover, the expression levels of the six significantly deregulated miRNAs in TAA plasma samples, miR-4732-3p, miR-6803-3p, miR-375-3p, miR-483-3p, miR-122-3p and miR-1255b-5p, were negligible in aortic tissue samples (Figure 1E).

3.2. Validation of Selected miRNAs in TAA Tissue and Plasma Samples by qRT-PCR

In order to corroborate the RNA sequencing-based predictions, we performed qRT-PCR analysis to examine the abundance of five selected miRNAs (mir-10a-5p and miR-155-5p exhibited the greatest up/down fold changes; miR-126-3p, mir-133a-3p and miR-148a-3p were implicated in TGF-β signaling routes, see below) in the independent group of 37 samples containing 20 non-TAA and 17 thoracic aortic aneurysm tissues (Supplementary Table S1). Our analysis validated the up- and downregulated expression of miR-10a-5p, miR-126-3p, miR-133a-3p and miR-155-5p, respectively, in the sex-undivided set of TAA tissue samples compared to the non-TAA group (Figure 2A, Supplementary Figure S2). Whereas, the difference in miR-148a-3p expression levels was significant among the groups only when stratifying by sex ($p = 0.0203$ for a male patient set). Interestingly, a significantly greater differential expression of miR-126-3p ($p = 0.0062$ vs. $p = 0.0225$ for sex-undivided set), miR-155-5p ($p = 0.0003$ vs. $p = 0.0017$) and miR-10a-5p ($p = 0.0001$ vs. $p = 0.0002$), except miR-133a-3p ($p = 0.0068$ vs. $p = 0.0031$), also was observed between 13 TAA and 13 normal aorta tissue samples from male patients showing sex-related miRNA expression variances in the TAA tissue. Because of the scarce representation of female samples (7 non-TAA vs. 4 TAA) the extent of involvement of these miRNAs in the thoracic aneurysm formation in female patients requires further analysis.

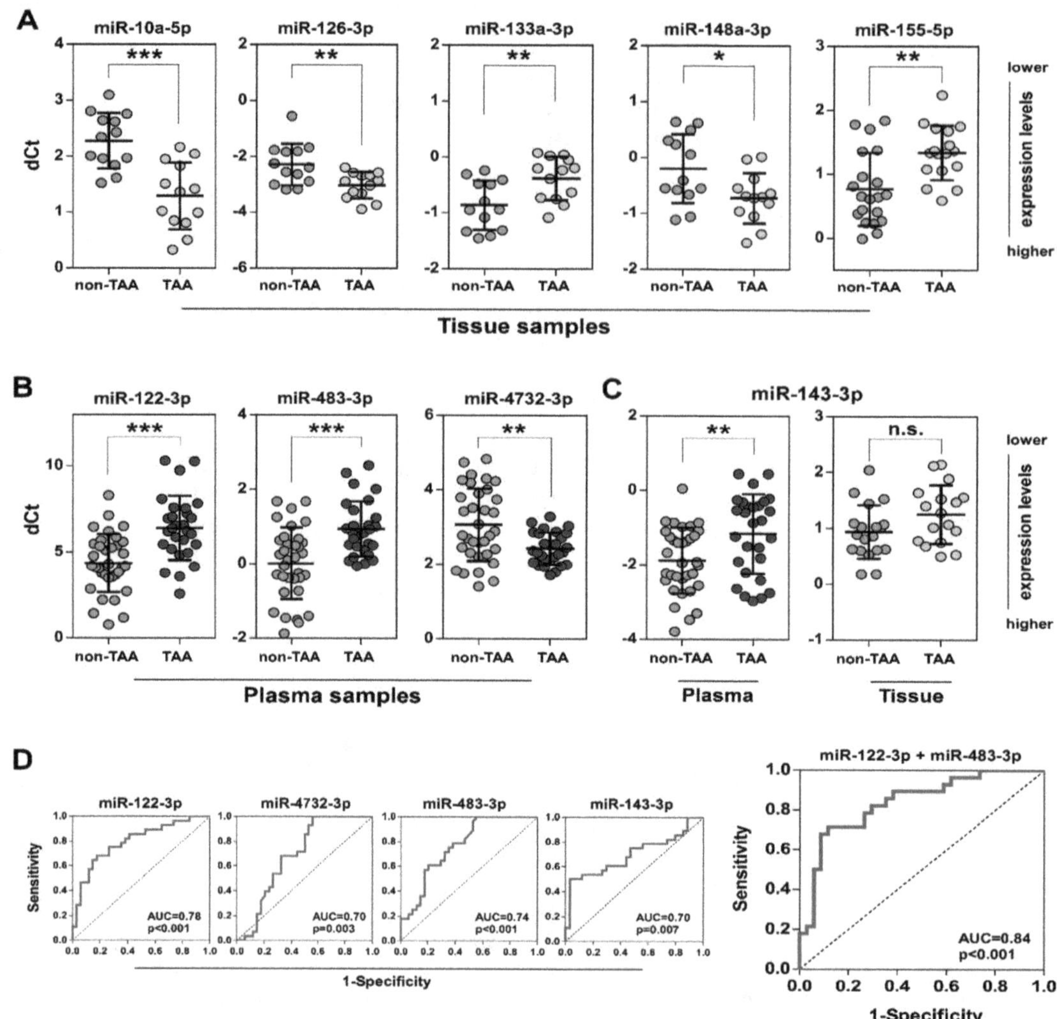

Figure 2. Validation of differentially expressed miRNAs in TAA tissue and plasma samples by qRT-PCR. qRT-PCR analysis was used for the comparison of relative miRNA expression levels between non-TAA and TAA groups in tissue (**A**) and plasma (**B**) both types (**C**) of samples. The cycle threshold (Ct) values of observed miRNAs were normalized to miR-152-3p and miR-185-5p for tissue and plasma samples, respectively, which were revealed as the most reliable endogenous controls according to miRNA-Seq data. Lines within boxes indicate relative miRNA expression median values; whiskers—5–95 percentile of the relative miRNA expression values. Significance between each group was evaluated using Student's t test and is shown as follows: n.s.—not significant; * $p < 0.05$; ** $p < 0.01$ and *** $p < 0.001$. (**D**) Diagnostic ROC curve analysis showing sensitivity and specificity of mir-122-3p, mir-483-3p, mir-4732-3p and mir-143-3p selected circulating miRNAs or the combination of mir-122-3p and mir-483-3p together. AUC denotes area under the ROC curve.

In contrast, the evaluation of the miRNA expression levels in 62 plasma samples (34 non-TAA vs. 28 TAA) demonstrated that all selected miRNAs, miR-4732-3p, miR-483-3p and miR-122-3p, exhibited statistically significant expression changes in TAA plasma samples compared to non-TAA group showing a good reliability of our miRNA-Seq data (Figure 2B). Of those, the difference of miR-122-3p expression levels was the most significant ($p < 0.0001$) between two plasma sample groups.

RNA-Seq analysis displayed that the difference of miR-143-3p expression was not statistically significant in TAA tissue samples compared to non-TAA. Consistently with this observation, a significant downregulation ($p = 0.0051$) was observed only in TAA plasma samples (Figure 2C) despite the decrement of miR-143-3p expression level in both TAA specimen groups compared to non-TAA group.

The diagnostic sensitivity and specificity of selected plasma circulating miRNAs which could serve as potential biomarkers of TAA was examined by ROC curve analysis (Figure 2D). The results demonstrated that miR-122-3p reached the most significant prognostic accuracy (AUC = 0.78, $p < 0.001$). Moreover, a combined analysis of miR-122-3p and miR-483-3p miRNAs showed even better diagnostic discrimination (AUC = 0.84, $p < 0.001$) indicating that these miRNAs could be applied as TAA biomarkers.

Finally, the statistical analysis showed no significant correlations between selected differential miRNAs, miR-10a-5p, miR-126-3p, mir-133a-3p miR-155-5p, miR-148a-3p, miR-122-3p, miR-483-3p, miR-4732-3p, miR-143-3p and chosen patient characteristics such as patients' age, aorta diameter, bicuspid (BAV)/tricuspid aortic valves (TAV)-associated aneurysms (data is not shown).

On the other hand, we revealed a significant moderate positive correlations between expression level of miR-126-3p and miR-148a-3p ($R = 0.67$) or miR-10a-5p ($R = 0.67$), miR-148a-3p and miR-10a-5p ($R = 0.49$), miR-133a-3p and miR-155-5p ($R = 0.67$) (Supplementary Table S2). Meanwhile, in plasma samples, the strongest correlation was observed between the expression of miR-122-3p and miR-483-3p ($R = 0.65$) (Supplementary Table S3).

3.3. *Functional Analysis of miRNA Target Genes Involved in TAA Development*

Next, we performed KEGG pathway enrichment analysis of dysregulated miRNA target genes to unravel the miRNA-mediated biological processes associated with TAA development. To provide the best set of relevant candidates for the bona fide miRNA-mRNA interactions, we evaluated combined scores from eight different miRNA target site prediction databases (see details in Methods). The examination identified 1133 target genes (exceeding combined score threshold value of 4) for group consisting of miRNAs which were differently expressed in TAA tissue (Supplementary File 3). The subsequent pathway enrichment analysis of the defined miRNA target sets revealed 48 KEGG categories significantly enriched in targeted genes (> 15 target genes in functional category, FDR < 0.05; Supplementary Table S4). In order to visualize the interconnection between signaling pathways regulated by miRNAs, we generated KEGG pathway network using Cytoscape plugin ClueGo. The network analysis clearly exposed three large functional clusters of KEGG categories closely related to immune response, cancer development and kinase signaling pathways, while any significant association of the remaining ten pathways to any other category was absent (Figure 3A, Supplementary Table S5). Transforming growth factor beta (*TGF-β*) signaling pathway, which plays a key role during aorta development and subsequent remodeling, was represented among these categories. To make a more detailed assessment of the miRNA-target interaction network, we additionally introduced target genes which were significantly related to differentially expressed miRNAs (target score > 4).

The expanded analysis revealed 17 target genes which could be potentially regulated by 9 out of 20 of miRNAs differentially expressed in TAA tissue (Figure 3B). Furthermore, our results defined two groups of genes sharing the similar functions which could be potentially affected by miRNAs - (i) *TGF-β* receptors and ligands and (ii) regulating *SMAD*s (r*SMAD*s) (Figure 3C, grey boxes). As shown above, the differential expression of two of them, miR-148a-3p and miR-155-5p, were additionally confirmed by qRT-PCR analysis. Moreover, miR-133a-3p, which was significantly downregulated in TAA tissue samples, has been previously described as a prominent indirect downregulator of Kruppel-like factor 4 (*KLF4*) [25]. According to these findings, we hypothesized that the miRNAs related to TAA could contribute significantly to critical changes in tissue remodeling in diseased aorta through of *TGF-β* signaling pathway: (i) leading to the functional dysregulation of the key regulators, *KLF4* and/or *MyoCD*, which determine the differentiation state of aorta smooth muscle cells (Figure 3C); (ii) the altered signaling balance between *TGF-β* receptors, ligands and r*SMAD*s could provoke alternative *MyoCD*-independent *TGF-β* signaling routes which could boost TAA development.

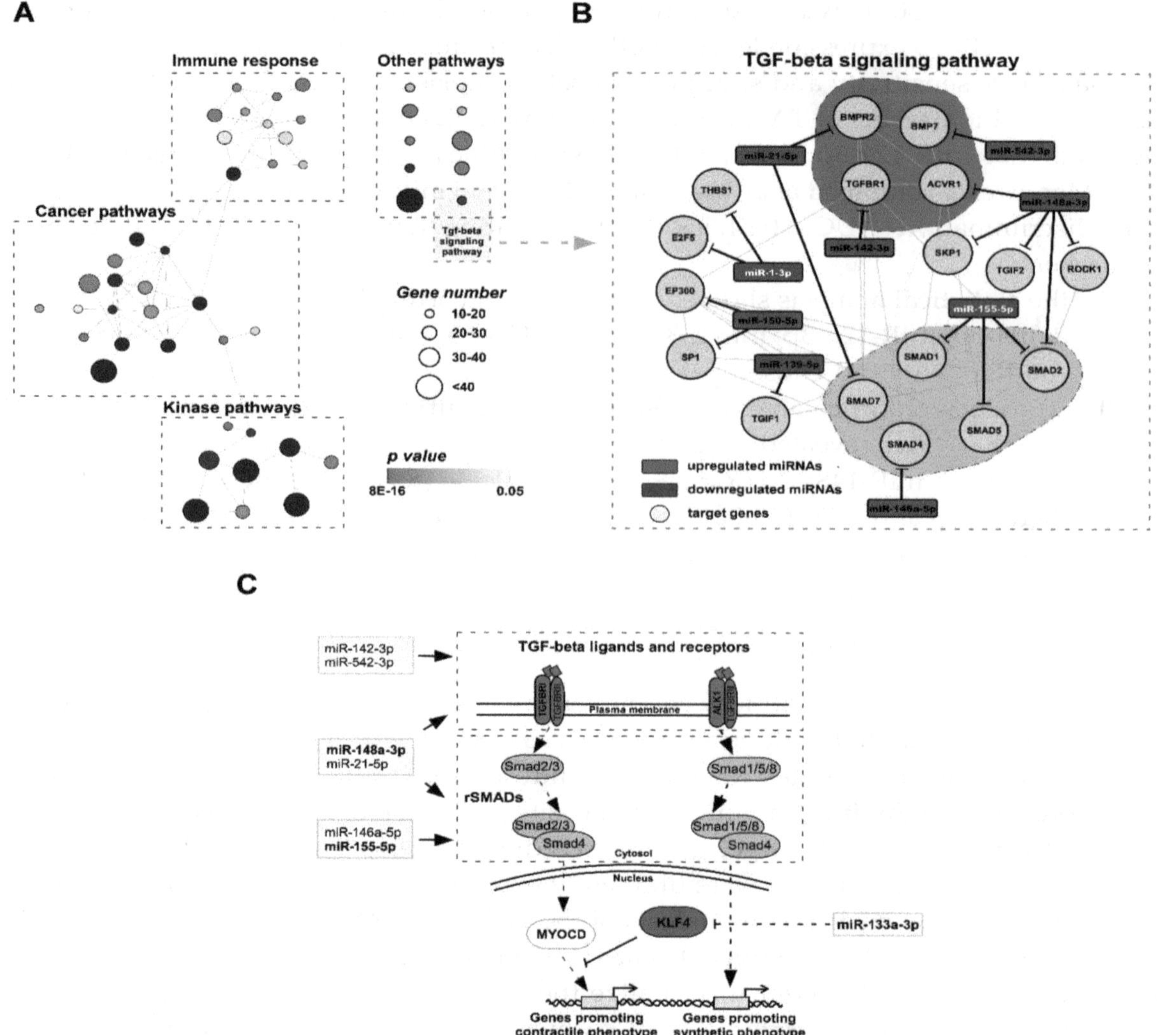

Figure 3. Functional analysis of target genes of miRNAs dysregulated in TAA. (**A**) Network analysis of 48 KEGG categories specified three clusters of closely related categories including immune response, cancer, kinase signaling pathways and ten separate groups that were not significantly associated with any other category. *TGF-β* signaling pathway is included in a grey box. The size of node represents gene number in particular, KEGG category, the node color – the significance level value of particular KEGG category. Edges indicate a statistically significant association between categories. (**B**) Expanded molecular network of miRNAs and their potential target genes involved in *TGF-β* signaling pathway. Grey nodes denote target genes, red and blue – upregulated and downregulated miRNAs, respectively. Dark orange area covers *TGF-β* ligands and receptors; light orange – regulatory *SMAD*s (r*SMAD*s). (**C**) Simplified hypothetical schema of *TGF-β* signal transduction in TAA tissue cells. miRNAs, which were differentially expressed in TAA tissue (grey boxes), could potentially disturb *TGF-β* signaling by targeting *TGF-β* ligands, receptors or r*SMAD*s leading to dysregulation of *MyoCD–KLF4* transcription regulator axis and further TAA progression.

3.4. Number of VSMCs Expressing KLF4 Dramatically Increases during TAA Development

To further explore the compelling connection of the reprogramed miRNA network with *TGF-β* signaling pathway, we assessed the mRNA expression levels of *TGF-β* receptors, *TGFBR1* and *ALK1* (also known as *ACVRL1*), and transcription factors, *MyoCD* and *KLF4*, in non-TAA (n=21) and TAA (n = 17) tissue samples (Supplementary Figure S3A). We observed a relevant elevation of *ALK1* gene transcription in TAA tissues (p = 0.0244) compared to non-TAA group of normal aortas but found no significant difference in cellular mRNA levels of *TGFBR1*, *KLF4*, and *MyoCD*. It is noteworthy that we revealed a moderate positive correlation between the changes in expression of *ALK1*, miR-10a-5p, miR-126-3p and miR-148a-5p (Supplementary Table S6; Supplementary Figure S4) suggesting a putative biological relationship between these miRNAs and *TGF-β* signaling pathway. Thus, the obtained data pointed out to a weak regulation of studied genes, except *ALK1*, on transcription or mRNA decay level. However, it has been reported that many human miRNAs control post-transcriptional processes at the protein translation stage [26]. Therefore, we further evaluated the protein expression levels of the selected genes in non-TAA and TAA tissue samples using immunohistochemical analysis (IHC) (Figure 4; Supplementary Figure S3B). The IHC analysis revealed higher expression of *ALK1* both in normal and TAA tissues (IHC score median = 4), whereas the expression levels of *TGFBR1* remained lower in both aortic sample groups (IHC score median = 2). However, the difference of expression levels of both *TGF-β* receptors remained insignificant between TAA and non-TAA specimens (Supplementary Figure S3B). In contrast, although the overall expression levels of *KLF4* were low in both groups of aortic samples, we detected a significant three-fold accumulation ($p = 0.0037$) of *KLF4* positive cells in TAA tissues compared to non-TAA group (Figure 4). Meanwhile, IHC analysis strongly supported upregulated expression of osteopontin ($p = 0.0311$), which is indicating shift of vascular smooth muscles from contraction to synthetic phenotype and is a positive marker of aortic aneurysms [27,28]. Finally, despite IHC results displaying high levels of *MyoCD* in both groups of samples (IHC score median = 6), a significant expression difference was absent between groups (Figure 4, lower panel).

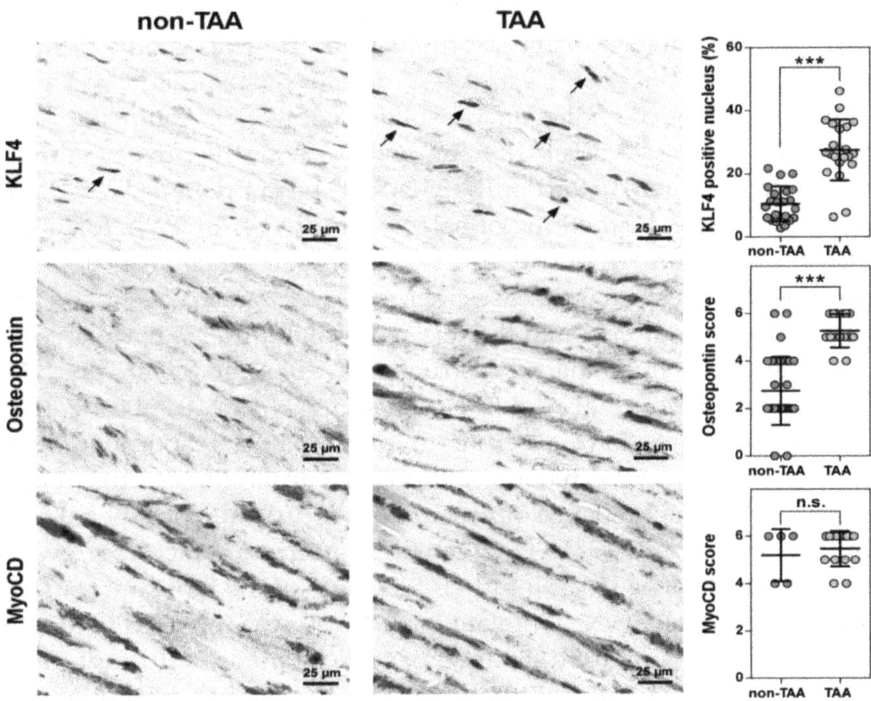

Figure 4. Immunohistochemical (IHC) analysis of KLF4, MyoCD, and osteopontin expression in non-TAA and TAA tissue samples. The abundance of proteins was examined by immunostaining and visualized with diaminobenzidine (brown). The sections were counterstained with hematoxylin (blue). Histological quantification of KLF4 was performed by counting KLF4 positive cell nucleus (black arrows; $n = 43$), whereas osteopontin ($n = 46$) and MyoCD ($n = 20$) by IHC score (graphs in right panel). Lines within boxes indicate KLF4 positive nucleus mean or MyoCD and osteopontin IHC score median values, whiskers – 5-95 percentile of KLF4 positive nucleus or MyoCD and osteopontin IHC score values. The histological data were assessed using Student's t test (for KLF4) or non-parametric Mann-Whitney U test (for MyoCD and osteopontin). The significance between each group is shown as follows: n.s.—not significant; * $p < 0.05$; ** $p < 0.01$, *** $p < 0.001$.

4. Discussion

Aneurysm is one of the most frequent diseases of the aorta [29]. The aortic aneurysms rarely cause any symptoms and thereby are commonly diagnosed incidentally. Consequently, the rupture or dissection of the aneurysm leads to lethal outcomes in over 15000 cases annually in the USA only [30]. Classification of aortic aneurysms is based on the anatomic location, with thoracic aortic aneurysms involving the ascending and descending aorta and abdominal aortic aneurysm [31]. The ascending aorta is derived from distinct embryonic origin defining some specific pathological aspects of aneurysms appearing in different locations [32]. The distinct disease entities at the molecular level may be regulated by specific, at least partially, miRNA networks. Previous studies have demonstrated that miRNAs play key roles during the formation of AAA by dysregulating VSMC homeostasis and extracellular matrix (ECM) composition or inducing vascular inflammatory response [33,34]. However, a global high-throughput miRNA-sequencing data of TAA tissue and plasma was still missing, despite some experimental data obtained by miRNA microarrays [19,20,35].

4.1. miRNA Expression Patterns in Tissues May Be Influenced by Aneurysmal Location and Sex

In the present study we determined a total of 20 miRNAs which were differentially expressed in ascending TAA tissues compared to non-aneurysmal group. A qRT-PCR testing further validated the differential expression of four selected miR-10a-5p, miR-133a-3p, miR-126-3p, miR-155-5p and miR-148a-3p in a larger set of independent samples supporting the reliability of miRNA-Seq results.

Despite a partial overlap (miR-126-3p, miR-155-5p and mir-133a-3p appeared to be involved in AAA [22,29,30]), our results confirmed previous assumptions indicating a quite distinct miRNA expression patterns between TAA and AAA tissues. This might be explained by different pathophysiological mechanism for ascending aneurysm development in comparison to AAA. The latter is most commonly caused by atherosclerosis [31]. In agreement with the present study, the dysregulated expression of miR-133a-3p, miR-126-3p and miR-155-5p has been previously associated with TAA [32]. However, the pathophysiological functions of selected miRNAs in TAA formation and how they modulate disease progression remain poorly understood. A significant upregulation of miR-155-5p was identified in various cardiovascular diseases including AAA and was linked to the inflammatory response in aortic wall. It was demonstrated that expression of miR-155 correlated with inflammatory macrophage response and extracellular matrix destruction in AAA model mice [33]. On the contrary, we identified miR-155-5p as the most strongly downregulated miRNA in TAA tissue. It might be explained by the absence of advanced atherosclerosis leading to inflammatory response in the studied ascending aorta samples obtained during aortic reconstruction. Meanwhile, vascular endothelium specific miR-126-3p is required for the maintenance of vascular integrity and endothelial cell homeostasis [34]. Reduced in proliferating VSMC miR-133a-3p switch on transcription factor *Sp1*, which activates *KLF4*, thus promoting synthetic phenotype [25,35]. miR-10a-5p, one of the most upregulated miRNAs in this study, and miR-148a-3p previously were not related to TAA. It was reported that increased miR-10a-5p expression leads to VSMC differentiation from embryonic stem cells through repression of histone deacetylase *HDAC4* [36]. Thus, we inferred that miR-10a-5p may be a potential modulator of VSMC phenotype as well.

We identified a positive correlation between expression levels of miR-126-3p and newly predicted TAA-related miR-10a-5p and miR-148a-3p (Supplementary Figure S4) indicating a possible functional or regulatory link between these miRNAs. Therefore, further studies of the molecular impact of miR-148a-3p and miR-10a-5p on TAA development is of interest.

An evaluation of sex-dependence revealed that miR-148a-3p varied significantly only in male TAA cohort (Supplementary Figure S1). Furthermore, miR-126-3p, miR-155-5p and miR-10a-5p expression changes were more statistically significant in male TAA patients. Notably, the incidence of TAA is more prevalent in males than females [4]. Moreover, previous reports emphasized relevant sex differences in the pathology of TAA, although underlying molecular mechanisms are unknown. Accordingly, aortic dilation rate was more than 3 times greater in women than in men [6]. This observation was associated with different levels of metalloproteinases *MMP2* and *MMP9*, inhibitory enzymes *TIMP1* and *TIMP2* and overall aortic stiffness highlighting a different ECM remodeling in female aortas [37]. Altogether, these findings suggest that sex-dependent physiological differences could be associated with different changes of miRNA levels in male aorta tissue during TAA development. Otherwise, a deregulation of miRNAs in sex-dependent manner could promote distinct pathways leading to different TAA progression and pathology rates in male patients.

4.2. Circulating miRNA Profile Does Not Match to Aneurysmal Signature of TAA Tissues

Herein we revealed 17 differentially expressed miRNAs in the TAA patients' plasma samples compared to the non-TAA group. The combination of two of them, miR-122-3p and miR-483-3p, allowed to distinguish TAA patients from non-TAA subjects suggesting a novel set of prognostic biomarkers for TAA non-invasive diagnostic. Notably, the majority of altered miRNAs were associated with TAA for the first time, and so far, have not been previously identified in AAA samples [22].

Suprisingly, the pattern of aneurysm-related alterations in TAA patients' plasma miRNA profile does not overlap with the tissue set (Figure 1D). Moreover, the expression of six miRNAs, which were among the most strongly deregulated in TAA plasma samples, was almost absent in TAA tissue. We can speculate that miRNA expression changes in TAA patient's plasma could be evoked by a complex physiological organismal response to the aortic aneurysm development passed by circulating miRNAs that are essential vehicles for organ-to-organ cross-talk between liver, pancreas, muscle, immune and endothelial cells [38]. For instance, miR-122, the most strongly downregulated miRNA in this study, is a key factor in liver development, homeostasis and metabolic functions [39]. The downregulation of miR-122 in the liver cells correlates with hepatic pathology [40], which could be further associated with metabolic syndrome and cardiovascular diseases [41]. In blood plasma, the downregulation of miR-122 was previously associated with other cardiovascular diseases including bicuspid aortic valve, myocardial infarction and cardiac arrest [42–44]. Thus, it seems that the dysregulation of circulating miR-122, highlighted in our study, is not TAA tissue-associated directly but rather is determined by response to the TAA. Meanwhile, an altered expression of mir-483-3p was associated with endothelial cell response to vascular injury [45].

4.3. miRNA Target Analysis Reveals KLF4 As a Key Factor for the TAA Development in vivo

Using bioinformatics approach, we exposed 48 KEGG pathways enriched in genes targeted by differentially expressed miRNAs in TAA tissue cells. Functional categories annotated by KEGG displayed overlapping among target genes which were mainly associated with the immune response, cancer, and kinase activity processes. We emphasized "*TGF-β* signaling pathway" as individual pathways of highest importance which could be involved in TAA development (Supplementary Table S5). Indeed, about half of differentially expressed miRNAs have predicted targets in 17 genes involved in *TGF-β* pathway. These miRNAs could interfere with the signal transduction by affecting two principal groups of target genes - *TGF-β* ligands/receptors and regulatory *SMAD*s (Figure 3C). Based on these findings, we hypothesized that the mis-expressed miRNAs could contribute significantly to critical changes in diseased aorta via alterations in components of *TGF-β* signaling pathway. It can lead to the functional dysregulation of the key downstream regulators, *KLF4* and/or *MyoCD*. On the other hand, the deregulated balance between *TGF-β* receptors, ligands and r*SMAD*s might trigger alternative *MyoCD*-independent *TGF-β* signaling routes promoting further TAA development [46]. As shown in Figure 3, a group of *TGF-β* receptors/r*SMAD*s-associated miRNAs was mis-regulated in TAA tissues. Previous reports revealed that deficiency of *SMAD4* and *TGFBR2* in VSMCs induced aortic dilation in TAA mice model indicating that the imbalance of TGF-β receptors and r*SMAD*s could promote TAA progression [47,48]. On the other hand, the overexpression and over-activation of *SMAD2* was *TGF-β* signaling independent in TAA tissue samples suggesting a functional dissociation between the Smad2 activation and activity of the *TGF-β* receptors [47,49]. A signaling switch from canonical *TGFBRI*/*Smad2*-dependent to *ALK1*/*Smad1/5/8* signaling was shown to activate genes related to synthetic VSMC phenotype in mice model [50]. In addition, previous report indicated that the differentiation state of VSMCs is controlled by miR-26a via suppression of *TGF-β* signaling molecules [51] demonstrating a link between the dysregulated miRNA expression and aberrant *TGF-β* signaling during TAA development.

Herein we demonstrated a significant upregulation of *ALK1* mRNA expression in TAA tissue cells compared to non-TAA. The expression of *ALK1* positively correlated with the levels of miR-126-3p, mir-10a-5p and miR-148a-3p indicating a functional connection between these miRNAs and *TGF-β* signaling. A follow-up IHC analysis revealed no significant changes in *ALK1* protein level in TAA tissues. However, the discrepancy between mRNA and protein assessments could be related to insufficient sensitivity of the immunohistochemistry approach that hamper the quantification of the modest changes at the protein level. Nevertheless, the main advantage of IHC analysis compared to other methods evaluating total levels of gene expression is the feasibility to visualize precisely the protein localization in individual cells of tissue. Thereby, the number of cells strongly expressing *KLF4* factor in the nucleus was shown to be nearly three-fold higher in TAA tissues compared to non-TAA (27% vs. 10%). Meanwhile, myocardin expression level appeared to be similar, although the precise estimation of the nuclear protein is encumbered by rather high myocardin abundance in cytoplasm. Thus, our *in vivo* data indicate that upregulation of *KLF4* does not directly abrogate the myocardin expression but rather regulates VSMC phenotypic transition from more differentiated contractile to synthetic by competing with myocardin-*SRF* (serum responce factor) complex for the contractile gene promoters [52]. Thus, *KLF4* is an important player in aortic aneurysm morphogenesis by regulating VSMC phenotypic switching [53]. We suggest that a marked reduction of miR-133a-3p *in vivo* could be associated with upregulated *KLF4* expression in one third of smooth muscle cells in the TAA tissues (Figure 3C). This supposition is supported by previous *in vitro* studies in rodent cell cultures [25,35] showing that VSMC phenotype switch could be regulated by miR-133a-3p via indirect repression of *KLF4*.

This study has some potential limitations: i) In order to thoroughly examine a homogenous etiological category of aneurysms, we have limited our investigation to the sporadic non-syndromic TAA cases. The samples of patients with severe atherosclerosis (calcified or ulcerating plagues), aortitis or phenotypic characteristics of the known genetic syndromes (Marfan, Ehlers Danlos, and other) were excluded, because these features can lead to skewed results. As a consequence of the abovementioned restrictions the total number of samples used in the analysis was limited. ii) Female sample size was small. A larger cohort of female specimens needs to be examined in the future to reliably corroborate sex-specific variances of miRNA signatures in TAA tissues. iii) We profiled miRNA from TAA and non-TAA samples which differed by age. However, the sequencing data was then validated by qRT-PCR performed on larger TAA and non-TAA groups of comparable age. iv) The control group included heart transplant donors, patients who underwent CABG and healthy volunteers. To diminish the impact of such diversity on the outcome of the study, a strict clinical testing was performed on the control group to confirm the normal measurements of ascending aorta.

5. Conclusions

Taken together, these observations point to a critical role of aberrant miRNAs expression in promoting TAA via imbalanced repression of *TGF-β* signaling pathway components and following deregulation of *KLF4* transcription axis in vivo. The miRNA-mediated gene expression regulatory networks elucidated herein in clinical samples have paved the ways to further in vitro studies of the miRNAs functions in controlling of VSMC phenotype switch. Moreover, co-expression analysis of selected miRNAs, *KLF4* and VSMC markers inside the cells should be performed in the future to extend our understanding of the miRNA-modulated gene activation shift during TAA development.

Author Contributions: Conceptualization, S.G., V.S., G.V.; methodology, S.G., V.S., V.P., D.Z.; software, R.R.; validation, S.G. and V.S.; formal analysis, S.G. and V.S.; investigation, S.G., V.S., V.P., G.Z., Z.K., R.B.; data curation, S.G. and V.S.; writing—original draft preparation, V.S. and G.V; writing—review and editing, V.L.; visualization, V.S. and V.P.; supervision, V.L. and G.V.; project administration, S.G., V.P., V.L. and G.V.; funding acquisition V.L. and G.V.

Acknowledgments: We thank Dovydas Gecys for technical assistance in preparing patients' aorta tissue and blood plasma samples.

References

1. Kuzmik, G.A.; Sang, A.X.; Elefteriades, J.A. Natural history of thoracic aortic aneurysms. *J. Vasc. Surg.* **2012**, *56*, 565–571. [CrossRef] [PubMed]
2. Elefteriades, J.A.; Farkas, E.A. Thoracic Aortic Aneurysm Clinically Pertinent Controversies and Uncertainties. *J. Am. Coll. Cardiol.* **2010**, *55*, 841–857. [CrossRef] [PubMed]
3. Quintana, R.A.; Taylor, W.R. Cellular Mechanisms of Aortic Aneurysm Formation. *Circ. Res.* **2019**, *124*, 607–618. [CrossRef] [PubMed]
4. Olsson, C.; Thelin, S.; Ståhle, E.; Ekbom, A.; Granath, F. Thoracic Aortic Aneurysm and Dissection. *Circulation* **2006**, *114*, 2611–2618. [CrossRef] [PubMed]
5. Von Allmen, R.S.; Anjum, A.; Powell, J.T. Incidence of Descending Aortic Pathology and Evaluation of the Impact of Thoracic Endovascular Aortic Repair: A Population-based Study in England and Wales from 1999 to 2010. *Eur. J. Vasc. Endovasc. Surg.* **2013**, *45*, 154–159. [CrossRef]
6. Cheung, K.; Boodhwani, M.; Chan, K.L.; Beauchesne, L.; Dick, A.; Coutinho, T. Thoracic Aortic Aneurysm Growth: Role of Sex and Aneurysm Etiology. *J. Am. Heart Assoc.* **2017**, *6*, e003792. [CrossRef]
7. Nicolini, F.; Vezzani, A.; Corradi, F.; Gherli, R.; Benassi, F.; Manca, T.; Gherli, T. Gender differences in outcomes after aortic aneurysm surgery should foster further research to improve screening and prevention programmes. *Eur. J. Prev. Cardiol.* **2018**, *25*, 32–41. [CrossRef]
8. Owens, G.K. Regulation of Differentiation of Vascular Smooth-Muscle Cells. *Physiol. Rev.* **1995**, *75*, 487–517. [CrossRef]
9. Owens, G.K.; Kumar, M.S.; Wamhoff, B.R. Molecular regulation of vascular smooth muscle cell differentiation in development and disease. *Physiol. Rev.* **2004**, *84*, 767–801. [CrossRef]
10. Wang, Z.G.; Wang, D.Z.; Pipes, G.C.T.; Olson, E.N. Myocardin is a master regulator of smooth muscle gene expression. *Proc. Natl. Acad. Sci. USA* **2003**, *100*, 7129–7134. [CrossRef]
11. Liu, Y.; Sinha, S.; McDonald, O.G.; Shang, Y.T.; Hoofnagle, M.H.; Owens, G.K. Kruppel-like factor 4 abrogates myocardin-induced activation of smooth muscle gene expression. *J. Biol. Chem.* **2005**, *280*, 9719–9727. [CrossRef] [PubMed]
12. Tang, Y.F.; Yang, X.H.; Friesel, R.E.; Vary, C.P.H.; Liaw, L. Mechanisms of TGF-beta-Induced Differentiation in Human Vascular Smooth Muscle Cells. *J. Vasc. Res.* **2011**, *48*, 485–494. [CrossRef] [PubMed]
13. Chuang, J.C.; Jones, P.A. Epigenetics and microRNAs. *Pediatr. Res.* **2007**, *61*, 24–29. [CrossRef] [PubMed]
14. Small, E.M.; Frost, R.J.A.; Olson, E.N. MicroRNAs Add a New Dimension to Cardiovascular Disease. *Circulation* **2010**, *121*, 1022–1032. [CrossRef]
15. Zhou, S.S.; Jin, J.P.; Wang, J.Q.; Zhang, Z.G.; Freedman, J.H.; Zheng, Y.; Cai, L. miRNAS in cardiovascular diseases: Potential biomarkers, therapeutic targets and challenges. *Acta Pharmacol. Sin.* **2018**, *39*, 1073–1084. [CrossRef] [PubMed]
16. Song, Z.F.; Li, G.H. Role of Specific MicroRNAs in Regulation of Vascular Smooth Muscle Cell Differentiation and the Response to Injury. *J. Cardiovasc. Transl. Res.* **2010**, *3*, 246–250. [CrossRef]

17. Merlet, E.; Atassi, F.; Motiani, R.K.; Mougenot, N.; Jacquet, A.; Nadaud, S.; Capiod, T.; Trebak, M.; Lompre, A.M.; Marchand, A. miR-424/322 regulates vascular smooth muscle cell phenotype and neointimal formation in the rat. *Cardiovasc. Res.* **2013**, *98*, 458–468. [CrossRef]
18. Dong, N.N.; Wang, W.; Tian, J.W.; Xie, Z.L.; Lv, B.; Dai, J.N.; Jiang, R.; Huang, D.; Fang, S.H.; Tian, J.T.; et al. MicroRNA-182 prevents vascular smooth muscle cell dedifferentiation via FGF9/PDGFR signaling. *Int. J. Mol. Med.* **2017**, *39*, 791–798. [CrossRef]
19. Jones, J.A.; Stroud, R.E.; O'Quinn, E.C.; Black, L.E.; Barth, J.L.; Elefteriades, J.A.; Bavaria, J.E.; Gorman, J.H.; Gorman, R.C.; Spinale, F.G.; et al. Selective MicroRNA Suppression in Human Thoracic Aneurysms Relationship of miR-29a to Aortic Size and Proteolytic Induction. *Circ-Cardiovasc. Genet.* **2011**, *4*, 605–613. [CrossRef]
20. Licholai, S.; Blaz, M.; Kapelak, B.; Sanak, M. Unbiased Profile of MicroRNA Expression in Ascending Aortic Aneurysm Tissue Appoints Molecular Pathways Contributing to the Pathology. *Ann. Thorac. Surg.* **2016**, *102*, 1245–1252. [CrossRef]
21. Boileau, A.; Lindsay, M.E.; Michel, J.B.; Devaux, Y. Epigenetics in Ascending Thoracic Aortic Aneurysm and Dissection. *Aorta* **2018**, *6*, 1–12. [CrossRef] [PubMed]
22. Moushi, A.; Michailidou, K.; Soteriou, M.; Cariolou, M.; Bashiardes, E. MicroRNAs as possible biomarkers for screening of aortic aneurysms: A systematic review and validation study. *Biomarkers* **2018**, *23*, 253–264. [CrossRef] [PubMed]
23. Raffort, J.; Lareyre, F.; Clement, M.; Mallat, Z. Micro-RNAs in abdominal aortic aneurysms: Insights from animal models and relevance to human disease. *Cardiovasc. Res.* **2016**, *110*, 165–177. [CrossRef]
24. Butkytė, S.; Čiupas, L.; Jakubauskienė, E.; Vilys, L.; Mocevicius, P.; Kanopka, A.; Vilkaitis, G. Splicing-dependent expression of microRNAs of mirtron origin in human digestive and excretory system cancer cells. *Clin. Epigenet.* **2016**, *8*, 33. [CrossRef] [PubMed]
25. Torella, D.; Iaconetti, C.; Catalucci, D.; Ellison Georgina, M.; Leone, A.; Waring Cheryl, D.; Bochicchio, A.; Vicinanza, C.; Aquila, I.; Curcio, A.; et al. MicroRNA-133 Controls Vascular Smooth Muscle Cell Phenotypic Switch In Vitro and Vascular Remodeling In Vivo. *Circ. Res.* **2011**, *109*, 880–893. [CrossRef] [PubMed]
26. Jonas, S.; Izaurralde, E. Towards a molecular understanding of microRNA-mediated gene silencing. *Nat. Rev. Genet.* **2015**, *16*, 421. [CrossRef] [PubMed]
27. Huusko, T.; Salonurmi, T.; Taskinen, P.; Liinamaa, J.; Juvonen, T.; Paakko, P.; Savolainen, M.; Kakko, S. Elevated messenger RNA expression and plasma protein levels of osteopontin and matrix metalloproteinase types 2 and 9 in patients with ascending aortic aneurysms. *J. Thorac. Cardiovasc. Surg.* **2013**, *145*, 1117–1123. [CrossRef]
28. Lesauskaite, V.; Tanganelli, P.; Sassi, C.; Neri, E.; Diciolla, F.; Ivanoviene, L.; Epistolato, M.C.; Lalinga, A.V.; Alessandrini, C.; Spina, D. Smooth muscle cells of the media in the dilatative pathology of ascending thoracic aorta: Morphology, immunoreactivity for osteopontin, matrix metalloproteinases, and their inhibitors. *Hum. Pathol.* **2001**, *32*, 1003–1011. [CrossRef]
29. Spin, J.M.; Li, D.Y.; Maegdefessel, L.; Tsao, P.S. Non-coding RNAs in aneurysmal aortopathy. *Vascul. Pharmacol.* **2018**, *114*, 110–121. [CrossRef]
30. Li, Y.H.; Maegdefessel, L. Non-coding RNA Contribution to Thoracic and Abdominal Aortic Aneurysm Disease Development and Progression. *Front. Physiol.* **2017**, *8*, 429. [CrossRef]
31. Ruddy, J.M.; Jones, J.A.; Spinale, F.G.; Ikonomidis, J.S. Regional heterogeneity within the aorta: Relevance to aneurysm disease. *J. Thorac. Cardiovasc. Surg.* **2008**, *136*, 1123–1130. [CrossRef] [PubMed]
32. Venkatesh, P.; Phillippi, J.; Chukkapalli, S.; Rivera-Kweh, M.; Velsko, I.; Gleason, T.; VanRyzin, P.; Aalaei-Andabili, S.H.; Ghanta, R.K.; Beaver, T.; et al. Aneurysm-Specific miR-221 and miR-146a Participates in Human Thoracic and Abdominal Aortic Aneurysms. *Int. J. Mol. Sci.* **2017**, *18*, 875. [CrossRef] [PubMed]
33. Zhang, Z.; Liang, K.; Zou, G.; Chen, X.; Shi, S.; Wang, G.; Zhang, K.; Li, K.; Zhai, S. Inhibition of miR-155 attenuates abdominal aortic aneurysm in mice by regulating macrophage-mediated inflammation. *Biosci. Rep.* **2018**, 38. [CrossRef] [PubMed]
34. Welten, S.M.J.; Goossens, E.A.C.; Quax, P.H.A.; Nossent, A.Y. The multifactorial nature of microRNAs in vascular remodelling. *Cardiovasc. Res.* **2016**, *110*, 6–22. [CrossRef] [PubMed]
35. Deaton, R.A.; Gan, Q.; Owens, G.K. Sp1-dependent activation of KLF4 is required for PDGF-BB-induced phenotypic modulation of smooth muscle. *Am. J. Physiol. Heart Circ. Physiol.* **2009**, *296*, H1027–H1037. [CrossRef] [PubMed]

36. Huang, H.R.; Xie, C.Q.; Sun, X.; Ritchie, R.P.; Zhang, J.F.; Chen, Y.E. miR-10a Contributes to Retinoid Acid-induced Smooth Muscle Cell Differentiation. *J. Biol. Chem.* **2010**, *285*, 9383–9389. [CrossRef] [PubMed]
37. Sokolis, D.P.; Iliopoulos, D.C. Impaired mechanics and matrix metalloproteinases/inhibitors expression in female ascending thoracic aortic aneurysms. *J. Mech. Behav. Biomed.* **2014**, *34*, 154–164. [CrossRef]
38. Guay, C.; Regazzi, R. Exosomes as new players in metabolic organ cross-talk. *Diabetes Obes. Metab.* **2017**, *19*, 137–146. [CrossRef] [PubMed]
39. Hu, J.; Xu, Y.; Hao, J.; Wang, S.; Li, C.; Meng, S. MiR-122 in hepatic function and liver diseases. *Protein Cell* **2012**, *3*, 364–371. [CrossRef]
40. Bandiera, S.; Pfeffer, S.; Baumert, T.F.; Zeisel, M.B. miR-122–A key factor and therapeutic target in liver disease. *J. Hepatol.* **2015**, *62*, 448–457. [CrossRef]
41. Olijhoek, J.K.; van der Graaf, Y.; Banga, J.-D.; Algra, A.; Rabelink, T.J.; Visseren, F.L. The Metabolic Syndrome is associated with advanced vascular damage in patients with coronary heart disease, stroke, peripheral arterial disease or abdominal aortic aneurysm. *Eur. Heart J.* **2004**, *25*, 342–348. [CrossRef] [PubMed]
42. D'Alessandra, Y.; Devanna, P.; Limana, F.; Straino, S.; Di Carlo, A.; Brambilla, P.G.; Rubino, M.; Carena, M.C.; Spazzafumo, L.; De Simone, M.; et al. Circulating microRNAs are new and sensitive biomarkers of myocardial infarction. *Eur. Heart J.* **2010**, *31*, 2765–2773. [CrossRef] [PubMed]
43. Devaux, Y.; Salgado-Somoza, A.; Dankiewicz, J.; Boileau, A.; Stammet, P.; Schritz, A.; Zhang, L.; Vausort, M.; Gilje, P.; Erlinge, D.; et al. Incremental Value of Circulating MiR-122-5p to Predict Outcome after Out of Hospital Cardiac Arrest. *Theranostics* **2017**, *7*, 2555–2564. [CrossRef] [PubMed]
44. Martínez-Micaelo, N.; Beltrán-Debón, R.; Baiges, I.; Faiges, M.; Alegret, J.M. Specific circulating microRNA signature of bicuspid aortic valve disease. *J. Transl. Med.* **2017**, *15*, 76. [CrossRef] [PubMed]
45. Kraenkel, N.; Kuschnerus, K.; Briand, S.; Luescher, T.F.; Landmesser, U. miR-483 impairs endothelial homeostasis and response to vascular injury: Upregulation by high-glucose and in patients with type-2 diabetes. *Eur. Heart J.* **2013**, *34*, 762. [CrossRef]
46. Takeda, N.; Hara, H.; Fujiwara, T.; Kanaya, T.; Maemura, S.; Komuro, I. TGF-β Signaling-Related Genes and Thoracic Aortic Aneurysms and Dissections. *Int. J. Mol. Sci.* **2018**, *19*, 2125. [CrossRef]
47. Zhang, P.; Hou, S.Y.; Chen, J.C.; Zhang, J.S.; Lin, F.Y.; Ju, R.J.; Cheng, X.; Ma, X.W.; Song, Y.; Zhang, Y.Y.; et al. Smad4 Deficiency in Smooth Muscle Cells Initiates the Formation of Aortic Aneurysm. *Circ. Res.* **2016**, *118*, 388–399. [CrossRef] [PubMed]
48. Li, W.; Li, Q.L.; Jiao, Y.; Qin, L.F.; Ali, R.; Zhou, J.; Ferruzzi, J.; Kim, R.W.; Geirsson, A.; Dietz, H.C.; et al. Tgfbr2 disruption in postnatal smooth muscle impairs aortic wall homeostasis. *J. Clin. Investig.* **2014**, *124*, 755–767. [CrossRef]
49. Gomez, D.; Coyet, A.; Ollivier, V.; Jeunemaitre, X.; Jondeau, G.; Michel, J.B.; Vranckx, R. Epigenetic control of vascular smooth muscle cells in Marfan and non-Marfan thoracic aortic aneurysms. *Cardiovasc. Res.* **2011**, *89*, 446–456. [CrossRef]
50. Jones, J.A.; Barbour, J.R.; Stroud, R.E.; Bouges, S.; Stephens, S.L.; Spinale, F.G.; Ikonomidis, J.S. Altered Transforming Growth Factor-Beta Signaling in a Murine Model of Thoracic Aortic Aneurysm. *J. Vasc. Res.* **2008**, *45*, 457–468. [CrossRef]
51. Leeper, N.J.; Raiesdana, A.; Kojima, Y.; Chun, H.J.; Azuma, J.; Maegdefessel, L.; Kundu, R.K.; Quertermous, T.; Tsao, P.S.; Spin, J.M. MicroRNA-26a is a novel regulator of vascular smooth muscle cell function. *J. Cell. Physiol.* **2011**, *226*, 1035–1043. [CrossRef] [PubMed]
52. Frismantiene, A.; Philippova, M.; Erne, P.; Resink, T.J. Smooth muscle cell-driven vascular diseases and molecular mechanisms of VSMC plasticity. *Cell. Signal.* **2018**, *52*, 48–64. [CrossRef] [PubMed]
53. Salmon, M.; Johnston, W.F.; Woo, A.; Pope, N.H.; Su, G.; Upchurch, G.R.; Owens, G.K.; Ailawadi, G. KLF4 Regulates Abdominal Aortic Aneurysm Morphology and Deletion Attenuates Aneurysm Formation. *Circulation* **2013**, *128*, S163–S174. [CrossRef] [PubMed]

7

Pregnancy Associated Plasma Protein-A as a Cardiovascular Risk Marker in Patients with Stable Coronary Heart Disease During 10 Years Follow-Up—A CLARICOR Trial Sub-Study

Erik Nilsson [1,2,*], Jens Kastrup [3], Ahmad Sajadieh [4], Gorm Boje Jensen [5], Erik Kjøller [6,11], Hans Jørn Kolmos [7], Jonas Wuopio [8], Christoph Nowak [9], Anders Larsson [10], Janus Christian Jakobsen [11,12], Per Winkel [11], Christian Gluud [11], Kasper K Iversen [6], Johan Ärnlöv [9,13] and Axel C. Carlsson [9]

1 Department of Medical Epidemiology and Biostatistics, Karolinska Institutet, 17177 Stockholm, Sweden
2 School of Medical Sciences, Örebro University, 70182 Örebro, Sweden
3 Department of Cardiology, Rigshospitalet University of Copenhagen, 2100 Copenhagen, Denmark; jens.kastrup@regionh.dk
4 Department of Cardiology, Copenhagen University Hospital of Bispebjerg and Frederiksberg, 2000 Frederiksberg, Denmark; ahmad.sajadieh@regionh.dk
5 Department of Cardiology, Hvidovre Hospital University of Copenhagen, 2650 Hvidovre, Denmark; gorm.boje.jensen.01@regionh.dk
6 Department of Cardiology S, Herlev Hospital University of Copenhagen, 2730 Herlev, Denmark; kjoller@dadlnet.dk (E.K.); kasper.karmark.iversen@regionh.dk (K.K.I.)
7 Department of Clinical Microbiology, Odense University Hospital, 5000 Odense, Denmark; h.j.kolmos@dadlnet.dk
8 Department of Medicine, Mora County Hospital, 79251 Mora, Sweden; jonas.wuopio@ltdalarna.se
9 Division for Family Medicine and Primary Care, Department of Neurobiology, Care Sciences and Society, Karolinska Institutet, 14183 Huddinge, Sweden; christoph.nowak@ki.se (C.N.); axelcefam@hotmail.com (A.C.C.)
10 Department of Medical Sciences, Uppsala University, 75185 Uppsala, Sweden; anders.larsson@akademiska.se
11 Copenhagen Trial Unit, Centre for Clinical Intervention Research, Rigshospitalet, Copenhagen University Hospital, 2100 Copenhagen, Denmark; janus.jakobsen@ctu.dk (J.C.J.); per.winkel@ctu.dk (P.W.); christian.gluud@ctu.dk (C.G.)
12 Department of Cardiology, Holbæk Hospital, 4300 Holbæk, Denmark
13 School of Health and Social Studies, Dalarna University, 79131 Falun, Sweden; johan.arnlov@ki.se
* Correspondence: erik.alfred.nilsson@gmail.com

Abstract: Elevated pregnancy-associated plasma protein A (PAPP-A) is associated with mortality in acute coronary syndromes. Few studies have assessed PAPP-A in stable coronary artery disease (CAD) and results are conflicting. We assessed the 10-year prognostic relevance of PAPP-A levels in stable CAD. The CLARICOR trial was a randomized controlled clinical trial including outpatients with stable CAD, randomized to clarithromycin versus placebo. The placebo group constituted our discovery cohort (n = 1.996) and the clarithromycin group the replication cohort (n = 1.975). The composite primary outcome was first occurrence of cardiovascular event or death. In the discovery cohort, incidence rates (IR) for the composite outcome were higher in those with elevated PAPP-A (IR 12.72, 95% Confidence Interval (CI) 11.0–14.7 events/100 years) compared to lower PAPP-A (IR 8.78, 8.25–9.34), with comparable results in the replication cohort. Elevated PAPP-A was associated with increased risk of the composite outcome in both cohorts (discovery Hazard Ratio (HR) 1.45, 95% CI 1.24–1.70; replication HR 1.29, 95% CI 1.10–1.52). In models adjusted for established risk factors, these trends were attenuated. Elevated PAPP-A was associated with higher all-cause mortality in both cohorts. We conclude that elevated PAPP-A levels are associated with increased long-term mortality in stable CAD, but do not improve long-term prediction of death or cardiovascular events when added to established predictors.

Keywords: pregnancy-associated plasma protein-A; coronary artery disease; cohort studies; biomarkers

---

1. Introduction

Pregnancy-associated plasma protein-A (PAPP-A) is a cell membrane-bound metalloproteinase which regulates local availability of insulin-like growth factor 1 (IGF-1) [1]. It has been evaluated as a prognostic biomarker in acute coronary syndromes [2–11], where elevated levels are associated with increased risk of death. However, this association may be confounded by heparin treatment causing elevated PAPP-A levels in vivo through release of PAPP-A attached to cell membranes [12]. Further, PAPP-A levels predict cardiovascular events in troponin-negative patients with suspected acute coronary syndrome [3] and higher levels of circulating PAPP-A are associated with more extensive coronary artery disease [13] as well as with plaque inflammation and echogenicity [14]. In chronic stable angina pectoris PAPP-A has been less extensively studied and is associated with outcomes in some studies [15–18] but not all [19]. Studies with long-term follow-up are scarce.

PAPP-A regulates downstream growth hormone effects in the paracellular environment by cleaving insulin-like growth factor binding protein 4 (IGFBP4) bound to insulin-like growth factor 1 (IGF-1), thereby making IGF-1 available to its receptor. Since PAPP-A is normally bound to the cell membrane and not abundantly expressed, increased plasma levels in the absence of heparin treatment may represent up-regulation due to inflammation or tissue damage, in combination with escape into the circulation [20–22].

The present study is part of the larger PREdictors for MAjor Cardiovascular outcomes in stable ischemic heart disease (PREMAC) study, which aimed to identify biochemical predictors of cardiovascular events and all-cause mortality in persons with stable coronary artery disease (CAD) utilizing data originating from the CLARICOR (clarithromycin for patients with stable coronary heart disease) trial [23]. In the CLARICOR Trial, patients were randomized to clarithromycin or placebo and the main outcomes consisted of myocardial infarction (AMI), unstable angina pectoris (UAP), cardiovascular mortality, and all-cause mortality. In a previous report on the same cohort, elevated PAPP-A, defined as values ≥ 4 μ/mL, was found to predict risk of death and myocardial infarction during medium term (median 2.8 years) follow up [17]. The aim of the present study was to assess the predictive power of elevated PAPP-A levels for the 10-year outcomes in stable CAD.

2. Experimental Section

The PREMAC study focused on the presence of predictors of cardiovascular events and all-cause mortality in persons with stable CAD and included a detailed statistical analysis plan [23]. Biomarker assessment was performed using stored biobank samples from the CLARICOR trial [24] and outcome data was retrieved from public registers. The CLARICOR trial was approved by local ethics committees and regulatory authorities (Regional Ethics Committee HB 2009/015 and KF 01-076/99; the Danish Data Protection Agency 1999–1200–174 and 2012–41–0757; and the Danish Medicines Agency 2612–975).

2.1. Patient Selection

The CLARICOR trial was a randomized, placebo-controlled trial with blinded outcome assessment including outpatients with stable CAD. All patients discharged from wards or outpatient clinics in the Copenhagen area in Denmark with a diagnosis of acute myocardial infarction or unstable angina pectoris during the years 1993–1999 who were alive and aged 18–85 years old in 1999 (n = 13.702) were invited to a screening interview at one of five cardiology centers. Of the 6116 (44.6%) patients accepting the invitation, 1567 (25.6%) were excluded, 177 (2.9%) chose not to participate, and the remaining 4372 (71.5%) were randomized to oral clarithromycin 500 mg once daily for 2 weeks (n = 2.172) vs. placebo (n = 2.200) during the winter 1999–2000. Exclusion criteria of the CLARICOR trial were: AMI or UAP within the previous 3 months, percutaneous transluminal coronary angioplasty and coronary bypass surgery within the previous 6 months, impaired renal or hepatic function, congestive heart failure (New York Heart Association (NYHA) IV classification of heart failure), active malignancy, incapacity to manage own affairs, breast feeding, and possible pregnancy. In the CLARICOR trial, clarithromycin was found to increase both the risk of cardiovascular and all-cause mortality [24–27].

The patients randomized to placebo in the CLARICOR study were included as the discovery cohort in the present study, while those randomized to clarithromycin formed the replication cohort. We excluded participants with missing data in any of the variables, leaving n = 1.996 (92%) in the discovery cohort, and n = 1.975 (90%) in the replication cohort.

2.2. Baseline Data

During enrollment interviews, smoking status, current medication, and known hypertension or diabetes were noted. Information concerning sex, age, and history of myocardial infarction or unstable angina pectoris were extracted from local hospital files. Blood samples were collected at each of the study sites immediately before randomization, using blood collection tubes without additives. Serum was prepared according to normal hospital routine with approximately coagulation for 30 min and centrifugation at 1500 g for 10 min. Serum was frozen on the day of collection at −20 °C and at −80 °C after transportation to the central laboratory facility. Storage problems were the only noteworthy cause of missing data. Estimated glomerular filtration rate (eGFR) was calculated using the creatinine-based Chronic Kidney Disease Epidemiology Collaboration (CKD-EPI) formula [28]. Smoking status was categorized as never, former, or current smoker. No physical investigations were made at randomization interview; nor were any longitudinal predictor information collected during follow-up.

2.3. Pregnancy-Associated Plasma Protein A Levels

The PAPP-A levels measured in a previous study were used in the present study [17]. The enzyme-linked immunosorbent assay used for quantification of PAPP-A has been described in detail previously [17,29]. The detection limit was 4 mIU/L. The intra-assay coefficient of variation was 2.0% at 71.7 mIU/L and 5.7% at 10.4 mIU/L, with corresponding inter-assay coefficients of variation of 6.4% and 8.7%, respectively. Elevated serum PAPP-A was defined as values at or above 4 mIU/L, based on levels in healthy blood donors [29]. Note that although the CLARICOR trial data did not include information on heparin use, study participants were outpatients with stable CAD and heparin is not used in this setting.

2.4. Outcomes

Follow-up was until 31 December 2009 where the official permissions expired. Outcome data was procured from national patient registries. These are mandatory for inpatient care and all events diagnosed and coded during hospital admission are therefore detected, resulting in virtually no loss to follow-up. Vital status was retrieved from the Danish Central Civil Register, cause of death from the National Register of Causes of Death, and hospital admissions from the Danish National Patient Register (NPR), which covers all hospital admissions. These registries have almost complete coverage [30]. By trial protocol, events during the first 2.6 years of follow-up were adjudicated by a blinded committee, previously described in detail [23,24]. For the 10-year studies, registry outcomes were used after verifying that the results were consistent with those based on adjudication data [30,31].

The Danish 10-digit central person registration (CPR) number is used at all contacts with the health care system. At discharge from hospital, at least one action diagnosis (A diagnosis) specifying the main reason for the admission is noted in the NPR. These A diagnoses, and in case of death the 'underlying cause of death' code (in the official terminology of the National Register of Causes of Death), was used for classifying outcomes according to the 10th revision of the International Statistical Classification of Diseases and Related Health Problems (ICD-10) coding system as follows: AMI (I21.0–23.9), UAP (I20.0 and I24.8–24.9), cerebrovascular disease (CeVD) (I60.0–64.9 and G45.0–46.8), cardiovascular death (I00.0–99.9 unless already covered), and death due to non-cardiovascular disease (A00.0–T98.3 unless already covered). A composite outcome was defined as AMI, UAP, CeVD, or death due to any cause. Follow-up time was censored at occurrence of an outcome, death, or end of follow-up (31st December 2009 giving a median possible survival time of 10 years ± 3 months after randomization).

2.5. Statistical Analysis

Incidence rates (IR) were calculated using only the first occurrence of an event and the time to event or censoring at end of study was used in the denominator. We used Cox proportional hazards model for the statistical analysis. Multivariable models were adjusted according to the pre-specified analysis plan, for clinical predictors (sex, age at randomization, smoking history, history of myocardial infarction, hypertension, and diabetes), medical treatment (acetylsalicylic acid, beta-blocker, calcium-antagonist, angiotensin-converting enzyme (ACE)-inhibitor, long lasting nitrate, diuretic, digoxin, statin, and anti-arrhythmic drugs), and standard biochemical predictors (log-transformed high-sensitivity-reactive protein (CRP), glomerular filtration rate (GFR) estimated by creatinine, triglycerides, total cholesterol, high-density lipoprotein (HDL) cholesterol, low-density lipoprotein (LDL) cholesterol, apolipoprotein A1, and apolipoprotein B). Standard predictors adjusted for in multivariable models are listed in Appendix A. Triglycerides and total cholesterol were log transformed.

As the proportional hazard's assumption was violated for age at entry for all-cause death and the composite outcome (Bonferroni adjusted $p < 0.0044$ for all-cause mortality; and $p < 0.00056$ for the composite outcome), we excluded age from all models for these two outcomes. In order to provide additional insights into the potential influence of age on these associations, we conducted multivariable logistic regression models (including age as a co-variate since the proportional hazard assumption is not a requisite for these analyses).

3. Results

Baseline characteristics of the discovery and replication cohorts are presented in Table 1 They showed no major differences between the cohorts. The proportion of participants with elevated PAPP-A levels was 13% (n = 263) in the discovery cohort and 12% (n = 244) in the replication cohort.

Table 2 displays outcomes by PAPP-A level. In the discovery cohort, the composite outcome was more common among those who elevated PAPP-A, compared to those with low PAPP-A levels (72% compared to 59%), with a corresponding difference in incidence rates ($p < 0.0001$). The same pattern was seen in the replication cohort.

Table 1. Baseline characteristics of the two study cohorts.

Variable	Discovery Cohort	Replication Cohort
Number of participants	1996	1975
PAPP-A ≥ 4 mIU/L	263 (13)	244 (12)
Female	623 (31)	602 (30)
Age at entry, years	65 ± 10	65 ± 10
CRP, mg/L	5.25 ± 7.7	5.76 ± 9.3
Apolipoprotein A1, mg/dL	1.70 ± 0.34	1.70 ± 0.36
Apolipoprotein, mg/dL	1.21 ± 0.32	1.21 ± 0.33
eGFR, mL/min	76.3 ± 20	76.5 ± 19
Diabetes mellitus	299 (15)	301 (15)
Hypertension	805 (40)	790 (40)
Never smoked	394 (20)	339 (17)
Former smoker	925 (46)	903 (46)
Current smoker	677 (34)	735 (37)
History of myocardial infarction	635 (32)	640 (32)
Statin treatment	822 (41)	812 (41)
Aspirin treatment	1763 (88)	1733 (88)
Beta blocker treatment	619 (31)	589 (30)
Calcium antagonist treatment	702 (35)	680 (34)
ACE inhibitor treatment	522 (26)	552 (28)
Long-acting nitrate treatment	412 (21)	411 (21)
Diuretics treatment	690 (35)	698 (35)
Digoxin treatment	115 (6)	138 (7)
Antiarrhythmic treatment	42 (2)	46 (2)

Baseline characteristics in the discovery (placebo) and replication (clarithromycin) cohorts, presented as mean ± standard deviation for continuous variables and *n* (%) for categorical variables. Abbreviations: PAPP-A: pregnancy-associated plasma protein A; CRP: high sensitivity C-reactive protein; eGFR: estimated glomerular filtration rate; ACE: angiotensin converting enzyme.

Table 2. Incidence rates of the composite outcome by PAPP-A level.

PAPP-A Category	Variable	Discovery Cohort	Replication Cohort
PAPP-A ≥ 4 mIU/L	*N*	263	244
	Outcomes, *N* (%)	189 (72)	168 (69)
	IR, per 100 years	12.72	12.04
	95% CI	11.0–14.7	10.35–14.01
PAPP-A < 4 mIU/L	*N*	1733	1731
	Outcomes, *N* (%)	1015 (59)	1052 (61)
	IR per 100 years	8.78	9.38
	95% CI	8.25–9.34	8.83–9.96

The composite outcome was defined as acute myocardial infarction, unstable angina pectoris, cerebrovascular disease, or death due to any cause. Outcomes (with % of participants at risk) is the number of persons experiencing the composite outcome during 10-years follow-up. Incidence rates (IR) were calculated using only the first occurrence of the outcome during follow-up. Abbreviations: PAPP-A: pregnancy-associated plasma protein A; CI, Confidence Interval.

In the survival analysis (Table 3), Cox proportional hazards models adjusted for sex (model A) showed that PAPP-A ≥ 4 μ/mL was associated with an increased risk of the composite outcome in the discovery cohort and, less markedly, in the replication cohort; with adjustment for a large number of other risk factors (model B, see Table 3), comprising comorbidities and biochemical markers, these risk trends were attenuated in the discovery cohort and disappeared in the replication cohort.

Table 3. Risk of composite outcome associated with the binary covariate elevated PAPP-A.

Variable	Discovery Cohort		Replication Cohort	
	Model A	**Model B**	**Model A**	**Model B**
Hazard ratio	1.45	1.29	1.28	1.06
95% CI	1.24–1.70	1.10–1.52	1.08–1.50	0.89–1.25
p-value	< 0.001	< 0.001	0.003	0.51

Cox proportional hazards models are applied to the composite outcome defined as acute myocardial infarction, unstable angina pectoris, cerebrovascular disease, or death due to any cause. Model A was adjusted for sex. Model B was adjusted for established risk factors and co-morbidities, standard biochemical predictors, and treatments as listed in Appendix A. All models in this table are shown without adjustments for age at entry. Abbreviations: PAPP-A, pregnancy-associated plasma protein A.

Comparable results, with elevated PAPP-A being associated with increased risk of the composite outcome in the discovery cohort, but not in the replication cohort, were found in adjusted logistic regression models (Table S1) where age was also included in the multivariable model. We found no interaction between sex and PAPP-A on mortality ($p = 0.22$) or on the composite outcome ($p = 0.17$).

The association between PAPP-A ≥ 4 mIU/L and other outcomes is shown in Table S2. Elevated PAPP-A was associated with higher all-cause mortality in the discovery cohort, an association that remained in the fully adjusted analysis as well as in a logistic regression that included age as a predictor variable (Table S1). These findings were reproduced in the replication cohort.

Interestingly, these secondary analyses suggest that PAPP-A elevation is at least as strong a predictor for non-cardiovascular as for cardiovascular death (Table S2).

We also evaluated the predictive utility of PAPP-A in the group of placebo-treated patients when added to a large number of standard predictors (Table S3). Adding elevated PAPP-A as a predictor produced no visible improvements (apart from a slight numerical instability).

4. Discussion

Our main finding is that PAPP-A levels ≥ 4 mIU/L are associated with increased long-term risk of composite adverse outcome as well as all-cause mortality in patients with stable CAD. Although the association to all-cause mortality remained after extensive multivariable adjustment, the association to the composite outcome was not reproduced in our replication cohort when adjusted for many other risk factors. This may indicate that the placebo group and the clarithromycin treated group (the replication group) are not completely compatible in that clarithromycin was found to increase mortality [24–27]. It may also indicate that the association between PAPP-A and outcomes is confounded by some of these other risk factors, for example diabetes [20,32]. Over-adjustment may also be a problem in this context [33]. Our choice of covariates in the various multivariate analyses was mandated by the choice made for the Cox analyses of the placebo-treated patients described in the pre-specified analysis plan.

The growth hormone (GH) axis and PAPP-A has been implicated in the progression of atherosclerosis. Locally, insulin-like growth factor 1 (IGF-1) promotes multiple mechanisms involved in plaque formation and an association between PAPP-A and atherosclerosis has been demonstrated [2,34]. PAPP-A is found in atherosclerotic plaques on cell-types involved in the atherosclerotic process, including vascular smooth muscle cells, endothelial cells and macrophages [1], its expression is elevated in vulnerable plaques [2]. PAPP-A activity is related to atherosclerotic lesion size in rodents [35,36] and higher levels of circulating PAPP-A are associated with more extensive coronary artery disease in humans [13].

Reduced PAPP-A activity is associated with diminished vascular cell proliferation in response to injury, reduced plaque area and less luminal occlusion in atherosclerosis [37]. Conversely, increased PAPP-A activity is associated with proliferation of vascular smooth muscle cells [34]. Regulation of vascular smooth muscle cell proliferation could therefore be a mechanism by which PAPP-A influences the atherosclerotic process. PAPP-A could also be linked to atherosclerosis through modulating the effects of IGF-1 on lipid-, glucose-, and protein metabolism [38,39].

However, the exact mechanism by which PAPP-A is involved (causally or as a by-product) in the promotion of atherosclerosis remains elusive, in part as a result of conflicting findings on the effects of IGF-1 action on the vasculature [40]. Notably, the relationship between serum levels of IGF-1 and PAPP-A and local IGF-1 activity is unclear and may for example be dependent on body composition, inflammation, or conditions such as diabetes mellitus or obesity [40]. Circulating levels are therefore not necessarily directly related to the hypothesized pathophysiological mechanisms by which IGF-1 and PAPP-A are implicated in development of coronary artery disease. Consequently, the association between PAPP-A and mortality described in the present study may be related to other factors than cardiovascular disease progression. Indeed, we did not find any clear association with cardiovascular outcomes and it should be noted that the IGF-1 system including PAPP-A may for example be related to development of cancer [41]. There was in our results consistently no association between elevated PAPP-A and myocardial infarction, UAP, or stroke, although there was an association to cardiovascular mortality in the minimally adjusted analysis in the replication cohort.

The association between PAPP-A levels and outcomes in stable CAD has been studied previously. In 103 stable CAD patients, with a median follow-up of 4.9 years, higher PAPP-A was associated with increased mortality as well as the composite outcome of death and acute coronary syndrome [15]. Interestingly, but potentially problematic [33], those authors adjusted their estimates for the extent of coronary atherosclerosis, which could be considered an intermediate in the hypothesized causal pathway between PAPP-A and cardiovascular events. In another cohort study, including 534 patients with stable CAD and 393 patients with acute coronary syndrome, with a median follow-up time of 5.0 years, the authors found no association to cardiovascular mortality in the subgroup stable CAD, but higher PAPP-A was associated with increased cardiovascular mortality in the overall cohort as well as in the acute coronary syndrome (ACS) subgroup [19]. Although these results were adjusted for several conventional predictors, there was no adjustment for age. In a previous study on the CLARICOR cohort participants, PAPP-A levels were studied in relation to medium-term outcomes [17]. Important differences in that study from the present study include a shorter follow-up (median 2.8 years), joining of the placebo and the treatment group in a single cohort, and differing definitions of the composite outcome. In line with our present results, the previous study found that elevated PAPP-A was associated with the composite outcome of myocardial infarction and death as well as all-cause mortality in adjusted analyses [17].

PAPP-A has also been studied in ACS, but there is limited generalizability from these studies to the context of stable CAD. In troponin-negative patients with suspected ACS, PAPP-A predicted future cardiovascular events [3], although we are uncertain if PAPP-A was sampled before administration of heparin. Others found that PAPP-A predicted cardiovascular events in ACS and it seems that PAPP-A was sampled after heparin infusion, indicating that the PAPP-A levels included PAPP-A released from the cell membrane during heparin treatment [6]. In that study, PAPP-A predicted outcomes in TnT-negative patients. Furthermore, differences in stable versus acute CAD may have support in PAPP-A physiology since chronic and transient PAPP-A expression may have differing effects on neointimal formation following vascular injury [42].

Our present study has several strengths: a large study sample, detailed characterization of the participants, longitudinal study design, 10 years follow-up, and a replication of all analyses in the clarithromycin group of the trial. As far as we know, there are no other large cohort studies on associations between PAPP-A levels in patients with stable CAD. National Danish registers are known to be of high completeness and accuracy [30], but a small number of non-fatal events can be missed when participants are hospitalized abroad. Results in our study are likely valid for patients with stable CAD as ascertained at the baseline interview and it remains to be shown if similar risks are seen for other relevant patient groups, such as patients with acute symptoms or patients during recovery from a major event.

Limitations are the unknown generalizability to other ethnic groups and to those unlikely to volunteer to participate in studies. Distortion by the active intervention with clarithromycin cannot be excluded, although we saw similar associations as to those in the placebo cohort. As regards the replication cohort, with its previously described surplus of unfavorable cardiovascular outcomes [26,27,43], we noted that elevated PAPP-A here tended to lose its unfavorable implications. Such interaction, if present, would imply that the harmful effect of clarithromycin was more marked in those with low PAPP-A levels. However, the trend nowhere came close to statistical significance. Nor do we have any theoretical arguments in favor thereof. Another limitation is that there was no data on heparin treatment at baseline. However, as the participants in our study had no indication for heparin, it is unlikely that this lack of data would have any substantial influence on our results and conclusions. In addition, there was no data on left ventricular ejection fraction, although this may be partially or completely compensated by other covariables included in the analyses, as age, sex, hypertension, prior acute myocardial infarction, creatinine, diuretics, and digoxin are related to left ventricular ejection fraction [44].

5. Conclusions

Elevated PAPP-A levels are associated with increased long-term mortality in stable CAD, but they do not improve long-term prediction of composite outcome of death or cardiovascular events when added to established predictors.

Author Contributions: Conceptualization, C.G. and A.S.; methodology, C.G., J.C.J., C.N., A.L., E.N., J.Ä., J.K., P.W., E.K., and J.W.; validation, C.G.; formal analysis, E.N., A.C.C., and P.W.; investigation, C.G., J.K., G.B.J., and K.K.I.; resources, C.G.; data curation, C.G. and P.W.; supervision, C.G., J.C.J. and J.Ä.; project administration, C.G. and G.B.J.; funding acquisition, C.G. and K.K.I.; software, P.W.; visualization, not applicable; writing—original draft preparation, E.N., A.C.C., and J.Ä.; writing—review and editing, All authors. All authors have read and agreed to the published version of the manuscript.

Acknowledgments: We thank the CLARICOR trial participants. We thank the investigators and other staff involved in the first phases of the CLARICOR trial: Bodil Als-Nielsen, Morten Damgaard, Jørgen Fischer Hansen, Stig Hansen, Olav H. Helø, Per Hildebrandt, Jørgen Hilden, Inga Lind, Henrik Nielsen, Lars Petersen, Christian M. Jespersen, Maria Skoog, and Jane Lindschou.

Appendix A

Predictors Adjusted for in Multivariable Models

Predictors were pre-specified in the study protocol. Standard predictors adjusted for in multivariable models are listed below. Note that age at entry was omitted from Cox regression analyses due to violation of proportional hazard assumption when all-cause mortality and the composite outcome was analyzed.

Clinical predictors were: sex, age at entry, smoking history, history of myocardial infarction as opposed to angina only, hypertension, and diabetes.

Standard biochemical predictors were: Log-transformed high-sensitivity C-reactive protein (CRP), estimated glomerular filtration rate (eGFR) estimated by creatinine, triglycerides and lipoproteins (total cholesterol, high density lipoprotein (HDL) cholesterol, low density lipoprotein (LDL) cholesterol, apolipoprotein A1, and apolipoprotein B).

The current medical treatment was included as proxy predictors because information about post infarction heart failure and post-infarction angina pectoris are not available to us: Aspirin (Yes/No), beta-blocker (Yes/No), calcium antagonist (Yes/No), ACE inhibitor (Yes/No), long lasting nitrate (Yes/No), diuretic (Yes/No), digoxin (Yes/No), statin (Yes/No), and anti-arrhythmic drugs (Yes/No).

References

1. Steffensen, L.B.; Conover, C.A.; Oxvig, C. PAPP-A and the IGF system in atherosclerosis: what's up, what's down? *Am. J. Physiol. Heart Circ. Physiol.* **2019**, *317*, H1039–H1049. [CrossRef]
2. Bayes-Genis, A.; Conover, C.A.; Overgaard, M.T.; Bailey, K.R.; Christiansen, M.; Holmes, D.R.J.; Virmani, R.; Oxvig, C.; Schwartz, R.S. Pregnancy-associated plasma protein A as a marker of acute coronary syndromes. *N. Engl. J. Med.* **2001**, *345*, 1022–1029. [CrossRef]
3. Lund, J.; Qin, Q.-P.; Ilva, T.; Pettersson, K.; Voipio-Pulkki, L.-M.; Porela, P.; Pulkki, K. Circulating pregnancy-associated plasma protein a predicts outcome in patients with acute coronary syndrome but no troponin i elevation. *Circulation* **2003**, *108*, 1924–1926. [CrossRef]
4. Qin, Q.-P.; Kokkala, S.; Lund, J.; Tamm, N.; Voipio-Pulkki, L.-M.; Pettersson, K. Molecular distinction of circulating pregnancy-associated plasma protein a in myocardial infarction and pregnancy. *Clin. Chem.* **2005**, *51*, 75–83. [CrossRef] [PubMed]
5. Heeschen, C.; Dimmeler, S.; Hamm, C.W.; Fichtlscherer, S.; Simoons, M.L.; Zeiher, A.M. Pregnancy-associated plasma protein-a levels in patients with acute coronary syndromes: Comparison with markers of systemic inflammation, platelet activation, and myocardial necrosis. *J. Am. Coll. Cardiol.* **2005**, *45*, 229–237. [CrossRef]
6. Armstrong, E.J.; Morrow, D.A.; Sabatine, M.S. Inflammatory biomarkers in acute coronary syndromes: Part IV: Matrix metalloproteinases and biomarkers of platelet activation. *Circulation* **2006**, *113*, e382–e385. [CrossRef]
7. Body, R.; Ferguson, C. Towards evidence-based emergency medicine: Best bets from the manchester royal infirmary. Pregnancy-associated plasma protein A: A novel cardiac marker with promise. *Emerg. Med. J.* **2006**, *23*, 875–877. [CrossRef] [PubMed]
8. Lund, J.; Qin, Q.-P.; Ilva, T.; Nikus, K.; Eskola, M.; Porela, P.; Kokkala, S.; Pulkki, K.; Pettersson, K.; Voipio-Pulkki, L.-M. Pregnancy-associated plasma protein A: A biomarker in acute ST-elevation myocardial infarction (STEMI). *Ann. Med.* **2006**, *38*, 221–228. [CrossRef]
9. Bonaca, M.P.; Scirica, B.M.; Sabatine, M.S.; Jarolim, P.; Murphy, S.A.; Chamberlin, J.S.; Rhodes, D.W.; Southwick, P.C.; Braunwald, E.; Morrow, D.A. Prospective evaluation of pregnancy-associated plasma protein-a and outcomes in patients with acute coronary syndromes. *J. Am. Coll. Cardiol.* **2012**, *60*, 332–338. [CrossRef]
10. Parveen, N.; Subhakumari, K.N.; Krishnan, S. Pregnancy associated plasma protein-a (PAPP-A) levels in acute coronary syndrome: A case control study in a tertiary care centre. *Indian J. Clin. Biochem.* **2015**, *30*, 150–154. [CrossRef]
11. Daidoji, H.; Takahashi, H.; Otaki, Y.; Tamura, H.; Arimoto, T.; Shishido, T.; Miyashita, T.; Miyamoto, T.; Watanabe, T.; Kubota, I. A combination of plaque components analyzed by integrated backscatter intravascular ultrasound and serum pregnancy-associated plasma protein a levels predict the no-reflow phenomenon during percutaneous coronary intervention. *Catheter. Cardiovasc. Interv.* **2015**, *85*, 43–50. [CrossRef] [PubMed]
12. Iversen, K.; Teisner, A.; Dalager, S.; Olsen, K.E.; Floridon, C.; Teisner, B. Pregnancy associated plasma protein-a (PAPP-A) is not a marker of the vulnerable atherosclerotic plaque. *Clin. Biochem.* **2011**, *44*, 312–318. [CrossRef] [PubMed]
13. Cosin-Sales, J.; Kaski, J.C.; Christiansen, M.; Kaminski, P.; Oxvig, C.; Overgaard, M.T.; Cole, D.; Holt, D.W. Relationship among pregnancy associated plasma protein-a levels, clinical characteristics, and coronary artery disease extent in patients with chronic stable angina pectoris. *Eur. Heart J.* **2005**, *26*, 2093–2098. [CrossRef] [PubMed]
14. Consuegra-Sanchez, L.; Fredericks, S.; Kaski, J.C. Pregnancy-associated plasma protein-a (PAPP-A) and cardiovascular risk. *Atherosclerosis* **2009**, *203*, 346–352. [CrossRef] [PubMed]
15. Elesber, A.A.; Conover, C.A.; Denktas, A.E.; Lennon, R.J.; Holmes, D.R.J.; Overgaard, M.T.; Christiansen, M.; Oxvig, C.; Lerman, L.O.; Lerman, A. Prognostic value of circulating pregnancy-associated plasma protein levels in patients with chronic stable angina. *Eur. Heart J.* **2006**, *27*, 1678–1684. [CrossRef] [PubMed]
16. Consuegra-Sanchez, L.; Petrovic, I.; Cosin-Sales, J.; Holt, D.W.; Christiansen, M.; Kaski, J.C. Prognostic value of circulating pregnancy-associated plasma protein-a (PAPP-A) and proform of eosinophil major basic protein (pro-MBP) levels in patients with chronic stable angina pectoris. *Clin. Chim. Acta* **2008**, *391*, 18–23. [CrossRef]

17. Iversen, K.K.; Teisner, B.; Winkel, P.; Gluud, C.; Kjøller, E.; Kolmos, H.J.; Hildebrandt, P.R.; Hilden, J.; Kastrup, J. Pregnancy associated plasma protein-a as a marker for myocardial infarction and death in patients with stable coronary artery disease: A prognostic study within the claricor trial. *Atherosclerosis* **2011**, *214*, 203–208. [CrossRef]
18. Schulz, O.; Reinicke, M.; Kramer, J.; Berghofer, G.; Bensch, R.; Schimke, I.; Jaffe, A. Pregnancy-associated plasma protein A values in patients with stable cardiovascular disease: Use of a new monoclonal antibody-based assay. *Clin. Chim. Acta* **2011**, *412*, 880–886. [CrossRef]
19. Zengin, E.; Sinning, C.; Zeller, T.; Rupprecht, H.-J.; Schnabel, R.B.; Lackner, K.-J.; Blankenberg, S.; Westermann, D.; Bickel, C. The utility of pregnancy-associated plasma protein A for determination of prognosis in a cohort of patients with coronary artery disease. *Biomark. Med.* **2015**, *9*, 731–741. [CrossRef]
20. Oxvig, C. The role of PAPP-A in the IGF system: Location, location, location. *J. Cell Commun. Signal.* **2015**, *9*, 177–187. [CrossRef]
21. Bayes-Genis, A.; Schwartz, R.S.; Lewis, D.A.; Overgaard, M.T.; Christiansen, M.; Oxvig, C.; Ashai, K.; Holmes, D.R.J.; Conover, C.A. Insulin-like growth factor binding protein-4 protease produced by smooth muscle cells increases in the coronary artery after angioplasty. *Arterioscler. Thromb. Vasc. Biol.* **2001**, *21*, 335–341. [CrossRef] [PubMed]
22. Conover, C.A. Key questions and answers about pregnancy-associated plasma protein-A. *Trends Endocrinol. Metab.* **2012**, *23*, 242–249. [CrossRef] [PubMed]
23. Winkel, P.; Jakobsen, J.C.; Hilden, J.; Lange, T.; Jensen, G.B.; Kjøller, E.; Sajadieh, A.; Kastrup, J.; Kolmos, H.J.; Larsson, A.; et al. Predictors for major cardiovascular outcomes in stable ischaemic heart disease (Premac): Statistical analysis plan for data originating from the Claricor (clarithromycin for patients with stable coronary heart disease) trial. *Diagn. Progn. Res.* **2017**, *1*, 10. [CrossRef] [PubMed]
24. Jespersen, C.M.; Als-Nielsen, B.; Damgaard, M.; Hansen, J.F.; Hansen, S.; Helø, O.H.; Hildebrandt, P.; Hilden, J.; Jensen, G.B.; Kastrup, J.; et al. Randomised placebo controlled multicentre trial to assess short term clarithromycin for patients with stable coronary heart disease: Claricor trial. *BMJ* **2006**, *332*, 22–27. [CrossRef]
25. Gluud, C.; Als-Nielsen, B.; Damgaard, M.; Fischer Hansen, J.; Hansen, S.; Helø, O.H.; Hildebrandt, P.; Hilden, J.; Jensen, G.B.; Kastrup, J.; et al. Clarithromycin for 2 weeks for stable coronary heart disease: 6-year follow-up of the CLARICOR randomized trial and updated meta-analysis of antibiotics for coronary heart disease. *Cardiology* **2008**, *111*, 280–287. [CrossRef]
26. Winkel, P.; Hilden, J.; Fischer Hansen, J.; Hildebrandt, P.; Kastrup, J.; Kolmos, H.J.; Kjøller, E.; Jespersen, C.M.; Gluud, C.; Jensen, G.B.; et al. Excess sudden cardiac deaths after short-term clarithromycin administration in the CLARICOR trial: Why is this so, and why are statins protective? *Cardiology* **2011**, *118*, 63–67. [CrossRef]
27. Winkel, P.; Hilden, J.; Hansen, J.F.; Kastrup, J.; Kolmos, H.J.; Kjøller, E.; Jensen, G.B.; Skoog, M.; Lindschou, J.; Gluud, C.; et al. Clarithromycin for stable coronary heart disease increases all-cause and cardiovascular mortality and cerebrovascular morbidity over 10years in the CLARICOR randomised, blinded clinical trial. *Int. J. Cardiol.* **2015**, *182*, 459–465. [CrossRef]
28. Levey, A.S.; Stevens, L.A.; Schmid, C.H.; Zhang, Y.L.; Castro, A.F.; Feldman, H.I.; Kusek, J.W.; Eggers, P.; Van Lente, F.; Greene, T.; et al. A new equation to estimate glomerular filtration rate. *Ann. Intern. Med.* **2009**, *150*, 604–612. [CrossRef]
29. Rossen, M.; Iversen, K.; Teisner, A.; Teisner, B.; Kliem, A.; Grudzinskas, G. Optimisation of sandwich ELISA based on monoclonal antibodies for the specific measurement of pregnancy-associated plasma protein (PAPP-A) in acute coronary syndrome. *Clin. Biochem.* **2007**, *40*, 478–484. [CrossRef]
30. Kjøller, E.; Hilden, J.; Winkel, P.; Galatius, S.; Frandsen, N.J.; Jensen, G.B.; Fischer Hansen, J.; Kastrup, J.; Jespersen, C.M.; Hildebrandt, P.; et al. Agreement between public register and adjudication committee outcome in a cardiovascular randomized clinical trial. *Am. Heart J.* **2014**, *168*, 197–204. [CrossRef]
31. Kjoller, E.; Hilden, J.; Winkel, P.; Frandsen, N.J.; Galatius, S.; Jensen, G.; Kastrup, J.; Hansen, J.F.; Kolmos, H.J.; Jespersen, C.M.; et al. Good interobserver agreement was attainable on outcome adjudication in patients with stable coronary heart disease. *J. Clin. Epidemiol.* **2012**, *65*, 444–453. [CrossRef] [PubMed]
32. Pellitero, S.; Reverter, J.L.; Granada, M.L.; Pizarro, E.; Pastor, M.C.; Tassies, D.; Reverter, J.C.; Salinas, I.; Sanmarti, A. Association of the IGF1/pregnancy-associated plasma protein-a system and adipocytokine levels with the presence and the morphology of carotid plaques in type 2 diabetes mellitus patients with stable glycaemic control. *Eur. J. Endocrinol.* **2009**, *160*, 925–932. [CrossRef] [PubMed]

33. Schisterman, E.F.; Cole, S.R.; Platt, R.W. Overadjustment bias and unnecessary adjustment in epidemiologic studies. *Epidemiology* **2009**, *20*, 488–495. [CrossRef] [PubMed]
34. Resch, Z.T.; Simari, R.D.; Conover, C.A. Targeted disruption of the pregnancy-associated plasma protein-a gene is associated with diminished smooth muscle cell response to insulin-like growth factor-i and resistance to neointimal hyperplasia after vascular injury. *Endocrinology* **2006**, *147*, 5634–5640. [CrossRef]
35. Conover, C.A.; Mason, M.A.; Bale, L.K.; Harrington, S.C.; Nyegaard, M.; Oxvig, C.; Overgaard, M.T. Transgenic overexpression of pregnancy-associated plasma protein-a in murine arterial smooth muscle accelerates atherosclerotic lesion development. *Am. J. Physiol. Heart Circ. Physiol.* **2010**, *299*, H284–H291. [CrossRef]
36. Conover, C.A.; Bale, L.K.; Oxvig, C. Targeted inhibition of pregnancy-associated plasma protein-a activity reduces atherosclerotic plaque burden in mice. *J. Cardiovasc. Trans. Res.* **2016**, *9*, 77–79. [CrossRef]
37. Swindell, W.R.; Masternak, M.M.; Bartke, A. In vivo analysis of gene expression in long-lived mice lacking the pregnancy-associated plasma protein A (PappA) gene. *Exp. Gerontol.* **2010**, *45*, 366–374. [CrossRef]
38. Root, A. Growth hormone. *Pediatrics* **1965**, *36*, 940–950.
39. Palmeiro, C.R.; Anand, R.; Dardi, I.K.; Balasubramaniyam, N.; Schwarcz, M.D.; Weiss, I.A. Growth hormone and the cardiovascular system. *Cardiol. Rev.* **2012**, *20*, 197–207. [CrossRef]
40. Hjortebjerg, R. IGFBP-4 and PAPP-A in normal physiology and disease. *Growth Horm. IGF Res.* **2018**, *41*, 7–22. [CrossRef]
41. Guo, Y.; Bao, Y.; Guo, D.; Yang, W. Pregnancy-associated plasma protein a in cancer: Expression, oncogenic functions and regulation. *Am. J. Cancer. Res.* **2018**, *8*, 955–963. [PubMed]
42. Bale, L.K.; Resch, Z.T.; Harstad, S.L.; Overgaard, M.T.; Conover, C.A. Constitutive expression of pregnancy-associated plasma protein-a in arterial smooth muscle reduces the vascular response to injury in vivo. *Am. J. Physiol. Endocrinol. Metab.* **2013**, *304*, E139–E144. [CrossRef] [PubMed]
43. Mosholder, A.D.; Lee, J.Y.; Zhou, E.H.; Kang, E.M.; Ghosh, M.; Izem, R.; Major, J.M.; Graham, D.J. Long-term risk of acute myocardial infarction, stroke, and death with outpatient use of clarithromycin: A retrospective cohort study. *Am. J. Epidemiol.* **2018**, *187*, 786–792. [CrossRef] [PubMed]
44. Solomon, S.D.; Claggett, B.; Desai, A.S.; Packer, M.; Zile, M.; Swedberg, K.; Rouleau, J.L.; Shi, V.C.; Starling, R.C.; Kozan, Ö.; et al. Influence of ejection fraction on outcomes and efficacy of sacubitril/valsartan (LCZ696) in heart failure with reduced ejection fraction: The prospective comparison of arni with acei to determine impact on global mortality and morbidity in heart failure (PARADIGM-HF) trial. *Circ. Heart Fail.* **2016**, *9*, e002744. [CrossRef] [PubMed]

8

Multimarker Approach to Identify Patients with Coronary Artery Disease at High Risk for Subsequent Cardiac Adverse Events: The Multi-Biomarker Study

Georgiana-Aura Giurgea [1], Katrin Zlabinger [2], Alfred Gugerell [2], Dominika Lukovic [2], Bonni Syeda [2], Ljubica Mandic [2], Noemi Pavo [2], Julia Mester-Tonczar [2], Denise Traxler-Weidenauer [2], Andreas Spannbauer [2], Nina Kastner [2], Claudia Müller [2], Anahit Anvari [2], Jutta Bergler-Klein [2] and Mariann Gyöngyösi [2,*]

1 Department of Angiology, Internal Medicine II, Medical University of Vienna, 1090 Vienna, Austria; georgiana-aura.giurgea@meduniwien.ac.at

2 Department of Cardiology, Internal Medicine II, Medical University of Vienna, 1090 Vienna, Austria; katrin.zlabinger@meduniwien.ac.at (K.Z.); alfred.gugerell@meduniwien.ac.at (A.G.); dominika.lukovic@meduniwien.ac.at (D.L.); b.syeda@internist-nord.at (B.S.); ljubica.mandic@gmail.com (L.M.); noemi.pavo@meduniwien.ac.at (N.P.); julia.mester-tonczar@meduniwien.ac.at (J.M.-T.); denise.traxler-weidenauer@meduniwien.ac.at (D.T.-W.); andreas.spannbauer@meduniwien.ac.at (A.S.); nina.kastner@meduniwien.ac.at (N.K.); claudia.mueller@meduniwien.ac.at (C.M.); anahit.anvari@meduniwien.ac.at (A.A.); jutta.bergler-klein@meduniwien.ac.at (J.B.-K.)

* Correspondence: mariann.gyongyosi@meduniwien.ac.at

Abstract: In our prospective non-randomized, single-center cohort study (n = 161), we have evaluated a multimarker approach including S100 calcium binding protein A12 (S100A1), interleukin 1 like-receptor-4 (IL1R4), adrenomedullin, copeptin, neutrophil gelatinase-associated lipocalin (NGAL), soluble urokinase plasminogen activator receptor (suPAR), and ischemia modified albumin (IMA) in prediction of subsequent cardiac adverse events (AE) during 1-year follow-up in patients with coronary artery disease. The primary endpoint was to assess the combined discriminatory predictive value of the selected 7 biomarkers in prediction of AE (myocardial infarction, coronary revascularization, death, stroke, and hospitalization) by canonical discriminant function analysis. The main secondary endpoints were the levels of the 7 biomarkers in the groups with/without AE; comparison of the calculated discriminant score of the biomarkers with traditional logistic regression and C-statistics. The canonical correlation coefficient was 0.642, with a Wilk's lambda value of 0.78 and $p < 0.001$. By using the calculated discriminant equation with the weighted mean discriminant score (centroid), the sensitivity and specificity of our model were 79.4% and 74.3% in prediction of AE. These values were higher than that of the calculated C-statistics if traditional risk factors with/without biomarkers were used for AE prediction. In conclusion, canonical discriminant analysis of the multimarker approach is able to define the risk threshold at the individual patient level for personalized medicine.

Keywords: multimarker approach; adverse event; risk prediction; canonical discriminant analysis; C-statistics; coronary artery disease

1. Introduction

Cardiovascular mortality or morbidity risk scores are essential in primary and secondary prevention of cardiovascular adverse events (AE), and are mostly based on traditional cardiovascular risk factors, such as hypertension, diabetes mellitus, hyperlipidemia, smoking, and family history. Risk scores are created and calculated for patients with acute coronary syndrome: Thrombolysis in

Myocardial Infarction (TIMI), Platelet Glycoprotein IIb/IIIa in Unstable Angina: Receptor Suppression Using Integrilin (PURSUIT), the Global Registry of Acute Coronary Events (GRACE) [1], for stable angina pectoris: Framingham Risk Score [2], Vienna and Ludwigshafen Coronary Artery Disease (VILCAD) score [3], or for general patient population, such as the SCORE-European High Risk Chart [4]. Previous studies suggested, that biomarkers of inflammation, fibrinolysis or fibrin formation, endothelial function, oxidative stress, or renal or heart function parameter enhance the value of risk prediction and enable early intervention and prevention of subsequent cardiovascular adverse events (AE) [5]. Adding of routinely used biomarkers, such as troponin T or NT-pro-brain natriuretic peptide (pro-BNP) or blood cholesterol level to the traditional risk factors enhanced moderately the risk prediction in the individual patients [6]. Single or combined new biomarkers, such as copeptin, neutrophil gelatinase-associated lipocalin (NGAL), or soluble urokinase plasminogen activator receptor (suPAR) have been tested and validated in larger cohorts of patients, anticipating prognostic values of these biomarkers [7–9]. However, statistical association between biomarkers and onset of AEs in a large patient cohort is not necessarily useful for personalized risk stratification [10]. In contrast with single blood marker analysis, the multi-biomarker approach by using traditional or new circulating proteins might have the potential to enhance the risk stratification in individual patients.

We have selected 7 non-traditional biomarkers of different classes, possessing diagnostic or prognostic significance in forecasting of cardiovascular AEs, and combined them in a multi-biomarker approach to yield prognostic value for a single patient. The selected biomarkers were as follows: S100 calcium binding protein A12 (S100A1) and interleukin 1 like-receptor-4 (ST2, IL1R4) (markers of inflammation), adrenomedullin and copeptin (vasoactive markers), NGAL (tissue injury marker), suPAR (fibrinolysis marker), and ischemia modified albumin (IMA) (oxidative stress marker).

S100A12 protein is released from activated macrophages and has been proposed to contribute to the acceleration of atherosclerosis [11,12]. Midregional pro-adrenomedullin (MR-proADM, adrenomedullin) is a potent vasodilatatory peptide, and a marker of hemodynamic stress [13,14]. Copeptin, the C-terminal portion of the vasopressin prohormone, is released stoichiometrically with vasopressin in the neurohypophysis, and in combination with troponin T, improved the early risk stratification of patients presenting with acute chest pain [15]. NGAL is a marker of acute kidney injury but has also been associated with different cardiovascular diseases and elevated in patients with heart failure after myocardial infarction [16]. The suPAR is a plasma marker of low-grade inflammation that has been associated with cardiovascular risk [17,18]. IL1R4 is up-regulated in conditions with increased myocardial strain [19–23]. IMA is a sensitive biomarker of myocardial ischemia after percutaneous coronary intervention (PCI), or during coronary artery bypass surgery (CABG), and used for risk stratification tool for suspected acute coronary syndrome or as a prognostic marker in patients with cardiopulmonary resuscitation [24,25]. All of these biomarkers have been associated with cardiovascular events in patients with coronary artery disease (CAD).

The aim of the multi-biomarker study was to evaluate the multimarker approach for personalized medicine including the selected biomarkers S100A1, adrenomedullin, copeptin, NGAL, suPAR, IL1R4, and IMA in prediction of subsequent cardiac AEs during 1-year follow-up (FUP) in patients with CAD.

2. Materials and Methods

2.1. Study Design

The multi-biomarker study and biobank is a prospective non-randomized, single-center cohort study, including patients with either stable CAD or subacute myocardial infarction (AMI)—including ST-segment elevation myocardial infarction (STEMI) or non-STEMI (NSTEMI). Blood samples were taken to assess the discriminatory values of the single or multi-biomarker approach for prediction of major cardiac AE during the 1-year FUP period. The study was conducted at the Department of Cardiology, Medical University of Vienna in accordance with the Declaration of Helsinki (1975) and approved by the Ethics Committee of the Medical University of Vienna (EK Nr: 2011/1091 and 1276/2019). Written informed consent was obtained from all patients.

2.2. *Patient Population, Inclusion and Exclusion Criteria*

Patients with stable CAD and recent AMI were included. Stable CAD was defined as previously angiographical documented CAD, with/without previous PCI, AMI, CABG, with no angina pectoris or inducible myocardial ischemia at the time of the study inclusion, recruited in the outpatient clinic. Recent AMI was defined as current STEMI or NSTEMI after primary PCI, recruited in the internal ward before hospital discharge post-AMI. The mean time of blood collection in the AMI group was 2.4 ± 0.3 days post AMI-onset.

Inclusion criteria were proven CAD (stable CAD or recent AMI) in patients older than 19 years, and willing to participate in the study.

Exclusion criteria were known cancer, acute or chronic infective or auto-immune inflammatory diseases, hemodynamically significant valvular diseases, hypertrophic or restrictive cardiomyopathy, congenital heart disease, previous acute renal failure, major surgery within the last 3 months, liver diseases requiring treatment, inability or unwillingness to comply with the study protocol, and chronic renal failure with glomerular filtration rate (GFR) ≤ 40.

2.3. *Endpoints of the Study*

The primary endpoint of the study was to assess the combined discriminatory predictive value of the biomarkers S100A1, adrenomedullin, copeptin, NGAL, suPAR, IL1R4, and IMA in prediction of cardiac AE, defined as recurring myocardial infarction, coronary revascularization by PCI or CABG, death, stroke, hospitalization due to angina pectoris without revascularization or heart failure and implantation of pacemaker or automatic implantable cardioverter defibrillator /AICD/ due to malignant arrhythmias, in comparison with the usual logistic regression or C-statistics.

The secondary endpoints of the study were the levels of the 7 selected biomarkers in the subgroups of stable CAD (group CAD) and recent AMI (group AMI), association between the new biomarkers and NT-proBNP.

2.4. *Clinical Data Collection*

Baseline medical history (age, gender, presence of atherosclerotic risk factors, such as hypertension, diabetes mellitus, hyperlipidemia, smoking, previous AMI, PCI, CABG, peripheral and/or carotid artery disease), current medical treatment (daily regular dose of aspirin, clopidogrel, beta-blocker, ACE inhibitor or ARB), and transthoracic echocardiography (TTE) data (global left ventricular function expressed as wall motion score index) were recorded at the study inclusion and at the 1-year control clinical investigation.

At 1-year FUP, patients were invited to medical examination and TTE. The follow-up clinical history was documented, including the AEs.

2.5. *Laboratory Procedures*

Fasting venous blood samples were obtained into commercially available tubes. Serum and plasma aliquots were stored at −80 °C until biomarker assay. Troponin T, N-terminal-proBNP (NT-proBNP), and creatine kinase MB fraction (CK-MB) were assessed using a routine diagnostic analyzer in the hospital laboratory.

Biomarker concentrations in samples were measured by commercially available enzyme-linked immunosorbent assays (ELISA): S100A12 and copeptin from Cloud-Clone Corp. (Houston, TX, USA); suPAR, adrenomedullin and IMA from MyBioSource Inc. (San Diego, CA, USA); NGAL (Lipocalin 2) from ABCAM (Cambridge, UK) and IL1R4/ST2 from Sigma-Aldrich Co (St. Louis, MO, USA). All assays were performed according to the manufacturer's instructions.

2.6. Statistics

The statistical analysis was performed using SPSS® version 23 (SPSS Inc, Chicago, IL). Continuous parameters with normal or non-normal distribution were expressed as mean ± standard deviations or median with interquartile range, respectively. Categorical variables were listed as number and percentages. For all tests, two-sided analyses were used and the significance level was set at $p < 0.05$.

The predictive power of the biomarkers in classification of AEs was calculated by using canonical discriminant function analysis. The predictor (independent) variables were the 7 selected biomarkers and NT-proBNP. Wilk's lambda test was used to test the significance between the groups with/without AEs. Parameters with discriminatory function <0.3 (non-significant correlation with the other parameter with low discriminatory function between the groups) were stepwise excluded from the further discriminant function model. A discriminant score was calculated by using weighted combination of the biomarkers with >3 discriminatory function. The means and SDs of the discriminant scores and the weighted mean score cut-off values between the groups (event yes/no) were calculated and described as centroid. Sensitivity and specificity of the discriminatory score were determined from the classification results. To confirm the correctness of the scoring, individual patient discriminant scores were calculated, and the mean scores of the groups (AE or non-AE) were compared by 2-sided Student *t*-test.

Multivariate binary logistic regression analysis was performed to analyze the traditional risk factors, supplemented with the biomarkers predictive for subsequent cardiac AE. Continuous parameters were transformed to binary parameter using the quadratic difference between supposed predictive value (75% interquartile value) and observed binary outcome (0 for no event, 1 for event) for each patient. The following parameters were included into the analysis: male gender, age, presence of atherosclerotic risk factors (diabetes mellitus, hypertension, smoking, hyperlipidemia), all 7 selected biomarkers, and NT-proBNP. C-statistics was performed to predict risk and sensitivity and specificity of all included clinical and biomarker risk factors.

Linear regression analysis was used to search association between NT-proBNP (as established prognostic marker) and the 7 selected biomarkers: S100A1, adrenomedullin, copeptin, NGAL, suPAR, IL1R4, and IMA.

3. Results

A total of 181 patients were included in the study. Due to comorbidities possibly or definitively influencing the blood levels of the selected 7 biomarkers, such as moderate to severe acute or chronic renal failure, or malignant or other chronic disease diagnosed after study inclusion, 20 patients were excluded from the biomarker measurement study. Therefore, blood levels of the 7 selected biomarkers were measured in 161 patients and these 161 patients were included in the further analyses.

3.1. Clinical Events during the 1-Year FUP

In total, 48 cardiac AEs occurred. Four patients died, 8 patients experienced re-AMI, and 23 patients were hospitalized for heart failure or angina pectoris, or implantation of pacemaker or automatic implantable cardioverter defibrillator. Coronary revascularization was performed in 13 patients.

Table 1 lists the patient characteristics, and the baseline blood levels of biomarkers in all patients, and the groups AE and non-AE. Patients with adverse event at the follow-up had more often diabetes mellitus and previous bypass surgery, and more patients were smokers. NGAL, suPAR, and IL1R4 were significantly higher in group AE, however, large scatter of the data was observed.

Table 1. Clinical and laboratory parameters of patients with coronary artery disease with/without cardiac adverse events (AE) during the 1-year follow-up.

Clinical and Laboratory Parameter	All Patients $n = 161$	Group AE $n = 48$	Group Non-AE $n = 113$	p Value between Groups
Male gender n (%)	126 (78.3%)	35 (72.9%)	91 (80.5%)	0.301
Age (y; mean ± SD)	67.0 ± 11.9	70.4 ± 11.1	65.6 ± 12.0	0.017
Diabetes mellitus n (%)	41 (25.5%)	18 (37.5%)	23 (20.4%)	0.030
Hypertension n (%)	129 (80.1%)	41 (85.4%)	88 (77.9%)	0.388
Hyperlipidemia n (%)	117 (72.7%)	37 (77.1%)	80 (70.8%)	0.447
Smoking n (%)	58 (36.0%)	26 (55.3%)	32 (28.3%)	0.011
Previous MI n (%)	83 (51.6%)	29 (60.4%)	54 (47.8%)	0.295
Previous PCI n (%)	85 (52.8%)	22 (45.8%)	63 (55.8%)	0.301
Previous CABG n (%)	31 (19.3%)	17 (35.4%)	14 (12.4%)	0.002
PAD n (%)	20 (12.4%)	9 (18.8%)	11 (9.7%)	0.123
Carotid artery disease n (%)	28 (17.4%)	9 (18.8%)	19 (17.0%)	0.822
Aspirin (%)	161 (100%)	48 (100%)	113 (100%)	1
Clopidogrel n (%)	132 (82.0%)	38 (79.2%)	94 (83.2%)	0.408
Beta-blocker n (%)	152 (94.4%)	43 (89.6%)	109 (96.4%)	0.398
ACE-inhibitor/ARB n (%)	146 (90.7%)	42 (87.5%)	104 (92.0%)	0.780
NT-proBNP (median; Q) (pg/mL)	280 (232; 335)	282 (243; 507)	279 (232; 309)	0.224
Troponin T (ng/L) (median; Q) (ng/mL)	0.01 (0.01; 0.41)	0.01 (0.01; 0.04)	0.01 (0.01; 0.08)	0.313
Creatine kinase (U/L) (median; Q)	116 (66; 188)	88 (67; 177)	118 (66; 106)	0.541
Baseline WMSI (mean ± SD)	1.31 ± 0.46	1.22 ± 0.45	1.34 ± 0.47	0.115
Follow-up WMSI (mean ± SD)	1.31 ± 0.51	1.28 ± 0.51	1.32 ± 0.51	0.651
Selected biomarkers (Median, 25% and 75% Quartiles)				
S100A1(ng/mL)	5504 (0; 11858)	5311 (0; 14462)	5674 (0; 11327)	0.724
Adrenomedullin (ng/mL)	189 (146; 328)	178 (144; 279)	194 (150; 343)	0.187
Copeptin (pg/mL)	1049 (817; 1049)	938 (731; 1049)	1049 (844; 1049)	0.058
NGAL (pg/mL)	18.5 (11.0; 39.0)	40.3 (16.5; 57.7)	16.2 (9.9; 27.6)	<0.05
suPAR (ng/mL)	5.37 (3.70; 8.51)	9.18 (3.58; 11.99)	4.94 (3.70; 6.95)	<0.05
IL1R4 (pg/mL)	347 (211; 616)	542 (222; 769)	318 (193; 548)	<0.05
IMA (ng/mL)	167 (53; 219)	156 (34; 211)	178 (76; 221)	0.120

MI: myocardial infarction; PCI: percutaneous coronary intervention; CABG: coronary artery bypass graft surgery; PAD: peripheral artery disease; ACE: angiotensin converting enzyme; ARB: angiotensin receptor blocker; NT-proBNP: N-terminal pro-brain natriuretic peptide; WMSI: wall motion score index, S100A1: S100 calcium binding protein A12; NGAL: neutrophil gelatinase-associated lipocalin; suPAR: soluble urokinase plasminogen activator receptor; IL1R4: interleukin 1 like-receptor-4; IMA: ischemia modified albumin. Q: 25% and 75% quartiles.

3.2. Multimarker Approach for Prediction of Adverse Events

The structure matrix of the canonical discriminant analysis including all selected 7 biomarkers showed low (<0.3) Pearson correlation between S100A1, adrenomedullin, copeptin, and IMA and the other biomarkers, with a low sensitivity of 43.5% and high specificity of 94.5% in prediction of AE. In order to increase the sensitivity of the multiple biomarker testing, we have stepwise excluded biomarkers with low level of correlation between the other markers. Finally, including the factors with the strongest discriminant predictive power, NGAL, suPAR, and IL1R4, the canonical correlation coefficient was 0.496, with a Wilk's lambda value of 0.001, resulting in a discriminant model of:

$$\text{Discriminant score} = -2.01 + 0.025 \times \text{NGAL}_i + 0.130 \times \text{suPAR}_i + 0.001 \times \text{IL1R4}_i,$$

where i: individual value of the same patient.

The weighted mean discriminant score (cutting point, centroid) was 0.225 (Figure 1), resulting in a sensitivity of 79.4% and specificity of 74.3% in prediction of adverse event, if the calculated discriminant equation was used. Accordingly, 76.9% of patients have been correctly classified to groups AE or non-AE if the calculated scores were used in the individual patient level. Patients with AEs had significantly higher discriminant value (calculated from the discriminant equation) as compared with patients without events (Figure 1).

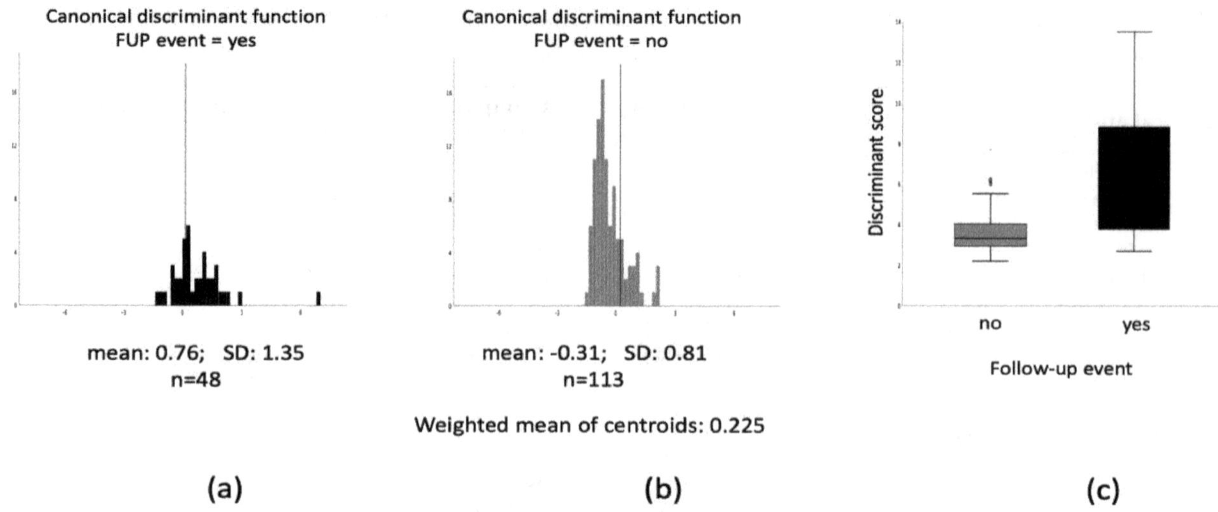

Figure 1. Discriminant scores, weighted mean of centroids, and C-statistics of patients experiencing cardiovascular adverse events. (**a**) and (**b**) discriminant score values of patients with (**a**) or without (**b**) adverse events at the 1-year follow-up (FUP); (**c**) mean (SD) discriminant scores of patients with or without adverse events at the FUP.

Interestingly, including NT-proBNP into the model did not enhance the power of the analysis, e.g., it did not increase the sensitivity/specificity values of the event prediction, most probably due to the significant association between NT-proBNP and NGAL or suPAR or IL1R4, respectively (Figure 2).

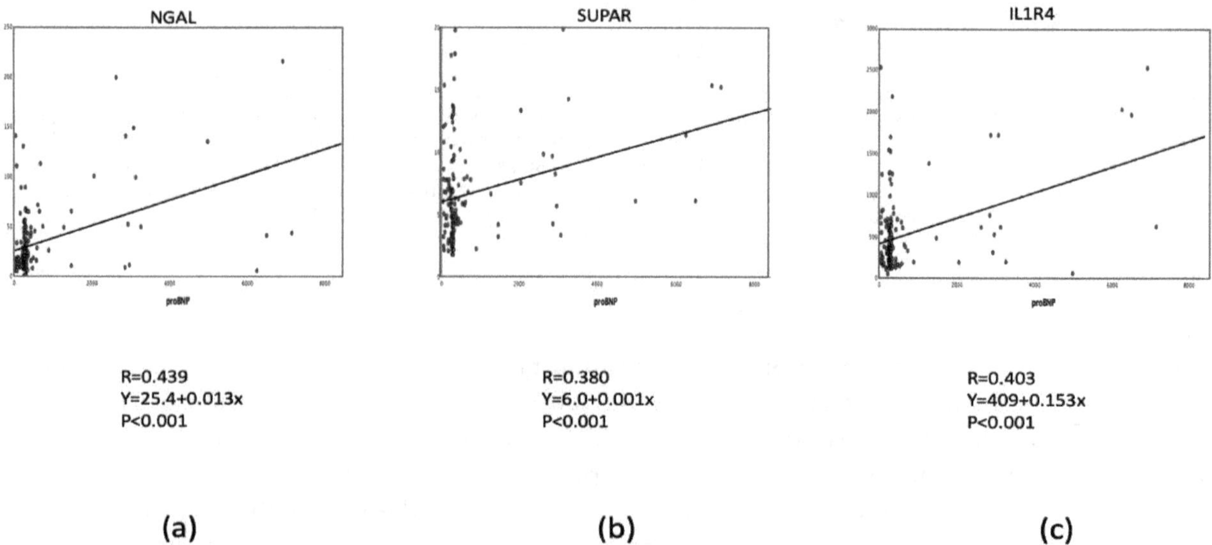

Figure 2. Significant correlation between N-terminal-pro-brain natriuretic peptide (NT-proBNP) (pg/mL) and new biomarkers with (**a**) neutrophil gelatinase-associated lipocalin (NGAL) (pg/mL); (**b**) soluble urokinase plasminogen activator receptor (SUPAR) (ng/mL); (**c**) interleukin 1 like-receptor-4 (ST2, IL1R4) (pg/mL).

3.3. Risk Prediction Including Clinical Variables by Using Logistic Regression and C-Statistics

Binary logistic regression analysis including the traditional risk factors (age, male gender, diabetes, hypertension, hyperlipidemia, and smoking) could not reveal any significant predictors for adverse events. C-statistics revealed a C value (area under the curve of ROC analysis) of 0.58, with no significant prediction value for AEs (Figure 3).

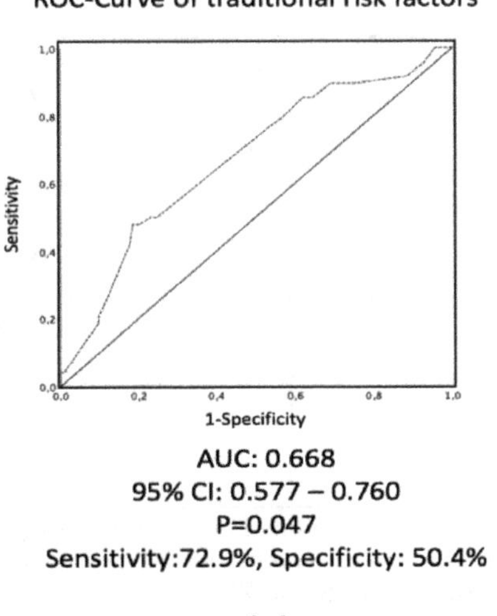

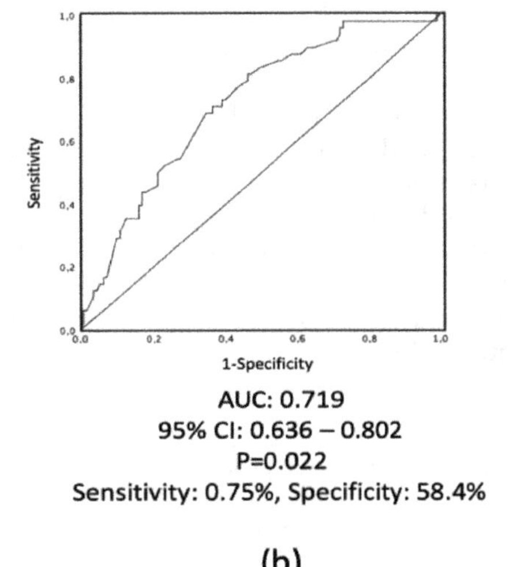

(a) (b)

Figure 3. C-statistics and receiver operator characteristics (ROC) curves of predictive adverse events of patients experiencing cardiovascular adverse events. (**a**) ROC curve analysis if traditional risk factors (male gender, older age, diabetes, hypertension, hyperlipidemia, and smoking) were included into the analysis; (**b**) ROC curve if 7 biomarkers and NT-proBNP were additionally included into the analysis of traditional risk factors.

Entering of the selected 7 biomarkers and NT-proBNP into the logistic regression analysis containing also the traditional risk factors did not result in any significant predictors. However, adding the 8 biomarkers increased moderately but significantly the prediction of AEs by a C value of 0.668 ($p = 0.047$) (Figure 3) in the C-statistics, with an optimized sensitivity and specificity values of 72.9% and 50.4%.

3.4. Diagnostic Value of Selected Biomarkers in Recent AMI

Patients were classified into subgroups CAD ($n = 39$) and AMI ($n = 42$). Table 2 lists the baseline clinical variables of the subgroups. Patients in the group CAD had a higher incidence of previous AMI and PCI. Patients in the AMI group had higher NT-proBNP, CK, and TnT 2.4 ± 0.3 days post AMI onset.

Table 2. Clinical and laboratory parameters of subgroup of patients with stable coronary artery disease (subgroup CAD) or with recent acute myocardial infarction (subgroup AMI).

Clinical and Laboratory Parameter	Subgroup CAD $n = 111$	Subgroup AMI $n = 50$	p Value between the Groups
Male gender n (%)	89 (80.2%)	37 (74.0%)	0.412
Age (y; mean ± SD)	68.4 ± 11.5	64.0 ± 12.3	0.036
Diabetes mellitus n (%)	34 (30.6%)	7 (14.0%)	0.031
Hypertension n (%)	92 (82.9%)	37 (74.0%)	0.205
Hyperlipidemia n (%)	77 (69.4%)	40 (80.0%)	0.185
Smoking n (%)	34 (30.6%)	24 (48.0%)	0.167
Previous MI n (%)	71 (64.0%)	12 (24.0%)	<0.001
Previous PCI n (%)	74 (66.7%)	11 (22.0%)	<0.001
Previous CABG n (%)	25 (22.5%)	6 (12.0%)	0.135
PAD n (%)	15 (13.5%)	5 (10.0%)	0.614
Carotid artery disease n (%)	23 (20.7%)	5 (10%)	0.117
Aspirin n (%)	111 (100%)	50 (100%)	1
Clopidogrel n (%)	92 (82.9%)	40 (80.0%)	0.666
Beta-blocker n (%)	102 (91.9%)	50 (100%)	0.863
ACE-inhibitor/ARB n (%)	102 (91.9%)	44 (88.0%)	0.814

Table 2. *Cont.*

Clinical and Laboratory Parameter	Subgroup CAD $n = 111$	Subgroup AMI $n = 50$	p Value between the Groups
NT-proBNP (median; Q) (pg/mL)	278 (241; 301)	359 (182; 881)	0.029
Troponin T (ng/L) (median; Q) (ng/mL)	0.01 (0.01; 0.01)	0.26 (0.04; 2.33)	<0.001
Creatine kinase (U/L) (median; Q)	85 (55; 137)	248 (131; 569)	<0.001
Baseline WMSI (mean ± SD)	1.29 ± 0.43	1.34 ± 0.54	0.611
Follow-up WMSI (mean ± SD)	1.29 ± 0.46	1.34 ± 0.64	0.716
FUP events n (%)	30 (27.0%)	18 (36.0%)	0.268
Hospitalization n (%)	16 (14.4%)	7 (14.0%)	
Acute MI n (%)	6 (5.4%)	2 (4.0%)	
Revascularization n (%)	6 (5.4%)	7 (14%)	
Death n (%)	2 (1.8%)	2 (4.0%)	

MI: myocardial infarction; PCI: percutaneous coronary intervention; ACBP: aorto-coronary bypass surgery; PAD: peripheral artery disease; ACE: angiotensin converting enzyme; ARB: angiotensin receptor blocker; NT-proBNP: N-terminal pro-brain natriuretic peptide; WMSI: wall motion score index; Q: 25% and 75% quartiles.

Table 2 and Figure 4 shows the blood levels of biomarkers. Beside the significantly elevated NT-proBNP value in the AMI group, from the 7 new biomarkers, only suPAR showed a trend towards higher value in the AMI group.

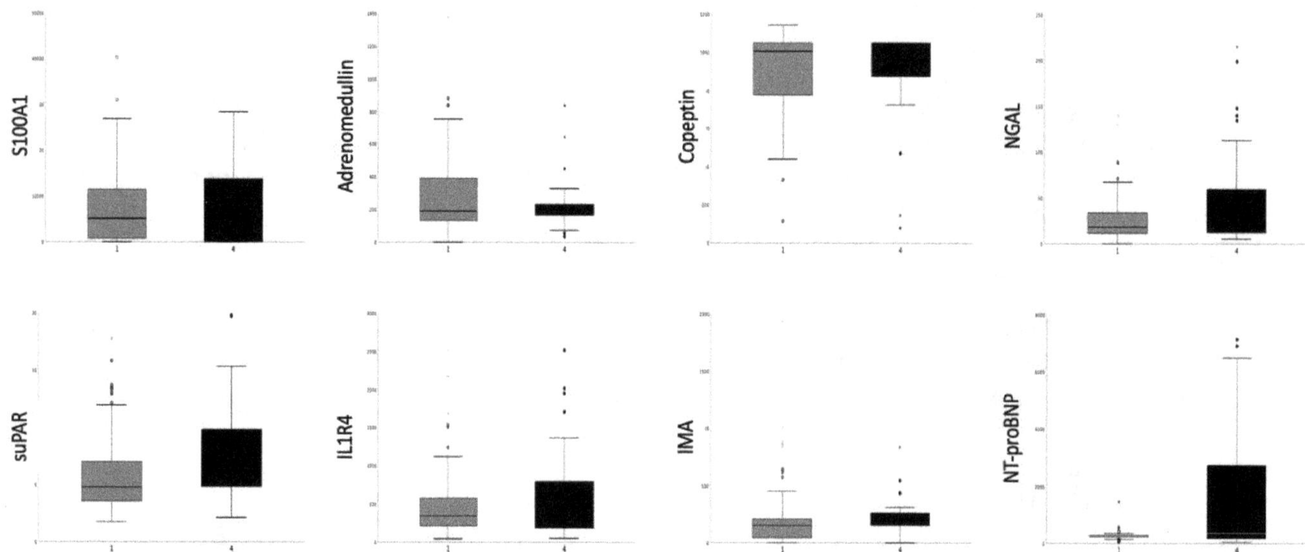

Figure 4. Blood levels of biomarkers of patients with stable coronary artery disease (subgroup CAD) or with recent acute myocardial infarction (subgroup AMI). S100 calcium binding protein A12 (S100A1) (ng/mL), adrenomedullin (ng/mL), copeptin (pg/mL), neutrophil gelatinase-associated lipocalin (NGAL) (pg/mL), soluble urokinase plasminogen activator receptor (suPAR) (ng/mL), interleukin 1 like-receptor-4 (ST2, IL1R4) (pg/mL), ischemia modified albumin (IMA) ng/mL), N-terminal-pro-brain natriuretic peptide (NT-proBNP) (pg/mL). No significant differences between the subgroups.

4. Discussion

To our knowledge, this is the first study to use the multi-biomarker approach by using the absolute values of the blood biomarkers, by using canonical discriminant analysis. Our study demonstrated, that (1) canonical discriminant analysis of the multimarker approach is able to define risk threshold in the individual single patient level; (2) the weighted mean discriminant score (cutting point, centroid) resulted in a sensitivity of 79.4% and specificity of 74.3% in prediction of adverse event, if calculated discriminant equation was used, with 76.9% of patients classified correctly to groups AE or non-AE; (3) classical C-statistics for adverse event prediction including the traditional risk factors (age, male gender, diabetes, hypertension, hyperlipidemia, and smoking) and 8 biomarkers revealed a C value of 0.719 ($p = 0.022$), with a sensitivity and specificity values of 75.0% and 58.4%; (4) canonical discriminant analysis using the absolute values of biomarkers of coronary artery disease has a better sensitivity and specificity in prediction of adverse events than the usual logistic regression or C-statistics in a single patient level. Additionally, our study revealed low diagnostic value of the selected 7 biomarkers in patients with recent AMI.

We have selected different class biomarkers (inflammation, vasoactive, fibrinolysis, oxidative stress, and tissue injury), since the biomarker of the same or similar classes may have coincidental information, failing to give additive values in event prediction. Additionally, a limited number of non-correlative markers may better improve the risk stratification than a larger number of biomarkers acting in the similar biological pathway. Most probably, this might be the reason, why the additive biomarker NT-proBNP did not improve the sensitivity/specificity values in our study, since NT-proBNP showed a significant correlation with all 3 biomarkers entered into the discriminant equation.

Previous studies investigating the role of multiple biomarkers in patients with or without CAD have demonstrated only modest improvement in predictive accuracy, by using C-statistic, if biomarkers were added to traditional clinical risk factors [26,27]. C-statistics are commonly applied to quantify and evaluate the risk score in patients with predefined AEs [28]. In C-statistics, a receiver operating characteristic (ROC) curve displays the diagnostic capacity of a binary classification system. In contrast discriminant analysis, it is allowed to utilize the continuous absolute values of the measured parameters without compulsory transformation of the continuous variables to categorical ones. Therefore, this analysis type may separate the groups by the most exact way and discard parameters mathematically which have less prediction value in the group classification. We did not include the established clinical risk factors into our discriminant model, because (1) dichotomy variables might weaken the prediction of AEs in our mathematical model; (2) the control of the cardiovascular risk factors via first and second prevention and guided therapies modify the course of heart diseases, effectively balancing the pre-existing risk; and (3) presence of multiple risk factors influences the co-incident risk factors, such as diabetic nephropathy results in hypertension, or male patients have higher risk for event in younger age than woman in similar age.

The sensitivity and specificity values of our discriminant model were 79.4.% and 74.3%, below the expected prediction values of over 80%, even if Wilk's lambda statistic value was significant. This is probably due to the heterogeneous patient population. We recognized a large scatter of the blood levels of the individual biomarkers, raising methodological concerns of the available ELISA kits.

The usual multivariate binary logistic regression model including the traditional risk factors did not reveal any significant predictors, even not, if the biomarkers (7 selected and NT-proBNP) were included into the model with mandatory transformation of the continuous variables to categorical ones. In contrast, C-statistics presented non-significant predictor values of the traditional risk factors, but adding the 8 biomarkers to the model improved the prediction significantly, albeit moderately. However, this latter approach still presented a less predictive accuracy with less optimal sensitivity and specificity values. The discrepancies between the outcomes of the logistic regression and C-statistics indicate the inconsistencies in statistical results, if individual patient risk prediction is required.

Our study has some limitations. There are several biomarkers associated with autoimmune diseases (such as copeptin with multiple sclerosis, NGAL, and systemic lupus erythematosus), therefore we have excluded patients with autoimmune disorders from our study [29,30]. We have also excluded patients with moderate or severe renal failure, because circulating levels of several biomarkers (copeptin, NT-proBNP, NGAL) are influenced by chronic kidney disease, independent from the coronary artery disease. Most of the assumptions needed for the correct calculation of the discriminant analysis were fulfilled, e.g., independent cases, within-group variance-co-variance matrices are equal across the groups; categorical parameter is used for group variable. However, some predictor variables do not have multivariate normal distribution, but our analysis including 161 patients is robust enough to overcome this assumption, and has high sensitivity and specificity to balance the outliers. As usual, in academic studies, our patient collective is heterogeneous, with a relatively small effect size in terms of AEs. However, a multimarker approach with calculated discriminant scores might be helpful for individual patient stratification, and improves the risk calculation at the individual patient level. Measuring more biomarkers would definitively increase in cost, with eventually only minor additive value in risk prediction.

5. Conclusions

Our canonical discriminatory model with multimarker approach is able to define a risk threshold at the individual patient level, additive to the conventional risk stratifications as part of personalized medicine in cardiology.

Author Contributions: Conceptualization, G.-A.G., B.S., J.B.-K., and M.G.; methodology, A.G., D.L., L.M., J.M.-T., and N.K.; validation, G.-A.G., N.P., D.T.-W., and J.B.-K.; formal analysis, K.Z., A.G., L.M., J.M.-T., D.T.-W., A.S., N.K., C.M., A.A., and M.G.; investigation, A.-G.G., B.S., L.M., J.B.-K., and M.G.; data curation, A.-G.G., K.Z., D.L., B.S., L.M., J.B.-K., C.M., A.A., and M.G.; writing—original draft preparation, G.-A.G., J.B.-K., and M.G.; writing—review and editing, K.Z., A.G., A.S., D.L., B.S., L.M., N.P., J.M.-T., D.T.-W., and N.K.; supervision, A.S.; project administration, G.-A.G., B.S., C.M., A.A., and L.M. All authors have read and agreed to the published version of the manuscript.

References

1. Morrow, D.A. Cardiovascular risk prediction in patients with stable and unstable coronary heart disease. *Circulation* **2010**, *121*, 2681–2691. [CrossRef]
2. Schnabel, R.B.; Sullivan, L.M.; Levy, D.; Pencina, M.J.; Massaro, J.M.; D'Agostino, R.B., Sr.; Newton-Cheh, C.; Yamamoto, J.F.; Magnani, J.W.; Tadros, T.M.; et al. Development of a risk score for atrial fibrillation (Framingham Heart Study): A community-based cohort study. *Lancet* **2009**, *373*, 739–745. [CrossRef]
3. Goliasch, G.; Kleber, M.E.; Richter, B.; Plischke, M.; Hoke, M.; Haschemi, A.; Marculescu, R.; Endler, G.; Grammer, T.B.; Pilz, S.; et al. Routinely available biomarkers improve prediction of long-term mortality in stable coronary artery disease: The Vienna and Ludwigshafen Coronary Artery Disease (VILCAD) risk score. *Eur. Heart J.* **2012**, *33*, 2282–2289. [CrossRef] [PubMed]
4. Conroy, R.M.; Pyörälä, K.; Fitzgerald, A.P.; Sans, S.; Menotti, A.; De Backer, G.; De Bacquer, D.; Ducimetière, P.; Jousilahti, P.; Keil, U.; et al. SCORE project group. Estimation of ten-year risk of fatal cardiovascular disease in Europe: The SCORE project. *Eur. Heart J.* **2003**, *24*, 987–1003. [CrossRef]
5. Meeuwsen, J.A.L.; Wesseling, M.; Hoefer, I.E.; de Jager, S.C.A. Prognostic value of circulating inflammatory cells in patients with stable and acute coronary artery disease. *Front. Cardiovasc. Med.* **2017**, *4*, 44. [CrossRef] [PubMed]
6. Tang, W.H. Contemporary challenges in translating biomarker evidence into clinical practice. *J. Am. Coll. Cardiol.* **2010**, *55*, 2077–2079. [CrossRef]
7. Reichlin, T.; Hochholzer, W.; Stelzig, C.; Laule, K.; Freidank, H.; Morgenthaler, N.G.; Bergmann, A.; Potocki, M.; Noveanu, M.; Breidthardt, T.; et al. Incremental value of copeptin for rapid rule out of acute myocardial infarction. *J. Am. Coll. Cardiol.* **2009**, *54*, 60–68. [CrossRef]
8. Nakada, Y.; Kawakami, R.; Matsui, M.; Ueda, T.; Nakano, T.; Takitsume, A.; Nakagawa, H.; Nishida, T.; Onoue, K.; Soeda, T.; et al. Prognostic value of urinary neutrophil gelatinase-associated lipocalin on the first day of admission for adverse events in patients with acute decompensated heart failure. *J. Am. Heart Assoc.* **2017**, *6*. [CrossRef] [PubMed]
9. Sehestedt, T.; Lyngbaek, S.; Eugen-Olsen, J.; Jeppesen, J.; Andersen, O.; Hansen, T.W.; Linneberg, A.; Jørgensen, T.; Haugaard, S.B.; Olsen, M.H.; et al. Soluble urokinase plasminogen activator receptor is associated with subclinical organ damage and cardiovascular events. *Atherosclerosis* **2011**, *216*, 237–243. [CrossRef]
10. Wang, T.J. Multiple biomarkers for predicting cardiovascular events: Lessons learned. *J. Am. Coll. Cardiol.* **2010**, *55*, 2092–2095. [CrossRef]

11. Mori, Y.; Kosaki, A.; Kishimoto, N.; Kimura, T.; Iida, K.; Fukui, M.; Nakajima, F.; Nagahara, M.; Urakami, M.; Iwasaka, T.; et al. Increased plasma S100A12 (EN-RAGE) levels in hemodialysis patients with atherosclerosis. *Am. J. Nephrol.* **2009**, *29*, 18–24. [CrossRef] [PubMed]
12. Shiotsu, Y.; Mori, Y.; Nishimura, M.; Sakoda, C.; Tokoro, T.; Hatta, T.; Maki, N.; Iida, K.; Iwamoto, N.; Ono, T.; et al. Plasma S100A12 level is associated with cardiovascular disease in hemodialysis patients. *Clin. J. Am. Soc. Nephrol.* **2011**, *6*, 718–723. [CrossRef]
13. Khan, S.Q.; O'Brien, R.J.; Struck, J.; Quinn, P.; Morgenthaler, N.; Squire, I.; Davies, J.; Bergmann, A.; Ng, L.L. Prognostic value of midregional pro-adrenomedullin in patients with acute myocardial infarction: The LAMP (Leicester Acute Myocardial Infarction Peptide) study. *J. Am. Coll. Cardiol.* **2007**, *49*, 1525–1532. [CrossRef]
14. Wild, P.S.; Schnabel, R.B.; Lubos, E.; Zeller, T.; Sinning, C.R.; Keller, T.; Tzikas, S.; Lackner, K.J.; Peetz, D.; Rupprecht, H.J.; et al. Midregional proadrenomedullin for prediction of cardiovascular events in coronary artery disease: Results from the AtheroGene study. *Clin. Chem.* **2012**, *58*, 226–236. [CrossRef] [PubMed]
15. Keller, T.; Tzikas, S.; Zeller, T.; Czyz, E.; Lillpopp, L.; Ojeda, F.M.; Roth, A.; Bickel, C.; Baldus, S.; Sinning, C.R.; et al. Copeptin improves early diagnosis of acute myocardial infarction. *J. Am. Coll. Cardiol.* **2010**, *55*, 2096–2106. [CrossRef] [PubMed]
16. Yndestad, A.; Landro, L.; Ueland, T.; Dahl, C.P.; Flo, T.H.; Vinge, L.E.; Espevik, T.; Frøland, S.S.; Husberg, C.; Christensen, G.; et al. Increased systemic and myocardial expression of neutrophil gelatinase-associated lipocalin in clinical and experimental heart failure. *Eur. Heart J.* **2009**, *30*, 1229–1236. [CrossRef] [PubMed]
17. Eugen-Olsen, J.; Andersen, O.; Linneberg, A.; Ladelund, S.; Hansen, T.W.; Langkilde, A.; Petersen, J.; Pielak, T.; Møller, L.N.; Jeppesen, J.; et al. Circulating soluble urokinase plasminogen activator receptor predicts cancer, cardiovascular disease, diabetes and mortality in the general population. *J. Intern. Med.* **2010**, *268*, 296–308. [CrossRef]
18. Koller, L.; Stojkovic, S.; Richter, B.; Sulzgruber, P.; Potolidis, C.; Liebhart, F.; Mörtl, D.; Berger, R.; Goliasch, G.; Wojta, J.; et al. Soluble urokinase-type plasminogen activator receptor improves risk prediction in patients with chronic heart failure. *JACC Heart Fail.* **2017**, *5*, 268–277. [CrossRef]
19. Dieplinger, B.; Mueller, T. Soluble ST2 in heart failure. *ClinChimActa* **2015**, *443*, 57–70. [CrossRef]
20. Sabatine, M.S.; Morrow, D.A.; Higgins, L.J.; MacGillivray, C.; Guo, W.; Bode, C.; Rifai, N.; Cannon, C.P.; Gerszten, R.E.; Lee, R.T.; et al. Complementary roles for biomarkers of biomechanical strain ST2 and N-terminal prohormone B-type natriuretic peptide in patients with ST-elevation myocardial infarction. *Circulation* **2008**, *117*, 1936–1944. [CrossRef] [PubMed]
21. Dhillon, O.S.; Narayan, H.K.; Quinn, P.A.; Squire, I.B.; Davies, J.E.; Ng, L.L. Interleukin 33 and ST2 in non-ST-elevation myocardial infarction: Comparison with Global Registry of Acute Coronary Events Risk Scoring and NT-proBNP. *Am. Heart J.* **2011**, *161*, 1163–1170. [CrossRef] [PubMed]
22. Eggers, K.M.; Armstrong, P.W.; Califf, R.M.; Simoons, M.L.; Venge, P.; Wallentin, L.; James, S.K. ST2 and mortality in non-ST-segment elevation acute coronary syndrome. *Am. Heart J.* **2010**, *159*, 788–794. [CrossRef]
23. Dieplinger, B.; Egger, M.; Haltmayer, M.; Kleber, M.E.; Scharnagl, H.; Silbernagel, G.; de Boer, R.A.; Maerz, W.; Mueller, T. Increased soluble ST2 predicts long-term mortality in patients with stable coronary artery disease: Results from the Ludwigshafen risk and cardiovascular health study. *Clin. Chem.* **2014**, *60*, 530–540. [CrossRef] [PubMed]
24. Turedi, S.; Gunduz, A.; Mentese, A.; Dasdibi, B.; Karahan, S.C.; Sahin, A.; Tuten, G.; Kopuz, M.; Alver, A. Investigation of the possibility of using ischemia-modified albumin as a novel and early prognostic marker in cardiac arrest patients after cardiopulmonary resuscitation. *Resuscitation* **2009**, *80*, 994–999. [CrossRef] [PubMed]
25. Kanko, M.; Yavuz, S.; Duman, C.; Hosten, T.; Oner, E.; Berki, T. Ischemia-modified albumin use as a prognostic factor in coronary bypass surgery. *J. Cardiothorac. Surg.* **2012**, *7*, 3. [CrossRef] [PubMed]
26. Kim, H.C.; Greenland, P.; Rossouw, J.E.; Manson, J.E.; Cochrane, B.B.; Lasser, N.L.; Limacher, M.C.; Lloyd-Jones, D.M.; Margolis, K.L.; Robinson, J.G. Multimarker prediction of coronary heart disease risk. *J. Am. Coll. Cardiol.* **2010**, *55*, 2080–2091. [CrossRef] [PubMed]
27. Wang, T.J.; Gona, P.; Larson, M.G.; Tofler, G.H.; Levy, D.; Newton-Cheh, C.; Jacques, P.F.; Rifai, N.; Selhub, J.; Robins, S.J.; et al. Multiple biomarkers for the prediction of first major cardiovascular events and death. *N. Engl. J. Med.* **2006**, *355*, 2631–2639. [CrossRef] [PubMed]
28. Uno, H.; Cai, T.; Pencina, M.J.v.; D'Agostino, R.B.; Wei, L.J. On the C-statistics for evaluating overall adequacy of risk prediction procedures with censored survival data. *Stat. Med.* **2011**, *30*, 1105–1117. [CrossRef]

29. Baranowska-Bik, A.; Kochanowski, J.; Uchman, D.; Litwiniuk, A.; Kalisz, M.; Martynska, L.; Wolinska-Witort, E.; Baranowska, B.; Bik, W. Association of copeptin and cortisol in newly diagnosed multiple sclerosis patients. *J. Neuroimmunol.* **2015**, *282*, 21–24. [CrossRef] [PubMed]
30. Gómez-Puerta, J.A.; Ortiz-Reyes, B.; Urrego, T.; Vanegas-García, A.L.; Muñoz, C.H.; González, L.A.; Cervera, R.; Vásquez, G. Urinary neutrophil gelatinase-associated lipocalin and monocyte chemoattractant protein 1 as biomarkers for lupus nephritis in Colombian SLE patients. *Lupus* **2018**, *27*, 637–646. [CrossRef]

9

Growth Differentiation Factor-8 (GDF8)/Myostatin is a Predictor of Troponin I Peak and a Marker of Clinical Severity after Acute Myocardial Infarction

Alexandre Meloux [1,2], Luc Rochette [1], Maud Maza [1,2], Florence Bichat [1,2], Laura Tribouillard [2], Yves Cottin [1,2], Marianne Zeller [1] and Catherine Vergely [1,*]

1 Laboratoire Physiopathologie et Epidémiologie Cérébro-Cardiovasculaires (PEC2, EA 7460), Université de Bourgogne-Franche-Comté, UFR des Sciences de Santé; 7 Bd Jeanne d'Arc, 21000 Dijon, France; alexandre.meloux@u-bourgogne.fr (A.M.); luc.rochette@u-bourgogne.fr (L.R.); maud.maza@chu-dijon.fr (M.M.); florence.bichat@chu-dijon.fr (F.B.); yves.cottin@chu-dijon.fr (Y.C.); marianne.zeller@u-bourgogne.fr (M.Z.)

2 Department of Cardiology, University Hospital of Dijon, 21000 Dijon, France; laura.tribouillard@chu-dijon.fr

* Correspondence: cvergely@u-bourgogne.fr

Abstract: Objective: Growth differentiation factor-8 (GDF8), also known as myostatin, is a member of the transforming growth factor-β superfamily that inhibits skeletal muscle growth. We aimed to investigate the association between GDF8 and peak troponin I levels after acute myocardial infarction (AMI). Methods: All consecutive patients admitted from June 2016 to February 2018 for type 1 AMI in the Coronary Care Unit of University Hospital of Dijon Bourgogne (France) were included in our prospective study. Blood samples were harvested on admission, and serum levels of GDF8 were measured using a commercially available enzyme-linked immunosorbent assay kit. Results: Among the 296 patients with type 1 AMI, median age was 68 years and 27% were women. GDF8 levels (median (IQR) = 2375 ng/L) were negatively correlated with age, sex and diabetes ($p < 0.001$ for all). GDF8 levels were higher in patients with in-hospital ventricular tachycardia or fibrillation (VT/VF) than those without in-hospital VT/VF. GDF8 was positively correlated with troponin I peak (r = 0.247; $p < 0.001$). In multivariate linear regression analysis, log GDF8 (OR: 21.59; 95% CI 34.08–119.05; $p < 0.001$) was an independent predictor of troponin I peak. Conclusions: These results suggest that GDF8 levels could reflect the extent of myocardial damage during AMI, similar to peak troponin I, which is currently used to estimate infarct size. Further studies are needed to elucidate the underlying mechanisms linking the GDF8 cytokine with troponin I levels.

Keywords: GDF8; myostatin; AMI; troponin

---

1. Introduction

Patients with acute myocardial infarction (AMI) have a high rate of mortality, and the risk of fatal events is highest in the first hours following onset. The severity of AMI, which is usually determined early on with the measurement of circulating troponins, has a major impact on the development of late AMI consequences such as heart failure. Therefore, precise and rapid assessment of the severity of AMI critically affects treatment choices and patient prognoses. Recently, there has been interest in the potential role of new biomarkers for the assessment of severity in the early stages of AMI, with a particular focus on NT-pro-natriuretic peptide (NT-proBNP), heart-type fatty acid binding protein (hFABP) and circulating cytokines such as growth differentiation factor-15 [1].

Growth differentiation factor-8 (GDF8), also known as myostatin, is a member of the transforming growth factor-β (TGF-β) superfamily. GDF8 shares many structural similarities with other members such as growth differentiation factor-11 [2,3]. GDF8 is mainly expressed in skeletal muscles, particularly during the development period but also in adulthood, and is considered a negative regulator of muscle growth [4]. Genetic inhibition of myostatin leads to an increase in skeletal muscle mass and triggers a hyper-muscular phenotype in mammals [5,6]. In the heart muscle, GDF8 is expressed in fetal and adult myocardium [7], and its expression is increased in cardiac diseases such as advanced heart failure [8] or congenital heart disease [9]. Following experimental myocardial infarction, GDF8 is up-regulated in cardiomyocytes surrounding the infarcted area [7] and its concentration rapidly increases in the circulation [10]. However, the role of GDF8 during the acute phase of AMI in humans is poorly understood.

The aim of our study was to evaluate GDF8/myostatin levels in patients admitted for AMI, and to investigate the associations between GDF8 and markers of AMI severity such as troponin.

2. Methods

2.1. Patients

The methods and design of the French Regional Observatoire des Infarctus de Côte-d'Or (RICO) survey have been previously described [11]. From June 2016 to February 2018, all consecutive patients admitted to the coronary care unit of the Dijon University Hospital (France) for type 1 AMI were prospectively included. Type 1 MI is defined as an acute atherothrombotic coronary event resulting in the formation of an intra-luminal thrombus (plaque rupture, ulceration, erosion or coronary dissection) [12]. The present study is in agreement with the ethical guidelines of the Declaration of Helsinki. All of the participants provided consent prior to inclusion, and the Ethics Committee of the University Hospital of Dijon approved the protocol (BIOCARDIS-2016–9205AAO034S02117).

2.2. Data Collection

Patient characteristics were obtained at hospital admission. These included cardiovascular risk factors and history, and clinical and biological data. Risk scores were calculated (GRACE score and SYNTAX score). Blood samples were collected on admission to measure serum C-reactive protein (CRP), creatinine, creatine kinase peak, troponin Ic peak, NT-proBNP, blood lipids, glucose and hemoglobin. eGFR was calculated using Chronic Kidney Disease-EPIdemiology Collaboration formula (CKD-EPI). Echocardiographic data such as left ventricular ejection fraction (LVEF) were recorded. Finally, in-hospital events were documented, including death, cardiovascular death, re-infarction, stroke, development of heart failure and ventricular tachycardia or fibrillation (VT/VF).

2.3. Determination of Serum GDF8

Blood samples were collected on admission from a vein in the arm, centrifuged at 4 °C to isolate the serum, and samples were stored at −80 °C until use. Median (IQR) time from symptom onset to blood sampling was 16(8–30) hours. Serum GDF8 was measured in duplicate using a commercially available Quantitine kit (DGDF80, R&D systems, MN). The minimum detectable concentration was 2.25 ng/L, and the coefficient of variation between duplicates did not exceed 10%.

2.4. Statistical Analysis

Dichotomous variables are expressed as n (%) and continuous variables as mean ± SD or median (interquartile range). A Kolmogorov–Smirnov test was performed to test the normality of continuous variables. For non-normally distributed variables (i.e., NT-proBNP), they were log transformed. The Mann-Whitney test or Student's t test was used to compare continuous data, and the Chi 2 test or Fisher's test was used for dichotomous data, as appropriate.

Pearson correlation analyses (for normally distributed variables) or Spearman correlation analyses (one or two non-Gaussian variables) were performed. The threshold for significance was set at 5%.

Bivariate linear regression analyses were used to adjust GDF8 with age.

Multivariate logistic regression models were built to estimate in-hospital VT/VF and troponin Ic peak based on significant variables in univariate analysis. The inclusion threshold was set at 5%.

SPSS version 12.0.1 (IBM Inc, Armonk, NY, USA) was used for all of the statistical tests.

3. Results

The baseline characteristics of the study population are shown in Table 1. Predictors of GDF8 are shown in Table 2. GDF8 levels were significantly associated with age, sex and diabetes. Clinical data showed an association with systolic and diastolic blood pressure, STEMI, heart failure and GRACE risk score. Moreover, GDF8 was strongly correlated with CRP, creatine kinase peak, troponin Ic peak, NT-proBNP and LDL-cholesterol, as well as creatinine clearance and acute statin medication.

Table 1. Baseline characteristics.

	N (%) or Median (IQR) N = 296
Risk factors	
Age, y	68 (58–78)
Female	81 (27%)
BMI, kg/m^2	26 (24–30), *n* = 295
Hypertension	178 (60%)
Diabetes	75 (25%)
Hypercholesterolemia	117 (40%)
Family history of CAD	74 (25%)
Current smoking	85 (29%)
Cardiovascular history	
CAD	53 (18%)
Stroke	17 (6%)
Chronic kidney disease	16 (5%)
Clinical data	
LVEF, %	55 (50–60), *n* = 294
LVEF <40%	22 (7%)
HR, bpm	76 (64–87), *n* = 283
SBP, mmHg	142 (123–165), *n* = 275
DBP, mmHg	82 (70–94), *n* = 274
STEMI	143 (48%)
HF	56 (19%)
GRACE risk score	141 (116–170), *n* = 268
ICU length of stay, *d*	3 (3–4), *n* = 290
Coronary angiography	294 (99%)
SYNTAX score	12 (7–18), *n* = 284
Multivessel disease	184 (63%)
Percutaneous coronary intervention	252 (86%)
Biological data	
GDF8 relative expression	2375.0 (1640.0–3346.7)
CRP > 3 mg/L	158 (54%)
Creatinine, μmol/L	79 (68–95), *n* = 295
eGFR CKD, mL/min	82.7 (65.9–95.5), *n* = 295
eGFR CKD < 45 mL/min	34 (12%)
CK peak, UI/L	583 (195–1483), *n* = 291
Troponin Ic peak, ng/mL	15.00 (3.21–70.00), *n* = 295
Nt-ProBNP, pg/mL	394 (93–1588), *n* = 295
LDL cholesterol, g/L	1.24 (0.92–1.53), *n* = 293
HDL cholesterol, g/L	0.50 (0.40–0.60), *n* = 293
Total cholesterol, g/L	2.06 (1.70–2.35), *n* = 293
Triglycerides, g/L	1.21 (0.84–1.76), *n* = 293
Glycemia, mmol/L	6.80 (5.80–8.63), *n* = 295

Table 1. *Cont.*

	N (%) or Median (IQR) N = 296
In-hospital events	
Death	7 (2%)
Cardiovascular death	6 (2%)
Recurrent MI	7 (2%)
Stroke	2 (1%)
HF	75 (26%)
VT or VF	10 (3%)
Chronic medications	
Antiplatelet therapy	24 (8%)
Aspirin	72 (24%)
ARB	63 (21%)
ACE inhibitor	58 (20%)
Statin	92 (31%)
Beta blocker	83 (28%)
Diuretic	57 (19%)
Acute medications	
Antiplatelet therapy	283 (96%)
Aspirin	290 (98%)
ARB	36 (12%)
ACE inhibitor	179 (60%)
Statin	270 (91%)
Beta blocker	207 (70%)
Diuretic	65 (22%)

Data are expressed as *n* (%) or median (25th and 75th percentiles). *n*: number; GDF8: growth differentiation factor 8; BMI: body mass index; CAD: coronary artery disease; LVEF: left ventricular ejection fraction; HR: heart rate; HF: Heart failure; SBP: systolic blood pressure; DBP: diastolic blood pressure; STEMI: ST segment elevation myocardial infarction; GRACE: Global Registry of Acute Coronary Events; ICU: Intensive Care Unit; CRP: C-reactive protein; CK: creatine kinase; NT-proBNP: N-terminal pro-brain natriuretic peptide; LDL: low density lipoprotein; HDL: high density lipoprotein; ARB: angiotensin receptor blockers; ACE: angiotensin converting enzyme.

Table 2. Association between GDF8 levels and study variables (*n* = 296).

		Patients (n = 296)	GDF8 Relative Expression or r	*p* Value
CV risk factors				
Age (years)		68 (58–78)	−0.26	<0.001
Female	Yes	81 (27)	2002 (1284–2785)	<0.001
	No	215 (73)	2554.9 (1759–3489)	
BMI (kg/m^2)		26 (24–30)	0.08	0.191
Hypertension	Yes	178 (60)	2247 (1532–3321)	0.063
	No	118 (40)	2585 (1756–3381)	
Diabetes	Yes	75 (25)	1946 (1429–2621)	<0.001
	No	221 (75)	2574 (1751–3526)	
Hypercholesterolemia	Yes	117 (40)	2501 (1697–3397)	0.396
	No	179 (60)	2311 (1621–3304)	
Current smoking	Yes	85 (29)	2482 (1689–3396)	0.306
	No	211 (71)	2256 (1633–3320)	
Cardiovascular history				
CAD	Yes	53 (18)	2209 (1477–2991)	0.189
	No	243 (82)	2426 (1688–3381)	
Stroke	Yes	17 (6)	1742 (1070–2636)	0.062
	No	279 (94)	2431 (1679–3372)	
Chronic kidney disease	Yes	16 (5)	2712 (1315–3416)	0.885
	No	280 (95)	2368 (1663–3346)	
Clinical data				

Table 2. *Cont.*

		Patients (n = 296)	GDF8 Relative Expression or r	*p* Value
LVEF		55 (50–60)	−0.05	0.396
HR (bpm)		76 (64–87)	−0.06	0.304
SBP (mmHg)		142 (123–165)	0.14	0.022
DBP (mmHg)		82 (70–94)	0.22	<0.001
STEMI	Yes	143 (48)	2748 (1802–3445)	0.001
	No	153 (52)	2141 (1519–2973)	
Heart failure	Yes	56 (19)	2018 (1252–2775)	0.006
	No	238 (81)	2511 (1695–3413)	
GRACE risk score		141 (116–170)	−0.22	<0.001
ICU stay length (days)		3 (3–4)	−0.01	0.877
Biological data				
CRP ≥ 3 mg/L	Yes	158 (54)	2102 (1471–3197)	<0.001
	No	136 (46)	2722 (1957–3525)	
Creatinine clearance (CKD EPI) (mL/min)		83 (66–96)	0.15	0.010
CK peak (UI/L)		583 (195–1493)	0.26	<0.001
Peak troponin Ic (ng/mL)		15 (3–70)	0.25	<0.001
NT-proBNP (pg/mL)		394 (93–1588)	−0.27	<0.001
Glucose (mmol/L)		7 (6–9)	−0.02	0.684
LDL cholesterol (g/L)		1.2 (0.9–1.5)	0.25	<0.001
HDL cholesterol (g/L)		0.5 (0.4–0.6)	0.07	0.211
Triglycerides (g/L)		1.2 (0.8–1.8)	0.02	0.773

Data are expressed as *n* (%) or median (25th and 75th percentiles). *n*: number; r: correlation coefficient; GDF8: growth differentiation factor 8; BMI: body mass index; CAD: coronary artery disease; LVEF: left ventricular ejection fraction; HR: heart rate; SBP: systolic blood pressure; DBP: diastolic blood pressure; STEMI: ST segment elevation myocardial infarction; GRACE: Global Registry of Acute Coronary Events; ICU: Intensive Care Unit; CRP: C-reactive protein; CK: creatine kinase; NT-proBNP: N-terminal pro-brain natriuretic peptide; LDL: low density lipoprotein; HDL: high density lipoprotein; ARB: angiotensin II receptor blockers; ACE inhibitors: angiotensin converting enzyme inhibitors.

3.1. Baseline Characteristics

Among the 296 included patients, eighty-one (27%) were female. The median age was 68 years, 178 (60%) had hypertension, 117 (40%) had hypercholesterolemia, 75 (25%) had diabetes and 85 (29%) are active smokers. Median GDF8 was 2375 (1640–3347) ng/L.

3.2. Associations between GDF8 Levels and in-Hospital Development of Ventricular Tachycardia or Fibrillation

Ten patients (3%) developed VT/VF during their hospital stay. GDF8 levels were higher in these patients than in those who did not experience VT/VF (2565 ± 75 vs. 3852 ± 642 ng/L, $p = 0.034$, Figure 1). To assess VT/VF risk, a GDF8 cut-off value of 2878 ng/L was established with a receiver operating characteristic (ROC) curve analysis. The value was rounded to 2800 ng/L to improve clinical relevance. The area under the curve (AUC) was 0.697 ($p = 0.034$) and the sensitivity and specificity were good (70% and 66%, respectively). Among patients with GDF8 > 2800 ng/L (112/296), the risk of developing in-hospital VT/VF was higher than in patients with GDF8 < 2800 ng/L (184/296) ($p = 0.046$). The other relevant biomarkers (CK and peak troponin Ic) showed similar associations with the outcome (VT/VF): the respective AUC were 0.717 ($p = 0.027$) and 0.698 ($p = 0.034$), and the cut-off values were 400.5 UI/L and 7.6 ng/mL. Sensitivity and specificity were respectively 100% and 44% for CK and 100% and 43% for peak troponin IC. Both CK and troponin Ic were significantly associated with VT/VF in logistic regression analysis (CK peak: OR (95% CI): 6.034 (1.684–21.621) and troponin Ic peak: OR (95% CI): 2.751 (1.079–7.019)).

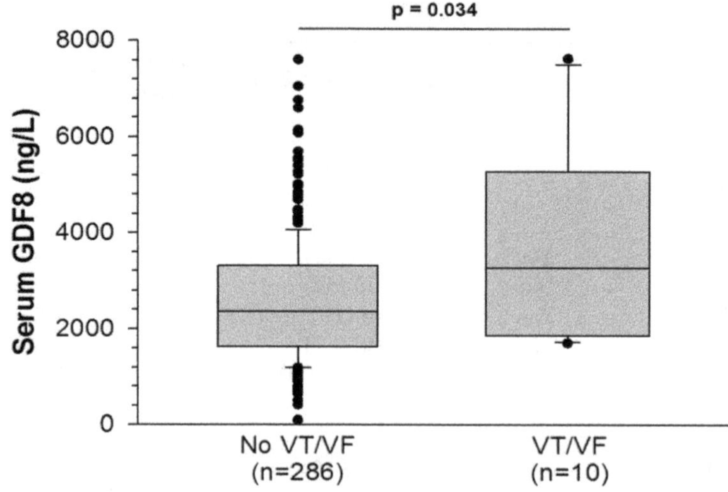

Figure 1. Serum growth differentiation factor-8 (GDF8) levels rise more in AMI patients with ventricular tachycardia or fibrillation (VT/VF) than AMI patients without VT/VF.

3.3. Associations between GDF8 Levels and Peak Troponin Ic

GDF8 was correlated with peak troponin Ic (r = 0.247; p <0.001). Patients with high (i.e., supramedian) GDF8 levels had a trend toward an increased risk of TV/FV compared with patients who had lower (i.e., inframedian) GDF8 levels (4.8% vs. 2%). Moreover, the troponin peak was much higher (X3) in patients with a supramedian GDF8 level, as shown in Table 3. In univariate analysis, diabetes (OR 11.82, 95% CI −3.49–43.03; $p = 0.095$), smoking (OR 11.34, 95% CI 0.78–45.40; $p = 0.043$), left ventricular ejection fraction <40% (OR 19.53, 95% CI 10.88–87.76; $p = 0.012$), GRACE risk score (OR 0.16, 95% CI 0.16–0.76; $p = 0.003$), and time to admission (OR 0.01, 95% CI −0.02–0.001; $p = 0.065$) and log GDF8 (OR 21.59, 95% CI 34.08–119.05; p <0.001) were associated with the prediction of troponin Ic peak. In multivariable analysis, log GDF8 remained associated to the prediction of troponin Ic peak, after adjustment for confounding factors (Table 4).

Table 3. Relevant outcomes according to high/low GDF8 levels (cutoff on median GDF8 value).

	GDF 8 ≤ 2400 ng/L N = 151	**GDF 8 > 2400 ng/L N = 145**	***p* Value**
In-hospital VF/VT	3 (2.0%)	7 (4.8%)	0.211
Troponin Ic peak, ng/mL	8.30 (2.10–36.00)	29.50 (4.22–92.75)	<0.001
LVEF, %	56 (50–60)	55 (50–60)	0.498

Table 4. Logistic regression analysis for prediction of troponin I peak.

	Univariate			**Multivariate**		
	OR	**95% CI**	***p* Value**	**OR**	**95% CI**	***p* Value**
Diabetes	11.82	−3.49–43.03	0.095	12.98	7.86–59.00	0.011
Smoking	11.34	0.78–45.40	0.043	13.19	10.32–62.28	0.006
LVEF > 40%	19.53	10.88–87.76	0.012	22.23	6.75–94.34	0.024
GRACE risk score	0.15	0.16–0.76	0.003	0.168	0.39–1.05	<0.001
Time to admission, per min	0.01	−0.02–0.00	0.065	0.01	−0.02–0.01	0.233
Log GDF8, per unit	21.59	34.08–119.05	<0.001	26.68	67.05–172.17	<0.001

LVEF: left ventricular ejection fraction; GRACE: Global Registry of Acute Coronary Events; NT-proBNP: N-terminal pro-brain natriuretic peptide; GDF8: growth differentiation factor 8; OR: odds ratio; CI: confidence interval.

4. Discussion

In our study, GDF8 levels were shown to be negatively associated with older age, and positively with female sex; these results corroborate existing clinical data. For instance, previous studies have shown that GDF8 levels were highest in men in their 20s and statistically declined throughout subsequent decades [13]. Indeed, in men, serum GDF8 increases slightly with age until 57 years and then decreases [14]. In both the "Heart and Soul" and the HUNT3 cohorts, GDF11/8 levels were lower in older participants [15]. In patients aged 60 years and older, a recent study has shown that women had higher GDF8 plasma levels than men and that the circulating plasma GDF8 was negatively associated with muscle function [16].

In the present work, we also observed correlations between GDF8 levels and traditional cardiovascular risk factors such as diabetes, increased systolic and diastolic blood pressure, increased LDL cholesterol and CRP. The role of GDF8 in regulating tissue glucose uptake has been documented both in experimental [17] and clinical studies [18,19]. Blocked GDF8 expression in mice resulted in increased insulin signaling and better insulin sensitivity in skeletal muscle [20]. Therefore, in patients with insulin resistance, GDF8 inactivation is a potential target for the prevention of risk factors associated with the development of ischemic cardiovascular diseases. The clinical data are sparse for hypertension, cholesterol levels and CRP, but one experimental study has demonstrated that GDF8 deletion in a mouse model of metabolic syndrome resulted in increased muscle mass and prevented an increase in blood pressure [21]. Inactivation of GDF8 in in *Ldlr-/-* mice was shown to protect against the development of insulin resistance, proatherogenic dyslipidemia and aortic atherogenesis [22].

The main findings of the present study involve the association of GDF8 with the markers of AMI severity such as ST-elevation myocardial infarction (STEMI), occurrence of complicating heart failure, GRACE risk score, CK peak, NT-proBNP, and troponin levels. In multivariable analysis, log GDF8 was associated with the prediction of troponin I peak, even after adjustment for age. Moreover, among patients with the highest GDF8 levels (>2800 ng/L), the risk of developing in-hospital VT/VF was higher. To our knowledge, this is the first time that GDF8 has been associated with clinical severity in the acute phase of MI. Previous studies in sheep found that GDF8 was expressed in the fetal and adult heart and was localized in the cardiomyocytes and Purkinje fibers [7]. Furthermore, after experimental myocardial infarction, GDF8 expression was upregulated in the cardiomyocytes surrounding the infarcted zone. Studies performed in mice have shown that GDF8 was upregulated in the heart as early as 10 min after coronary artery ligation, reaching peak expression in tissue between 24 h and 1 month following the acute event. In the serum of the mice, GDF8 levels also promptly and steadily increased [10]. Indeed, elevated circulating levels of GDF8 have been observed in several types of serious myocardial diseases such as anthracycline-induced cardiotoxicity [23] and in experimental [24–26] and clinical heart failure [8,9,27]. In particular, serum GDF8 levels were shown to have predictive value for the severity of chronic heart failure and to be a predictor of adverse prognosis in these patients [27]. In myocardial infarction, both the destruction of the cardiac tissue and the up-regulation of its expression may account for the elevated levels found in serum. Consequently, it has been suggested that the heart could function as an endocrine organ promoting skeletal or myocardial muscle wasting, inducing cardiac muscle weakness [25]. In fact, the absence of GDF8 in GDF8-deficient mice subjected to myocardial infarction seemed to protect the heart, possibly by limiting the extent of fibrosis and improving survival [28]. We suggest here that during the course of AMI, GDF8 is produced and released by the cardiac tissue proportionally to the severity of the ischemia. GDF levels may therefore be strongly associated with peak troponin, but also with the occurrence of complications such as heart failure or ventricular arrhythmias. Of course, the estimation of myocardial damage is complex and might not be only reflected by one circulating factor such as GDF8 and/or troponin peak. Hemodynamic measurements, expansion index, and other exams as such as magnetic resonance imaging are necessary to quantify the extent of the infarct, the myocardial tissue loss and fibrosis after AMI [29,30]. Further studies should be conducted to evaluate whether GDF8 could be a predictor of poor outcomes after AMI, in particular those related to skeletal or myocardial muscle wasting.

5. Study Limitations

The first limitation of our study is the small number of patients who developed VT/VF ($n = 10$), limiting statistical power. The second limitation is the monocentric nature of the study with a subsequent selection bias. However, the strong association between GDF8 and the prediction of troponin I peak was supported by results of univariate regression analysis ($p < 0.001$) and the enduring significance after adjustment for determinants ($p < 0.001$). In future, these preliminary results need to be confirmed in larger studies.

6. Conclusions

To conclude, our original results suggest that GDF8 levels could reflect the extent of myocardial damage during AMI, similar to peak troponin I, which is currently used to estimate infarct size. Further studies are needed to elucidate the underlying mechanisms linking the GDF8 cytokine with troponin I levels.

Author Contributions: Conceptualization, C.V., L.R. and M.Z.; Methodology, C.V. and M.Z.; Validation, M.Z.; Formal analysis, A.M. and M.M.; Investigation, Y.C., A.M., F.B. and L.T.; Resources, L.T. and F.B.; Writing—original draft preparation, A.M., C.V., L.R. and M.Z.; writing—review and editing, C.V., L.R. and M.Z.; Supervision, C.V.; Project administration, C.V.; Funding acquisition, C.V., M.Z. and Y.C. All authors have read and agreed to the published version of the manuscript.

Acknowledgments: The authors thank Suzanne Rankin for English revision of the manuscript, Ivan Porcherot and Morgane Laine for providing technical assistance.

References

1. Wollert, K.C.; Kempf, T.; Wallentin, L. Growth Differentiation Factor 15 as a Biomarker in Cardiovascular Disease. *Clin Chem.* **2017**, *63*, 140–151. [CrossRef] [PubMed]
2. Walker, R.G.; Poggioli, T.; Katsimpardi, L.; Buchanan, S.M.; Oh, J.; Wattrus, S.; Heidecker, B.; Fong, Y.W.; Rubin, L.L.; Ganz, P.; et al. Biochemistry and Biology of GDF11 and Myostatin: Similarities, Differences, and Questions for Future Investigation. *Circ. Res.* **2016**, *118*, 1125–1141. [CrossRef] [PubMed]
3. Rochette, L.; Zeller, M.; Cottin, Y.; Vergely, C. Growth and differentiation factor 11 (GDF11): Functions in the regulation of erythropoiesis and cardiac regeneration. *Pharmacol. Ther.* **2015**, *156*, 26–33. [CrossRef] [PubMed]
4. Argiles, J.M.; Orpi, M.; Busquets, S.; Lopez-Soriano, F.J. Myostatin: More than just a regulator of muscle mass. *Drug Discov. Today* **2012**, *17*, 702–709. [CrossRef]
5. McPherron, A.C.; Lee, S.J. Double muscling in cattle due to mutations in the myostatin gene. *Proc. Natl. Acad. Sci. USA* **1997**, *94*, 12457–12461. [CrossRef]
6. Mosher, D.S.; Quignon, P.; Bustamante, C.D.; Sutter, N.B.; Mellersh, C.S.; Parker, H.G.; Ostrander, E.A. A mutation in the myostatin gene increases muscle mass and enhances racing performance in heterozygote dogs. *PLoS Genet.* **2007**, *3*, e79. [CrossRef]
7. Sharma, M.; Kambadur, R.; Matthews, K.G.; Somers, W.G.; Devlin, G.P.; Conaglen, J.V.; Fowke, P.J.; Bass, J.J. Myostatin, a transforming growth factor-beta superfamily member, is expressed in heart muscle and is upregulated in cardiomyocytes after infarct. *J. Cell Physiol.* **1999**, *180*, 1–9. [CrossRef]
8. George, I.; Bish, L.T.; Kamalakkannan, G.; Petrilli, C.M.; Oz, M.C.; Naka, Y.; Lee Sweeney, H.; Maybaum, S. Myostatin activation in patients with advanced heart failure and after mechanical unloading. *Eur. J. Heart Fail.* **2010**, *12*, 444–453. [CrossRef]
9. Bish, L.T.; George, I.; Maybaum, S.; Yang, J.; Chen, J.M.; Sweeney, H.L. Myostatin is elevated in congenital heart disease and after mechanical unloading. *PLoS ONE* **2011**, *6*, e23818. [CrossRef]

10. Castillero, E.; Akashi, H.; Wang, C.; Najjar, M.; Ji, R.; Kennel, P.J.; Sweeney, H.L.; Schulze, P.C.; George, I. Cardiac myostatin upregulation occurs immediately after myocardial ischemia and is involved in skeletal muscle activation of atrophy. *Biochem. Biophys. Res. Commun.* **2015**, *457*, 106–111. [CrossRef]
11. Zeller, M.; Steg, P.G.; Ravisy, J.; Lorgis, L.; Laurent, Y.; Sicard, P.; Janin-Manificat, L.; Beer, J.C.; Makki, H.; Lagrost, A.C.; et al. Relation between body mass index, waist circumference, and death after acute myocardial infarction. *Circulation* **2008**, *118*, 482–490. [CrossRef] [PubMed]
12. Thygesen, K.; Alpert, J.S.; Jaffe, A.S.; Simoons, M.L.; Chaitman, B.R.; White, H.D. Third universal definition of myocardial infarction. *Circulation* **2012**, *126*, 2020–2035. [CrossRef] [PubMed]
13. Schafer, M.J.; Atkinson, E.J.; Vanderboom, P.M.; Kotajarvi, B.; White, T.A.; Moore, M.M.; Bruce, C.J.; Greason, K.L.; Suri, R.M.; Khosla, S.; et al. Quantification of GDF11 and Myostatin in Human Aging and Cardiovascular Disease. *Cell Metab.* **2016**, *23*, 1207–1215. [CrossRef] [PubMed]
14. Szulc, P.; Schoppet, M.; Goettsch, C.; Rauner, M.; Dschietzig, T.; Chapurlat, R.; Hofbauer, L.C. Endocrine and clinical correlates of myostatin serum concentration in men–the STRAMBO study. *J. Clin. Endocrinol. Metab.* **2012**, *97*, 3700–3708. [CrossRef]
15. Olson, K.A.; Beatty, A.L.; Heidecker, B.; Regan, M.C.; Brody, E.N.; Foreman, T.; Kato, S.; Mehler, R.E.; Singer, B.S.; Hveem, K.; et al. Association of growth differentiation factor 11/8, putative anti-ageing factor, with cardiovascular outcomes and overall mortality in humans: Analysis of the Heart and Soul and HUNT3 cohorts. *Eur. Heart J.* **2015**, *36*, 3426–3434. [CrossRef]
16. Fife, E.; Kostka, J.; Kroc, L.; Guligowska, A.; Piglowska, M.; Soltysik, B.; Kaufman-Szymczyk, A.; Fabianowska-Majewska, K.; Kostka, T. Relationship of muscle function to circulating myostatin, follistatin and GDF11 in older women and men. *BMC Geriatr.* **2018**, *18*, 200. [CrossRef]
17. Zhao, B.; Wall, R.J.; Yang, J. Transgenic expression of myostatin propeptide prevents diet-induced obesity and insulin resistance. *Biochem. Biophys. Res. Commun.* **2005**, *337*, 248–255. [CrossRef]
18. Brandt, C.; Nielsen, A.R.; Fischer, C.P.; Hansen, J.; Pedersen, B.K.; Plomgaard, P. Plasma and muscle myostatin in relation to type 2 diabetes. *PLoS ONE* **2012**, *7*, e37236. [CrossRef]
19. Hittel, D.S.; Berggren, J.R.; Shearer, J.; Boyle, K.; Houmard, J.A. Increased secretion and expression of myostatin in skeletal muscle from extremely obese women. *Diabetes* **2009**, *58*, 30–38. [CrossRef]
20. Zhang, C.; McFarlane, C.; Lokireddy, S.; Bonala, S.; Ge, X.; Masuda, S.; Gluckman, P.D.; Sharma, M.; Kambadur, R. Myostatin-deficient mice exhibit reduced insulin resistance through activating the AMP-activated protein kinase signalling pathway. *Diabetologia* **2011**, *54*, 1491–1501. [CrossRef]
21. Butcher, J.T.; Mintz, J.D.; Larion, S.; Qiu, S.; Ruan, L.; Fulton, D.J.; Stepp, D.W. Increased Muscle Mass Protects Against Hypertension and Renal Injury in Obesity. *J. Am. Heart Assoc.* **2018**, *7*, e009358. [CrossRef] [PubMed]
22. Tu, P.; Bhasin, S.; Hruz, P.W.; Herbst, K.L.; Castellani, L.W.; Hua, N.; Hamilton, J.A.; Guo, W. Genetic disruption of myostatin reduces the development of proatherogenic dyslipidemia and atherogenic lesions in Ldlr null mice. *Diabetes* **2009**, *58*, 1739–1748. [CrossRef] [PubMed]
23. Kesik, V.; Honca, T.; Gulgun, M.; Uysal, B.; Kurt, Y.G.; Cayci, T.; Babacan, O.; Gocgeldi, E.; Korkmazer, N. Myostatin as a Marker for Doxorubicin Induced Cardiac Damage. *Ann. Clin. Lab. Sci.* **2016**, *46*, 26–31. [PubMed]
24. Biesemann, N.; Mendler, L.; Wietelmann, A.; Hermann, S.; Schafers, M.; Kruger, M.; Boettger, T.; Borchardt, T.; Braun, T. Myostatin regulates energy homeostasis in the heart and prevents heart failure. *Circ. Res.* **2014**, *115*, 296–310. [CrossRef]
25. Heineke, J.; Auger-Messier, M.; Xu, J.; Sargent, M.; York, A.; Welle, S.; Molkentin, J.D. Genetic deletion of myostatin from the heart prevents skeletal muscle atrophy in heart failure. *Circulation* **2010**, *121*, 419–425. [CrossRef]
26. Damatto, R.L.; Lima, A.R.; Martinez, P.F.; Cezar, M.D.; Okoshi, K.; Okoshi, M.P. Myocardial myostatin in spontaneously hypertensive rats with heart failure. *Int. J. Cardiol.* **2016**, *215*, 384–387. [CrossRef]
27. Chen, P.; Liu, Z.; Luo, Y.; Chen, L.; Li, S.; Pan, Y.; Lei, X.; Wu, D.; Xu, D. Predictive value of serum myostatin for the severity and clinical outcome of heart failure. *Eur. J. Intern. Med.* **2019**, *64*, 33–40. [CrossRef]
28. Lim, S.; McMahon, C.D.; Matthews, K.G.; Devlin, G.P.; Elston, M.S.; Conaglen, J.V. Absence of Myostatin Improves Cardiac Function Following Myocardial Infarction. *Heart Lung Circ.* **2018**, *27*, 693–701. [CrossRef]

29. Flachskampf, F.A.; Schmid, M.; Rost, C.; Achenbach, S.; DeMaria, A.N.; Daniel, W.G. Cardiac imaging after myocardial infarction. *Eur. Heart J.* **2011**, *32*, 272–283. [CrossRef]
30. Ibanez, B.; James, S.; Agewall, S.; Antunes, M.J.; Bucciarelli-Ducci, C.; Bueno, H.; Caforio, A.L.P.; Crea, F.; Goudevenos, J.A.; Halvorsen, S.; et al. 2017 ESC Guidelines for the management of acute myocardial infarction in patients presenting with ST-segment elevation: The Task Force for the management of acute myocardial infarction in patients presenting with ST-segment elevation of the European Society of Cardiology (ESC). *Eur. Heart J.* **2018**, *39*, 119–177.

10

Expression of the Novel Cardiac Biomarkers sST2, GDF-15, suPAR and H-FABP in HFpEF Patients Compared to ICM, DCM and Controls

Peter Jirak [1,*,†], Rudin Pistulli [2,†], Michael Lichtenauer [1], Bernhard Wernly [1], Vera Paar [1], Lukas J. Motloch [1], Richard Rezar [1], Christian Jung [3], Uta C. Hoppe [1], P. Christian Schulze [4], Daniel Kretzschmar [4], Rüdiger C. Braun-Dullaeus [5] and Tarek Bekfani [5]

[1] Clinic of Internal Medicine II, Department of Cardiology, Paracelsus Medical University of Salzburg, 5020 Salzburg, Austria; m.lichtenauer@salk.at (M.L.); b.wernly@salk.at (B.W.); v.paar@salk.at (V.P.); l.motloch@salk.at (L.J.M.); r.rezar@salk.at (R.R.); u.hoppe@salk.at (U.C.H.)

[2] Division of Vascular Medicine, Department of Cardiology and Angiology, University Hospital Muenster, Albert-Schweitzer-Campus 1, Munster, North Rhine-Westphalia, 48149 Münster, Germany; Rudin.Pistulli@ukmuenster.de

[3] Division of Cardiology, Pulmonology, and Vascular Medicine, Medical Faculty, University Duesseldorf, 40225 Duesseldorf, Germany; Christian.Jung@med.uni-duesseldorf.de

[4] Department of Internal Medicine I, Division of Cardiology, Angiology, Pneumology and Intensive Medical Care, University Hospital Jena, Friedrich Schiller University Jena, 07740 Jena, Germany; Christian.Schulze@med.uni-jena.de (P.C.S.); daniel.kretzschmar@med.uni-jena.de (D.K.)

[5] Department of Internal Medicine I, Division of Cardiology, Angiology and Intensive Medical Care, University Hospital Magdeburg, Otto von Gericke University, Magdeburg, 39120 Magdeburg, Germany; r.braun-dullaeus@med.ovgu.de (R.C.B.-D.); tarek.bekfani@med.ovgu.de (T.B.)

* Correspondence: p.jirak@salk.at

† These authors contributed equally to the paper.

Abstract: Background: Heart failure with preserved ejection fraction (HFpEF) remains an ongoing therapeutic and diagnostic challenge to date. In this study we aimed for an analysis of the diagnostic potential of four novel cardiovascular biomarkers, GDF-15, H-FABP, sST2, and suPAR in HFpEF patients compared to controls as well as ICM, and DCM. Methods: In total, we included 252 stable outpatients and controls (77 DCM, 62 ICM, 18 HFpEF, and 95 controls) in the present study. All patients were in a non-decompensated state and on a stable treatment regimen. Serum samples were obtained and analyzed for GDF-15 (inflammation, remodeling), H-FABP (ischemia and subclinical ischemia), sST2 (inflammation, remodeling) and suPAR (inflammation, remodeling) by means of ELISA. Results: A significant elevation of GDF-15 was found for all heart failure entities compared to controls ($p < 0.005$). Similarly, H-FABP evidenced a significant elevation in all heart failure entities compared to the control group ($p < 0.0001$). Levels of sST2 were significantly elevated in ICM and DCM patients compared to the control group and HFpEF patients ($p < 0.0001$). Regarding suPAR, a significant elevation in ICM and DCM patients compared to the control group ($p < 0.0001$) and HFpEF patients ($p < 0.01$) was observed. An AUC analysis identified H-FABP (0.792, 95% CI 0.713–0.870) and GDF-15 (0.787, 95% CI 0.696–0.878) as paramount diagnostic biomarkers for HFpEF patients. Conclusion: Based on their differences in secretion patterns, novel cardiovascular biomarkers might represent a promising diagnostic tool for HFpEF in the future.

Keywords: HFpEF; heart failure; HFrEF; biomarker; sST2; suPAR; H-FABP; sST2

1. Introduction

With an overall prevalence of 2%, heart failure (HF) represents one of the leading causes of morbidity and mortality in the western world and thus also an important economic factor [1]. About 50% of all heart failure patients suffer from heart failure with preserved ejection fraction (HFpEF). HFpEF is characterized by a deterioration of cardiac relaxation resulting in an impaired diastolic filling of the left ventricle, mainly triggered by arterial hypertension along with obesity and metabolic disorders [2,3]. In contrast to heart failure with reduced ejection fraction (HFrEF), the left ventricular ejection fraction in HFpEF remains preserved [2,3].

The cellular processes involved in the development of HFpEF are heterogeneous. One of the most generally accepted hypotheses is that cellular hypertrophy combined with a reduction in cellular relaxation and an increase in tissue fibrosis could contribute strongly to the development of ventricular stiffening [4,5]. Furthermore, obesity, which is a very frequent co-morbidity of HF, leads to adipose tissue dysfunction along with elevated leptin levels and can trigger an upregulation of aldosterone, leading to sodium retention [6]. In consequence, higher levels of aldosterone trigger a volume expansion leading to increased filling pressures, thereby promoting cardiac remodeling, myocardial hypertrophy and fibrosis [6].

While numerous advancements have been made in the pharmacologic treatment of heart failure with reduced ejection fraction over the last decades (e.g., ARNIs), no evidence-based therapy for HFpEF patients exists to date [3,7]. Despite huge efforts, studies failed to show a significant prognostic benefit of pharmaceutical therapies in HFpEF, with the "PARAGON-Trial" as most prominent example [8]. Accordingly, the prognosis in HFpEF remains poor [9].

In addition to the lack of an evidence-based therapy, the actual diagnosis of HFpEF remains challenging and the precise diagnostic criteria are still matter of ongoing debates [9]. According to the current ESC guidelines, HFpEF is defined as a combination of: (I) Typical signs and symptoms of heart failure, (II) elevated levels of natriuretic peptides, (III) LVEF > 50%, (IV) evidence of diastolic dysfunction and/or structural heart disease (left ventricular hypertrophy or left atrial enlargement) [3]. Given the vague diagnostic criteria, the need for novel and additional diagnostic markers for HFpEF is evident.

In the last years, novel cardiac biomarkers have emerged as promising diagnostic tools for the assessment of different cardiovascular disease entities [10,11]. As a result to the complex pathophysiological background of most cardiovascular diseases, a multi-marker approach was reported as most effective for diagnosis, therapy monitoring and risk prediction due to the incorporation of different pathophysiologic processes covered by each respective marker [10,12].

Among the tested markers in previous studies, H-FABP (myocardial ischemia), sST-2 (myocardial strain and inflammation), GDF-15 (inflammation, remodeling), and suPAR (inflammation, remodeling) proved to be promising tools in achieving an improvement in the diagnosis and prognosis of cardiovascular diseases [13–16]. Accordingly, some of the listed markers are already included in the current guidelines and used in clinical routine [17].

Given the evident need for novel diagnostic tools in HFpEF we aimed for a head-to-head analysis of these four novel cardiovascular biomarkers in patients with heart failure with preserved ejection fraction compared to controls. Additionally, as the aforementioned markers are well studied in HFrEF patients, we aimed for a head-to-head analysis of HFpEF and HFrEF patients to put our findings into reference.

2. Experimental Section

The present study was conducted in accordance with the Universal Declaration of Helsinki and was approved by the local ethics committee at the University Hospital Jena, Germany. In total, we included 252 patients in this retrospective single-center study. Seventy-seven patients diagnosed with DCM, 62 patients with ICM, and 18 patients diagnosed with HFpEF were enrolled. Additionally, a control group of 95 patients was included. In these patients, coronary artery disease was excluded by coronary angiography. During visits in the outpatient ward, serum samples of all patients were obtained and analyzed for GDF-15, H-FABP, sST2, and suPAR.

The diagnosis of ICM, DCM and HFpEF was made according to the current guidelines of the European Society of Cardiology [3]. Clinical examination, assessment of medical history, laboratory analysis as well as transthoracic echocardiography was performed in all patients in the outpatient ward. Additionally, ICM and DCM patients underwent coronary angiography for diagnosis/exclusion of coronary artery disease. Controls also underwent coronary angiography because of suspected coronary artery disease and a relevant risk profile (hypertension, smoking etc.) and evidenced a rule out. All patients were in a stable, non-decompensated state at the timepoint of inclusion and clinical examination and were on a stable treatment regimen. Decompensated HF patients were not enrolled in this study. All examinations were performed by an experienced heart failure specialist. Laboratory analysis was conducted in all patients after informed consent. Serum samples were analyzed by means of ELISA and were stored at −80°C until measurements were conducted. Exclusion criteria were defined as: (I) Age under 18 years, (II) acute or chronic infections, (III) malignancies, (IV) advanced stages of renal failure (as indicated by a glomerular filtration rate less than 30 mL/min), (V) decompensated heart failure, (VI) hyperthyroidism, (VII) medication with immunosuppressive agents, and (VIII) recent acute coronary syndrome. For HFpEF patients a glomerular filtration rate under 60 ml/min was an exclusion criterion to rule out a potential cardiorenal confounder in this cohort.

2.1. Laboratory Analysis

Routine analysis of blood samples was performed at the Department of Clinical Chemistry (University Hospital Jena). The analyses comprised high-density lipoprotein (HDL; mmol/L), low density, lipoprotein (LDL; mmol/L), triglycerides (mmol/L), and C-reactive protein (CRP, mg/L) and hematological parameters. The glomerular filtration rate was calculated according to the CKD-EPI equation. Serum levels of sST2, GDF-15, suPAR, and H-FABP were measured using commercially available ELISA kits (DuoSet ELISA, DY523B, DY957, DY807, DY1678, and DFTA00, R&D Systems, Minneapolis, Minnesota, USA) in accordance with the instructions provided by R&D. ELISA analyses were performed at room temperature. In brief, 96-well plates were coated with the provided capture antibody according to the certificate of analysis and manufacturer's instructions. The multiwell plates were incubated overnight on a horizontal shaker. The next day, plates were washed using 0.5% Tween 20 (Carl Roth, Karlsruhe, Germany) in 1× phosphate buffered saline (PBS) and were then blocked with 1% bovine serum albumin (BSA; Carl Roth, Karlsruhe, Germany) in 1× PBS for one hour. After a further washing step, serum and the appropriate standard concentrations for sample quantification were added onto the wells and incubated for two hours. Again, the plate was washed and the provided biotin-labelled detection antibody was added to each well, followed by an incubation of another two hours. Thereafter, ELISA plates were washed again, before a provided streptavidin-horseradish-peroxidase (HRP) solution was added and incubated for 20 min. After a final washing step, the addition of the substrate tetramethylbenzidine (TMB; Sigma Aldrich, St. Louis, Missouri, USA) resulted in a blue color reaction which was stopped by adding 2 N sulfuric acid (H_2SO_4; Sigma Aldrich, St. Louis, Missouri, USA), changing the color to yellow. Optical density (OD) was measured at 450 nm on an ELISA microplate reader (iMark Microplate Absorbance Reader, Bio-Rad Laboratories, Wien Austria).

2.2. Statistical Analysis

Statistical analysis was performed using GraphPad-Prism software (GraphPad-Software, La Jolla, CA, USA), SPSS (22.0, SPSS Inc., Chicago, IL, USA) and MedCalc (19.1.3 MedCalc Software bv, Ostend, Belgium). The Kolmogorov-Smirnov test was used to assess normal distribution of parameters in the study population. Demographic parameters were compared by using ANOVA. Normally distributed parameters are given as mean + standard deviation. As biomarker concentrations were not normally distributed, they are given as median and inter-quartile range. Median values were compared using the Mann–Whitney-U test. Correlation analysis was performed using Spearman's rank-coefficient. Correction for multiple comparison was conducted using the Bonferroni–Holm method. ROC analysis was performed and AUCs were compared according to DeLong [18]. A $p < 0.05$ was considered as statistically significant.

3. Results

3.1. Baseline Characteristics

In total, the present study included 252 patients with a mean age of 62.6 years. While the distribution of male and female patients was quite balanced in HFpEF patients and controls, the HFrEF collective showed a significant higher number of male patients ($p < 0.001$). HFpEF patients were considerably older, compared to ICM, DCM, and controls ($p < 0.001$). Ejection fraction was significantly higher in patients with HFpEF compared to ICM and DCM patients ($p < 0.001$). BNP levels were significantly elevated in ICM ($p < 0.001$) and DCM ($p < 0.001$) compared to controls and HFpEF, while renal function was significantly impaired in the HFrEF collective ($p < 0.001$).

Regarding comorbidities, the rates of diabetes were evenly distributed in all three heart failure entities. Hypertension was present in similar rates in controls, HFpEF and ICM patients, with DCM patients showing significantly lower rates ($p < 0.001$). The rates of atrial fibrillation were significantly increased in HFpEF patients compared to all other entities ($p < 0.001$). With regards to medical therapy, HFrEF patients evidenced significantly higher rates beta-blockers, ACE-inhibitors and diuretics compared to HFpEF and controls ($p < 0.001$). Similarly, the rates of aldosterone antagonists were also higher in the HFrEF collective compared to HFpEF and controls ($p < 0.001$). Baseline characteristics are depicted in Tables 1 and 2

Table 1. Baseline Characteristics.

	Controls		HFpEF		ICM		DCM		Total		*p*-Value
	Mean	SD	Mean	SD	Mean	SD	Mean	SD	Mean	SD	
Age (y)	63.56	9.25	70.94	6.49	65.12	11.16	57.10	10.73	62.65	10.73	<0.0001
Height (m)	1.68	0.09	1.69	0.09	1.74	0.09	1.75	0.09	1.72	0.09	<0.0001
Weight (kg)	77.68	17.22	81.86	12.82	76.66	25.58	89.09	18.74	81.06	20.27	0.001
BMI	27.22	5.71	28.68	4.63	28.08	4.37	29.02	5.24	28.30	5.08	0.334
LVEF (%)	65.93	8.63	59.75	9.85	37.42	12.93	35.32	11.87	48.04	17.92	<0.0001
BNP (pg/mL)	73.74	86.08	165.22	162.54	435.75	488.22	684.64	866.83	430,10	646.27	<0.0001
Creatinine (μmol/L)	74.29	15.67	85.06	25.96	108.19	39.05	98.35	31.15	89.14	30.44	<0.0001
GFR (mL/min)	83.62	13.33	71.08	13.78	66.97	17.61	74.69	24.96	75.75	17.68	0.084
CRP (mg/L)	2.28	2.98	5.58	8.87	4.33	4.20	7.55	14.29	4.55	9.19	0.005
Hb (mmol/L)	8.79	0.56	8.16	0.87	8.51	0.94	8.92	0.91	8.67	0.91	0.005
LDL (mmol/L)	3.47	0.94	2.76	1.40	2.23	0.89	2.88	1.07	3.10	1.10	<0.0001
HDL (mmol/L)	1.49	0.41	1.29	0.35	0.99	0.22	1.15	0.31	1.32	0.40	<0.0001

Table 2. Concomitant diseases and medication.

	Controls	HFpEF	ICM	DCM	Total	*p*-Value
Sex (male)	36%	44%	86%	77%	61%	<0.0001
Diabetes	15%	39%	36%	38%	29%	0.003
Hypertension	77%	89%	78%	50%	70%	<0.001
Atrial Fibrillation	5%	50%	3%	18%	15%	<0.0001
Beta Blockers	39%	72%	100%	99%	76%	<0.0001
ACE-Inhibitors	59%	72%	96%	96%	82%	<0.0001
Loop-Diuretics	30%	56%	79%	91%	64%	<0.0001
MRA	2%	19%	61%	68%	43%	<0.0001

3.2. Biomarkers

GDF-15, evidenced a significant elevation for all heart failure entities compared to controls ($p < 0.005$) with no significant differences between the respective groups. For H-FABP, a significant elevation in all heart failure entities was observed compared to the control group ($p < 0.0001$). However, H-FABP levels were significantly higher in ICM and DCM patients compared to HFpEF ($p < 0.0001$). Levels of sST2 were significantly higher in ICM and DCM patients than in the control group ($p < 0.0001$). No significant differences between HFpEF patients and the control group were observed for sST2. Similar to sST2, levels of suPAR were significantly elevated in ICM and DCM patients compared to the control group ($p < 0.0001$) and HFpEF patients ($p < 0.01$). No significant differences between HFpEF patients and controls were observed. Biomarker levels are depicted in Table 3, comparisons of biomarker levels are depicted in Figure 1. In addition, a correction for multiple comparison was conducted by using the Bonferroni–Holm method. After correction for multiple testing, we found no changes in the statistical significance of our findings except for GDF-15 levels in controls vs. DCM. Correlation analysis of baseline characteristics and biomarkers of are given in the supplement Table S1. Results after multiple testing are given in the supplement Table S2. All biomarkers evidenced a significant correlation with BNP, Creatinine and CRP as well as an inverse correlation with ejection fraction.

Table 3. Levels of biomarkers.

	Controls		HFpEF		ICM		DCM	
	Median	**Interquartile Range**	**Median**	**Interquartile Range**	**Median**	**Interquartile Range**	**Median**	**Interquartile Range**
sST2 (pg/mL)	4999.00	2970.00	4318.00	2332.00	7869.00	5191.00	7010.00	5892.00
GDF-15 (pg/mL)	561.20	276.60	838.00	415.90	720.50	565.60	639.10	595.10
H-FABP (ng/mL)	0.00	0.60	0.82	0.53	1.66	3.59	1.94	1.83
suPAR (pg/mL)	2414.00	1280.00	2279.00	1753.00	3576.00	2567.00	3280.00	2349.00

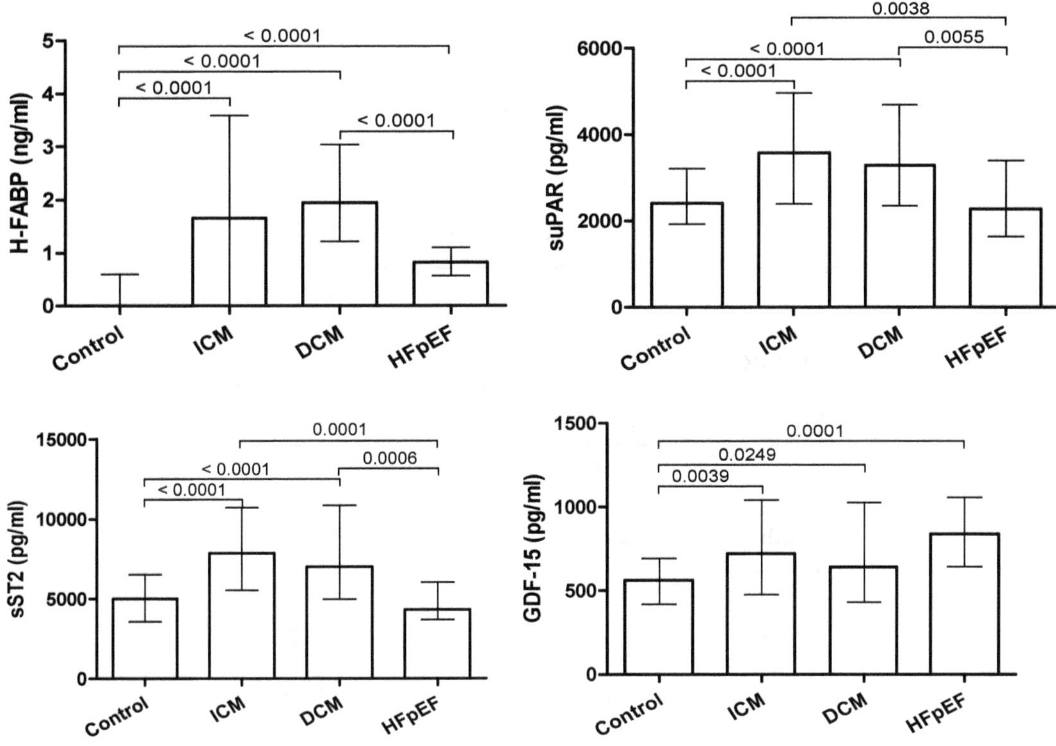

Figure 1. Comparison of biomarker levels between control group, HFpEF, ICM, and DCM patients (median + IQR).

3.3. *AUC-Analysis*

To evaluate the diagnostic potential of tested biomarkers in HFpEF, a ROC analysis was performed (Figure 2), and AUC was calculated for sST2, suPAR, GDF-15 and H-FABP plasma levels as diagnostic indicators for HFpEF patients. Our analysis identified H-FABP (0.792, 95% CI 0.713–0.870) and GDF-15 (0.787, 95% CI 0.696–0.878) as paramount diagnostic biom markers. In comparison, sST2 (0.567, 95%CI

0.294–0.572) and suPAR (0.543, 95% CI 0.298–0.616) evidenced a considerably lower AUC. The detailed results are depicted in Table 4. Additionally, we conducted a pairwise comparison of ROC curves according to DeLong et al. [18]. Here GDF-15 and H-FABP showed significantly higher AUCs compared to sST2 and suPAR respectively, while no significant difference between GDF-15 and H-FABP was observed. The detailed results are depicted in Table 5.

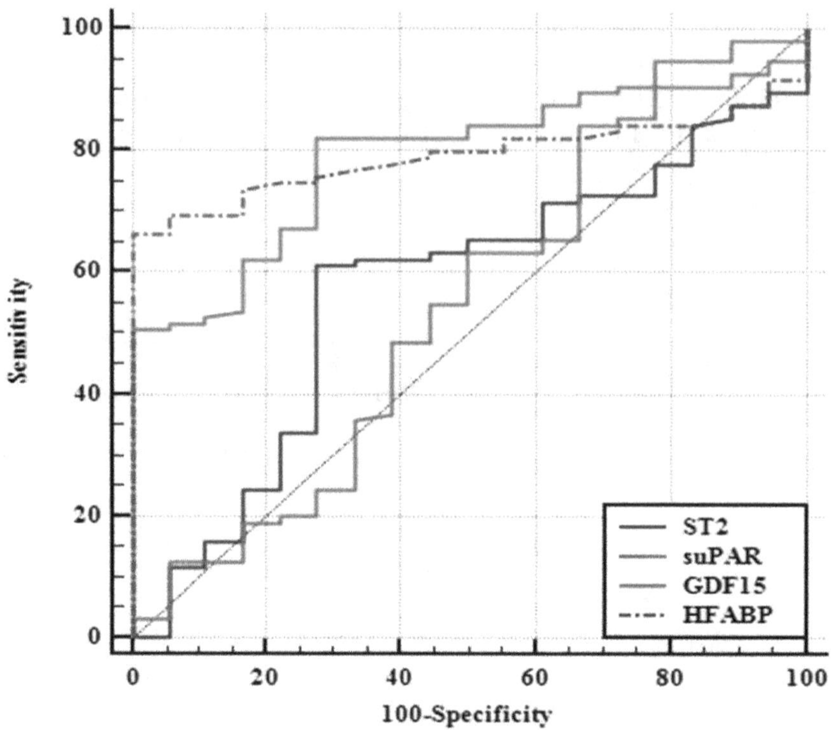

Figure 2. Receiver operating curve.

Table 4. AUC-Analysis.

Variable	AUC	SE [a]	95% CI [b]
ST2	0.567	0.0725	0.470 to 0.660
suPAR	0.543	0.0829	0.447 to 0.637
GDF15	0.787	0.0469	0.700 to 0.859
HFABP	0.792	0.0401	0.705 to 0.862

[a] DeLong et al., 1988; [b] Binomial exact

Table 5. Pairwise comparison of ROC curves.

ST2 ~ suPAR	
Difference between areas	0.0240
Standard Error [a]	0.112
95% Confidence Interval	−0.196 to 0.244
Z statistic	0.214
Significance level	$p = 0.8307$
ST2 ~ GDF15	
Difference between areas	0.220
Standard Error [a]	0.0999
95% Confidence Interval	0.0247 to 0.416
Z statistic	2.207
Significance level	$p = 0.0273$

Table 5. *Cont.*

ST2 ~ HFABP	
Difference between areas	0.225
Standard Error [a]	0.0830
95% Confidence Interval	0.0621 to 0.388
Z statistic	2.708
Significance level	$p = 0.0068$
suPAR ~ GDF15	
Difference between areas	0.244
Standard Error [a]	0.0996
95% Confidence Interval	0.0492 to 0.440
Z statistic	2.453
Significance level	$p = 0.0141$
suPAR ~ HFABP	
Difference between areas	0.249
Standard Error [a]	0.0983
95% Confidence Interval	0.0562 to 0.442
Z statistic	2.531
Significance level	$p = 0.0114$
GDF15 ~ HFABP	
Difference between areas	0.00439
Standard Error [a]	0.0563
95% Confidence Interval	−0.106 to 0.115
Z statistic	0.0779
Significance level	$p = 0.9379$

[a] DeLong et al., 1988.

4. Discussion

Despite the growing awareness, HFpEF remains a diagnostic and clinical challenge to date. This is partially related to its complex pathophysiology [9]. Given the increasing prevalence of HFpEF and the high rates of misdiagnosis, the need for new diagnostic tools is evident [5]. Accordingly, we aimed for a head-to-head analysis of four novel cardiovascular biomarkers and their diagnostic benefit in patients with HFpEF compared to controls to address this evident gap.

Regarding baseline characteristics we observed significant differences between the respective patient collectives. HFpEF patients were the oldest subgroup in our study, a finding that is typical for this disease entity and also matches former studies. A slow progression of myocardial fibrosis and remodeling with gradual diastolic impairment might explain the delayed onset of symptoms and consequently the higher age. Additionally, ICM and DCM patients evidenced worse renal function as well as decreased ejection fraction and significantly elevated BNP levels compared to HFpEF and controls. Moreover, HFpEF patients evidenced lower rates of a standard heart failure therapy, a finding which must be mainly attributed to the lack of an evidence-based therapy for HFpEF patients.

With regards to levels of GDF-15, a significant elevation was present in all three types of heart failure compared to controls. HFpEF patients provided the highest levels in the study collective, however without significant differences between HFpEF in comparison to HFrEF patients. While the detailed mechanisms involved in the GDF-15 pathway are not yet fully understood, it seems to be involved in the regulation of apoptosis, cell repair, and cell growth [15,19]. Accordingly, latest studies have also demonstrated a correlation between GDF-15 and atrial and myocardial fibrosis along with a prognostic impact in cardiovascular disease [20,21]. Additionally, GDF-15 is also involved in the regulatory processes of inflammatory pathways [22]. GDF-15 levels were shown to be significantly elevated in HFrEF in former studies [10]. However, the finding of an increase in GDF-15 in HFpEF patients represents a new aspect. The elevation might be attributed to the progressive myocardial fibrosis and remodeling involved in this disease entity, which could act as a trigger for the secretion of GDF-15. As GDF-15 has shown a significant prognostic impact in HFrEF patients, a similar prognostic value can be assumed for HFpEF patients. As potential surrogate for fibrosis burden, GDF-15 might also act as a monitoring parameter for HFpEF patients in the future.

H-FABP represents a highly sensitive marker for myocardial ischemia [23]. We observed a significant increase in all three heart failure entities. For HFrEF patients, an increase in H-FABP was reported in earlier studies and subclinical myocardial ischemia was proposed as the most probable cause for this finding [10]. Interestingly, based on our results it seems that subclinical ischemia is also present in HFpEF patients. A possible explanation might be a relative shortage in myocardial oxygen supply, based on various processes such as increased wall thickness of the left ventricle in this group of patients. Above all, due to the impaired ventricular filling, a relative shortage in blood supply is present [4]. Moreover, ventricular hypertrophy primarily triggered by arterial hypertension might add to this shortage [4]. Nevertheless, former studies have also shown a considerable prevalence of storage diseases such as amyloidosis and Morbus Fabry resulting in HFpEF [24]. Additionally, also an impairment in coronary microcirculation by means of coronary microvascular endothelial inflammation increasing resting tension through a reduction in nitric oxide bioavailability, cyclic guanosine monophosphate content and protein kinase G (PKG) activity found in HFpEF patients contributes to a shortage in myocardial oxygen supply [25]. Accordingly, based on these processes, H-FABP might prove a promising tool in the diagnosis and controlling the success of treatment of HFpEF patients, quantitating the amount of subclinical ischemia.

Regarding levels of sST2 we found a significant increase in ICM and DCM patients compared to controls and HFpEF, while no significant difference between HFpEF patients and the control group was observed. There are two isoforms of ST2, which both act as receptor to Interleukin-33: The membrane bound ST2L receptor responsible for potential cardioprotective effects, mediated trough IL-33 and the soluble ST2, which acts as a decoy receptor for IL-33 [26]. Due to its role as decoy receptor for the cardioprotective IL-33, sST2 constitutes a marker of increased cardiac strain and cardiac fibrosis and was also reported to be elevated in inflammatory diseases [26,27]. Moreover, studies have shown increased levels and a prognostic relevance of sST2 in HFrEF and acute coronary syndrome [14]. Accordingly, our findings regarding elevated concentrations of sST2 in ICM and DCM patients are consistent with former studies. However, contrary to our expectations, HFpEF patients evidenced low levels of sST2 similar to the control group. This finding also matches former studies, which reported lower levels of sST2 in HFpEF compared to HFrEF [28]. Further and bigger studies are required to verify these findings and help in explaining the underlying mechanisms of these results. Nevertheless, the process of fibrosis itself represents an important prognostic factor also for HFpEF patients [29]. Thus, despite the low levels, sST2 could potentially serve as monitoring parameter in HFpEF analogical to its application HFrEF patients due to the representation of fibrosis progression.

Similar to our findings on sST2, we found significantly elevated levels of suPAR in ICM and DCM patients compared to controls and HFpEF, while again no significant differences were observed between HFpEF patients and controls. The membrane bound uPAR is mainly expressed on the cell membrane of immunocompetent cells [30]. The soluble form (suPAR) is created through the cleavage and release of uPAR [30]. Correspondingly, suPAR represents a marker of inflammation and immune system activity [30,31]. A significant correlation of suPAR with myocardial infarction and HFrEF has been demonstrated [10,11]. The finding of increased suPAR levels in ICM and DCM patients might be mainly explained by a higher prevalence of inflammatory processes present in HFrEF, also triggered by further concomitant diseases. Further, especially larger studies should be performed to scrutinize for an explanation of these findings. To further analyze the diagnostic implications of biomarkers in HFpEF patients, we conducted an AUC analysis. Here we found considerably high values for GDF-15 and H-FABP in contrast to sST2 and suPAR. Additionally, to further evaluate the diagnostic potential of biomarkers in HFpEF patients, we conducted a pairwise comparison of ROCs. This further confirmed our previous findings of H-FABP and GDF-15 constituting paramount diagnostic markers for HFpEF. In contrast, sST2 and suPAR did not seem to have a major diagnostic benefit (see Table 2). Accordingly, with regards to HFpEF patients, GDF-15 and H-FABP represent the most promising markers for the future.

All biomarkers included in our study evidenced a significant correlation with creatinine, BNP and CRP as well as an inverse correlation with ejection fraction. Most importantly, the highly significant correlation with BNP and ejection fraction emphasizes their great potential as heart failure biomarkers. However, contrary to BNP, which is mainly secreted by cardiomyocytes in response to volume increase, novel biomarkers are involved in numerous different pathophysiologic processes, thus providing additive information to natriuretic peptides. These processes comprise subclinical ischemia and ischemic events (H-FABP) as well as cardiovascular remodeling and inflammatory processes (sST2, GDF-15 and suPAR) [11,12]. Since all these processes represent key factors in the development and progression of heart failure, novel biomarkers offer a promising opportunity to assess the impact of comorbidities on this regard [3,4]. Correspondingly, the involvement of novel biomarkers in inflammatory processes was also observed in our study, reflected by a significant correlation of all markers with CRP. In addition to novel biomarkers tested in our project, latest studies also proposed an analysis of micro-RNA expression patterns as a novel diagnostic approach in heart failure [32–34]. On this regard, De Rosa et al. could show, that transcoronary concentration gradients of circulating microRNAs could help to distinguish between different heart failure entities [33]. Similar to biomarkers in our study, circulating and exosomal micro-RNAs were also shown to correlate with clinical parameters such as left ventricular function in former studies [32,34]. In consequence, micro-RNA analysis might offer a great diagnostic benefit in the assessment of heart failure in the future. Moreover, micro-RNAs were also shown to provide diagnostic potential in other cardiovascular diseases as for example coronary artery disease and myocardial infarction [32,34]. However, while standardized testing kits for a clinical application of novel biomarkers are already available and their application is also represented in current guidelines, the diagnostic application of micro-RNA testing has yet to be implemented in clinical practice.

With regards to our findings, suggestions on the future role of H-FABP and GDF-15 in HFpEF are highly speculative due to the hypothesis generating character of our study. Nevertheless, since established testing kits are already available, their use in addition to already established markers such as BNP might be a useful approach for the future. Especially with regards to the pathophysiology in HFpEF, a combination of natriuretic peptides and novel markers seems reasonable, in order to target the different processes involved in this disease [9,19,23]. Taken together, novel biomarkers represent a promising diagnostic approach in HFpEF patients. Based on their expression patterns, they reflect different pathophysiological processes relevant in this disease entity and thus might enable a more precise diagnosis of HFpEF in the future.

5. Conclusions

In summary, novel cardiovascular biomarkers provide a considerable potential to add to the diagnostic process in HFpEF patients. While sST2 and suPAR did not show a relevant dynamic in HFpEF patients compared to controls, a significant difference was evident for H-FABP and GDF-15. These findings point towards a relevant role of subclinical ischemia in HFpEF patients and offer a new aspect in this complex pathophysiology. The increase in GDF-15 might be mainly induced by myocardial remodeling and fibrosis. Thus, GDF-15 could also offer a prognostic benefit in the future. However, cardiac biomarkers showed a lower overall expression in HFpEF patients compared to other heart failure entities, emphasizing the diagnostic challenges in HFpEF. Nevertheless, by combining the information of different pathophysiological processes by means of a multi-marker approach, novel biomarkers might be very useful in the identification of HFpEF patients in the future.

6. Limitations

The most important limitation of our study is the small sample size of the HFpEF cohort involved. This of course markedly limits the results of the current analyses. Moreover, the diagnostic criteria for HFpEF is a matter of ongoing debate and represents a clinical challenge as already mentioned above. Accordingly, the findings of the study must be interpreted with care. Additionally, the single-center and retrospective character must be taken into account. As no follow-up was performed, the dynamic of biomarkers in the progression of heart failure cannot be reflected. Moreover, our study does not include a comparison with already established markers as for example BNP. In consequence, direct comparison is limited. Despite the limitations mentioned above, the present study points out the potential benefits and advantages of the application of novel biomarkers in the diagnosis of heart failure and HFpEF. As our study suggests a diagnostic benefit in HFpEF patients, our results give rise to further investigation.

Author Contributions: Conceptualization: All authors, Methodology: P.J., M.L., B.W., V.P., T.B.; software, P.J., B.W., V.P., M.L.; validation, P.J., L.J.M., R.R., U.C.H.; formal analysis, P.J., B.W.; investigation, C.J., D.K., R.P.; resources, R.C.B.-D., T.B., P.C.S., D.K.; data curation, M.L., T.B., P.J., P.C.S., C.J., R.P.; writing—original draft preparation, P.J., M.L., T.B.; writing—review and editing, P.J., M.L., T.B., R.C.B.-D., R.P., R.R., L.J.M., Christian Jung; visualization, M.L., B.W.; supervision, M.L., T.B., P.C.S., C.J., U.C.H.; project administration, P.J., T.B.; All authors have read and agreed to the published version of the manuscript.

Acknowledgments: We want to thank Fitore Marmullaku for performing assays and analyses in the laboratory.

Abbreviations

AUC	area under the curve
BMI	body mass index
BNP	brain natriuretic peptide
CKD-EPI	Chronic Kidney Disease Epidemiology Collaboration
CRP	C-reactive protein
DCM	dilative cardiomyopathy
ESC	European society of cardiology
ELISA	enzyme-linked immunosorbent assay
GDF-15	growth differentiation factor-15
GFR	glomerular filtration rate
Hb	haemoglobin
H-FABP	heart-type fatty acid binding protein
HFpEF	heart failure with preserved ejection fraction
HFrEF	heart failure with reduced ejection fraction
HDL	high density lipoprotein
ICM	ischemic cardiomyopathy
IL-33	interleukin 33
LDL	low density lipoprotein
LVEF	left ventricular ejection fraction
MRA	mineralocorticoid receptor antagonist
NYHA	New York heart association
PKG	protein kinase G
ROC	receiver operating curve
sST2	soluble suppression of tumorigenicity 2
suPAR	soluble urokinase-type plasminogen activator receptor

References

1. Bleumink, G.S.; Knetsch, A.M.; Sturkenboom, M.C.J.M.; Straus, S.M.J.M.; Hofman, A.; Deckers, J.W.; Witteman, J.C.M.; Stricker, B.H.C. Quantifying the heart failure epidemic: Prevalence, incidence rate, lifetime risk and prognosis of heart failure The Rotterdam Study. *Eur. Heart J.* **2004**, *25*, 1614–1619. [CrossRef] [PubMed]
2. Redfield, M.M. Heart Failure with Preserved Ejection Fraction. *N. Engl. J. Med.* **2017**, *376*, 897. [CrossRef] [PubMed]
3. Ponikowski, P.; Voors, A.A.; Anker, S.D.; Bueno, H.; Cleland, J.G.F.; Coats, A.J.S.; Falk, V.; González-Juanatey, J.R.; Harjola, V.P.; Jankowska, E.A.; et al. 2016 ESC Guidelines for the diagnosis and treatment of acute and chronic heart failure: The Task Force for the diagnosis and treatment of acute and chronic heart failure of the European Society of Cardiology (ESC). Developed with the special contribution of the Heart Failure Association (HFA) of the ESC. *Eur. J. Heart Fail.* **2016**, *18*, 891–975. [PubMed]
4. Borlaug, B.A. The pathophysiology of heart failure with preserved ejection fraction. *Nat. Rev. Cardiol.* **2014**, *11*, 507–515. [CrossRef]
5. Gevaert, A.B.; Boen, J.R.A.; Segers, V.F.; van Craenenbroeck, E.M. Heart Failure With Preserved Ejection Fraction: A Review of Cardiac and Noncardiac Pathophysiology. *Front. Physiol.* **2019**, *10*, 638. [CrossRef]
6. Packer, M. Leptin-Aldosterone-Neprilysin Axis: Identification of Its Distinctive Role in the Pathogenesis of the Three Phenotypes of Heart Failure in People with Obesity. *Circulation* **2018**, *137*, 1614–1631. [CrossRef]
7. McMurray, J.J.; Packer, M.; Desai, A.S.; Gong, J.; Lefkowitz, M.P.; Rizkala, A.R. Angiotensin-neprilysin inhibition versus enalapril in heart failure. *N. Engl. J. Med.* **2014**, *371*, 993–1004. [CrossRef]
8. Solomon, S.D.; McMurray, J.J.V.; Anand, I.S.; Ge, J.; Lam, C.S.P.; Maggioni, A.P.; Martinez, F.; Packer, M.; Pfeffer, M.A.; Pieske, B.; et al. Angiotensin-Neprilysin Inhibition in Heart Failure with Preserved Ejection Fraction. *N. Engl. J. Med.* **2019**, *381*, 1609–1620. [CrossRef]
9. Lekavich, C.L.; Barksdale, D.J.; Neelon, V.; Wu, J. Heart failure preserved ejection fraction (HFpEF): An integrated and strategic review. *Heart Fail. Rev.* **2015**, *20*, 643–653. [CrossRef]
10. Lichtenauer, M.; Jirak, P.; Wernly, B.; Paar, V.; Rohm, I.; Jung, C.; Schernthaner, C.; Kraus, J.; Motloch, L.J.; Yilmaz, A.; et al. A comparative analysis of novel cardiovascular biomarkers in patients with chronic heart failure. *Eur. J. Intern. Med.* **2017**. [CrossRef]
11. Schernthaner, C.; Lichtenauer, M.; Wernly, B.; Paar, V.; Pistulli, R.; Rohm, I.; Jung, C.; Figulla, H.R.; Yilmaz, A.; Cadamuro, J.; et al. Multibiomarker analysis in patients with acute myocardial infarction. *Eur. J. Clin. Investig.* **2017**, *47*, 638–648. [CrossRef] [PubMed]
12. Jirak, P.; Fejzic, D.; Paar, V.; Wernly, B.; Pistulli, R.; Rohm, I.; Jung, C.; Hoppe, U.C.; Schulze, P.C.; Lichtenauer, M.; et al. Influences of Ivabradine treatment on serum levels of cardiac biomarkers sST2, GDF-15, suPAR and H-FABP in patients with chronic heart failure. *Acta Pharmacol. Sin.* **2018**, *39*, 1189–1196. [CrossRef] [PubMed]
13. Otaki, Y.; Watanabe, T.; Kubota, I. Heart-type fatty acid-binding protein in cardiovascular disease: A systemic review. *Clin. Chim. Acta* **2017**, *474*, 44–53. [CrossRef] [PubMed]
14. Pascual-Figal, D.A.; Lax, A.; Perez-Martinez, M.T.; Asensio-Lopez, M.D.; Sanchez-Mas, J. Clinical relevance of sST2 in cardiac diseases. *Clin. Chem. Lab. Med.* **2016**, *54*, 29–35. [CrossRef] [PubMed]
15. Wollert, K.C.; Kempf, T.; Wallentin, L. Growth Differentiation Factor 15 as a Biomarker in Cardiovascular Disease. *Clin. Chem.* **2017**, *63*, 140–151. [CrossRef]
16. Eugen-Olsen, J.; Giamarellos-Bourboulis, E.J. suPAR: The unspecific marker for disease presence, severity and prognosis. *Int. J. Antimicrob. Agents* **2015**, *46*, 31. [CrossRef]
17. Yancy, C.W.; Jessup, M.; Bozkurt, B.; Butler, J.; Casey, D.E.; Colvin, M.M.; Drazner, M.H.; Filippatos, G.S.; Fonarow, G.C.; Givertz, M.M.; et al. 2017 ACC/AHA/HFSA Focused Update of the 2013 ACCF/AHA Guideline for the Management of Heart Failure: A Report of the American College of Cardiology/American Heart Association Task Force on Clinical Practice Guidelines and the Heart Failure Society of America. *J. Am. Coll. Cardiol.* **2017**, *70*, 776–803.
18. DeLong, E.R.; DeLong, D.M.; Clarke-Pearson, D.L. Comparing the areas under two or more correlated receiver operating characteristic curves: A nonparametric approach. *Biometrics* **1988**, *44*, 837–845. [CrossRef]
19. Xu, X.; Li, Z.; Gao, W. Growth differentiation factor 15 in cardiovascular diseases: From bench to bedside. *Biomarkers* **2011**, *16*, 466–475. [CrossRef]

20. Zhou, Y.M.; Li, M.J.; Zhou, Y.L.; Ma, L.; Yi, X. Growth differentiation factor-15 (GDF-15), novel biomarker for assessing atrial fibrosis in patients with atrial fibrillation and rheumatic heart disease. *Int. J. Clin. Exp. Med.* **2015**, *8*, 21201–21207.
21. Farhan, S.; Freynhofer, M.K.; Brozovic, I.; Bruno, V.; Vogel, B.; Tentzeris, I.; Baumgartner-Parzer, S.; Huber, K.; Kautzky-Willer, A. Determinants of growth differentiation factor 15 in patients with stable and acute coronary artery disease. A prospective observational study. *Cardiovasc. Diabetol.* **2016**, *15*, 016–0375. [CrossRef]
22. Adela, R.; Banerjee, S.K. GDF-15 as a Target and Biomarker for Diabetes and Cardiovascular Diseases: A Translational Prospective. *J. Diabetes Res.* **2015**, *490842*, 27. [CrossRef]
23. Niizeki, T.; Takeishi, Y.; Arimoto, T.; Takabatake, N.; Nozaki, N.; Hirono, O.; Watanabe, T.; Nitobe, J.; Harada, M.; Suzuki, S. Heart-type fatty acid-binding protein is more sensitive than troponin T to detect the ongoing myocardial damage in chronic heart failure patients. *J. Card. Fail.* **2007**, *13*, 120–127. [CrossRef]
24. Seferovic, P.M.; Damman, K.; Harjola, V.P.; Mebazaa, A.; Brunner-La Rocca, H.P.; Martens, P.; Testani, J.M.; Tang, W.H.W.; Orso, F.; Rossignol, P.; et al. Heart failure in cardiomyopathies: A position paper from the Heart Failure Association of the European Society of Cardiology. *Eur. J. Heart Fail.* **2019**, *21*, 553–576. [CrossRef] [PubMed]
25. Paulus, W.J.; Tschope, C. A novel paradigm for heart failure with preserved ejection fraction: Comorbidities drive myocardial dysfunction and remodeling through coronary microvascular endothelial inflammation. *J. Am. Coll. Cardiol.* **2013**, *62*, 263–271. [CrossRef] [PubMed]
26. Sanada, S.; Hakuno, D.; Higgins, L.J.; Schreiter, E.R.; McKenzie, A.N.J.; Lee, R.T. IL-33 and ST2 comprise a critical biomechanically induced and cardioprotective signaling system. *J. Clin. Investig.* **2007**, *117*, 1538–1549. [CrossRef] [PubMed]
27. Griesenauer, B.; Paczesny, S. The ST2/IL-33 Axis in Immune Cells during Inflammatory Diseases. *Front. Immunol.* **2017**, *8*, 475. [CrossRef] [PubMed]
28. Najjar, E.; Faxén, U.L.; Hage, C.; Donal, E. ST2 in heart failure with preserved and reduced ejection fraction. *Scand. Cardiovasc. J.* **2019**, *53*, 21–27. [CrossRef] [PubMed]
29. Schelbert, E.B.; Fridman, Y.; Wong, T.C.; Abu Daya, H.; Piehler, K.M.; Kadakkal, A.; et al. Temporal Relation Between Myocardial Fibrosis and Heart Failure With Preserved Ejection Fraction: Association With Baseline Disease Severity and Subsequent Outcome. *JAMA Cardiol.* **2017**, *2*, 995–1006. [CrossRef]
30. Thuno, M.; Macho, B.; Eugen-Olsen, J. suPAR: The molecular crystal ball. *Dis. Markers* **2009**, *27*, 157–172. [CrossRef]
31. Hamie, L.; Daoud, G.; Nemer, G.; Nammour, T.; el Chediak, A.; Uthman, I.W.; Kibbi, A.G.; Eid, A.; Kurban, M. SuPAR, an emerging biomarker in kidney and inflammatory diseases. *Postgrad. Med. J.* **2018**, *94*, 517–524. [CrossRef] [PubMed]
32. De Rosa, S.; Curcio, A.; Indolfi, C. Emerging role of microRNAs in cardiovascular diseases. *Circ. J.* **2014**, *78*, 567–575. [CrossRef] [PubMed]
33. De Rosa, S.; Eposito, F.; Carella, C.; Strangio, A.; Ammirati, G.; Sabatino, J.; Abbate, F.G.; Iaconetti, C.; Liguori, V.; Pergola, V.; et al. Transcoronary concentration gradients of circulating microRNAs in heart failure. *Eur. J. Heart Fail.* **2018**, *20*, 1000–1010. [CrossRef] [PubMed]
34. Iaconetti, C.; Sorrentino, S.; De Rosa, S.; Indolfi, C. Exosomal miRNAs in Heart Disease. *Physiology* **2016**, *31*, 16–24. [CrossRef]

11

The Ser290Asn and Thr715Pro Polymorphisms of the *SELP* Gene are Associated with A Lower Risk of Developing Acute Coronary Syndrome and Low Soluble P-Selectin Levels in A Mexican Population

Gabriel Herrera-Maya [1,‡], Gilberto Vargas-Alarcón [1,‡], Oscar Pérez-Méndez [1], Rosalinda Posadas-Sánchez [2], Felipe Masso [3], Teresa Juárez-Cedillo [4], Galileo Escobedo [5], Andros Vázquez-Montero [1] and José Manuel Fragoso [1,*]

1 Department of Molecular Biology, Instituto Nacional de Cardiología Ignacio Chávez, Mexico City 14080, Mexico; mayadermata@ciencias.unam.mx (G.H.-M.); gvargas63@yahoo.com (G.V.-A.); opmendez@yahoo.com (O.P.M.); koapa_93and@hotmail.com (A.V.-M.)
2 Department of Endocrinology, Instituto Nacional de Cardiología Ignacio Chávez, Mexico City 14080, Mexico; rossy_posadas_s@yahoo.it
3 Laboratory of Translational Medicine, UNAM-INC Research Unit, Instituto Nacional de Cardiología, Ignacio Chávez, Mexico City 14080, Mexico; f_masso@yahoo.com
4 Commissioned of the Research Unit in Clinical Epidemiology, Hospital Regional No. 1, Dr. Carlos McGregor Sánchez Navarro, Instituto Mexicano del Seguro Social, Mexico City 14080, Mexico; terezillo@exalumno.unam.mx
5 Unit of the Experimental Medicine, Hospital General de Mexico, Dr. Eduardo Liceaga, Mexico City 14080, Mexico; gescobedog@msn.com
* Correspondence: mfragoso1275@yahoo.com.mx
† Running Head: SELP gene polymorphisms in acute coronary syndrome.
‡ The contributions by G. Herrera-Maya and G. Vargas-Alarcón are equal and the order of authorship is arbitrary.

Abstract: Recent studies have shown that P-selectin promotes the early formation of atherosclerotic plaque. The aim of the present study was to evaluate whether the *SELP* gene single nucleotide polymorphisms (SNPs) are associated with presence of acute coronary syndrome (ACS) and with plasma P-selectin levels in a case-control association study. The sample size was estimated for a statistical power of 80%. We genotyped three *SELP* (*SELP* Ser290Asn, *SELP* Leu599Val, and *SELP* Thr715Pro) SNPs using 5′ exonuclease TaqMan assays in 625 patients with ACS and 700 healthy controls. The associations were evaluated with logistic regressions under the co-dominant, dominant, recessive, over-dominant and additive inheritance models. The genotype contribution to the plasma P-selectin levels was evaluated by a Student's t-test. Under different models, the *SELP* Ser290Asn (OR = 0.59, $pC_{Co\text{-}Dominant} = 0.047$; OR = 0.59, $pC_{Dominant} = 0.014$; OR = 0.58, $pC_{Over\text{-}Dominant} = 0.061$, and OR = 0.62, $pC_{Additive} = 0.015$) and *SELP* Thr715Pro (OR = 0.61, $pC_{Dominant} = 0.028$; OR = 0.63, $pC_{Over\text{-}Dominant} = 0.044$, and OR = 0.62, $pC_{Additive} = 0.023$) SNPs were associated with a lower risk of ACS. In addition, these SNPs were associated with low plasma P-selectin levels. In summary, this study established that the *SELP* Ser290Asn and *SELP* Thr715Pro SNPs are associated with a lower risk of developing ACS and with decreased P-selectin levels in plasma in a Mexican population.

Keywords: acute coronary syndrome; P-selectin; genetics; polymorphisms; susceptibility

1. Introduction

Acute coronary syndrome (ACS) comprises a spectrum of obstructive coronary artery diseases that most commonly arise from plaque rupture and/or erosion, leaving the vulnerable lipid-rich core exposed to the circulation. As a result, platelets and the coagulation cascade are activated, leading to acute thrombotic occlusion [1,2]. This syndrome is a consequence of atherosclerosis associated with a strong inflammatory component, which is immune mediated by chemokines. These molecules have an important role in the development of atherosclerotic plaque [3–5]. P-selectin is a chemokine, which mediates lymphocyte and monocyte recruitment, rolling, and diapedesis to the areas of inflammation [4–6]. Experimental studies have shown that higher expression of SELP increases adhesion, monocytes rolling to the vascular wall, accumulation of oxidized low-density lipoproteins, and the early formation of atherosclerotic plaque and other inflammatory diseases [4–7].

P-selectin contains 17 exons and is encoded by the *SELP* gene located on chromosome 1q21-q24 spanning <50 kb [8]. Recently, three single nucleotide polymorphism (SNPs) in the *SELP* gene in the exons 7, 12, and 13 [positions *G1057A* Ser290Asn (rs6131), *G1980T* Leu599Val (rs6133), and *A2331C* Thr715Pro (rs6136)] have been associated with myocardial infarction, hypertension, coronary heart disease, lupus erythematosus, type 2 diabetes mellitus (T2DM), and atherosclerosis [8–13]. Nonetheless, the association between these SNPs and other inflammatory diseases, such as diabetic retinopathy and multiple sclerosis is controversial, with negative results [14,15].

Considering the prominent role of P-selectin as a key in the chain of events leading to atherosclerotic plaque formation, the aim of this study was to investigate the association of three *SELP* SNPs (Ser290Asn, Leu599Val and Thr715Pro) with the risk of developing ACS. Furthermore, we evaluated whether these SNPs were associated with plasma P-selectin levels in a Mexican population sample.

2. Subjects and Methods

2.1. Study Population

This case-control study was carried out at the Instituto Nacional de Cardiologia Ignacio Chavez. The sample size was calculated for unmatched cases and controls with OpenEpi software (http://www.openepi.com/SampleSize/SSCC.html) with a statistical power of 80% and an alpha error of 0.05. Using this criterion, we included 625 patients with ACS (82% men and 18% women with a mean age of 57.97 ± 10.5 years) who were diagnosed based on clinical characteristics, electrocardiographic changes and biochemical markers of cardiac necrosis, according to guidelines from the European Society of Cardiology (ESC) and American College of Cardiology (ACC) [16,17]. The exclusion criteria were (1) patients with clear inflammatory pathologies on admission, such as infection established by clinical, laboratory, or image investigations, and (2) patients with an autoimmune disease or cancer previously diagnosed or documented during their hospitalization. Moreover, we included 700 healthy controls (66% men and 34% women with a mean age of 54.37 ± 7.65 years) coming from the Genetics of Atherosclerosis Disease (GEA) Mexican study previously described by Rosalinda-Posadas et al [18]. All healthy controls were asymptomatic and apparently healthy individuals without a family history of CAD and with a negative calcium score, indicative of the absence of subclinical atherosclerosis [18]. The exclusion criteria included not only the use anti-dyslipidemic, anti-hypertensive, and anti-diabetic drugs at the time of the study, but also congestive heart failure, as well as liver, renal, thyroid or oncological disease. All GEA participants were unrelated and of self-reported Mexican ancestry (3 generations). A Mexican mestizo was defined as a person who (1) was born in Mexico and (2) is a descendant of the original autochthonous inhabitants and of individuals (Caucasian and/or African, mainly Spaniards) who migrated to America in or after the XVI century. This study was conducted according to the principles of the Declaration of Helsinki and was approved by the Ethics and Research committee of our institution (registration number: 17CI09012010). Written informed consent was obtained from all individuals enrolled in the study.

2.2. Laboratory Analyses

After a 12-h overnight fast, EDTA blood samples were drawn and centrifuged within 15 min after collection; the plasma was separated into aliquots and immediately analyzed or frozen at −80 °C until analysis. Cholesterol and triglyceride plasma concentrations were determined by enzymatic/colorimetric assays (Randox Laboratories, UK). The phosphotungstic acid-Mg^{2+} method was used to determine HDL-C concentrations. LDL-C was estimated in samples with a triglyceride level lower than 400 mg/dl, using the modified Friedewald formula [19]. Plasma lipid concentrations were determined within 24 h after blood sample collection. We followed the National Cholesterol Education Project (NCEP) Adult Treatment Panel (ATP III) guidelines and thus defined dyslipidemia with the following levels: cholesterol > 200 mg/dl, LDL-C > 130 mg/dl, HDL-C < 40 mg/dl, and triglyceride > 150 mg/dl (http://www.nhlbi.nih.gov/guidelines/cholesterol/atp3_rpt.htm). Type 2 diabetes mellitus (T2DM) was defined with a fasting glucose ≥ 126 mg/dL and was also considered when participants reported glucose-lowering treatment or a physician diagnosis of T2DM. Hypertension was defined by a systolic blood pressure ≥ 140 mmHg and/or diastolic blood pressure ≥ 90 mmHg, or the use of oral antihypertensive therapy [18].

2.3. Genetic Analysis

DNA extraction was performed from peripheral blood in agreement with the method of Lahiri and Nurnberger [20]. The *SELP G1057A* Ser290Asn, *SELP G1980T* Leu599Val, and *SELP A2331C* Thr715Pro SNPs were genotyped using 5′ exonuclease TaqMan assays on a 7900HT Fast Real-Time PCR system according to manufacturer's instructions (Applied Biosystems, foster City, CA, USA). In order to avoid genotyping errors, ten percent of the samples were determined twice; the results were concordant for all cases.

2.4. Determination of P-Selectin Levels

Samples were aliquoted and stored at −70 °C for further use. Plasma P-selectin levels were measured using a quantitative sandwich enzyme immunoassay technique (ELISA) kit in accordance with the manufacturer's instructions (Human P-Selectin/CD62P Quantikine ELISA Kit, R&D systems). The detection range was 0.8–50.00 ng/mL and the sensitivity was equal to the minimal detectable dose of this kit (≥ 0.121 ng/mL).

2.5. Functional Prediction Analysis

Two in silico programs, the ESEfinder (http://rulai.cshl.edu/cgi-bin/tools/ESE3/esefinder.cgi?process=home) and SNP Function Prediction (http://snpinfo.niehs.nih.gov/cgi-bin/snpinfo/snpfunc.cgi) were used to predict the possible functional effect of the *SELP* SNPs. Both programs (ESEfinder2.0 and SNPinfo) analyzed the localization of the SNPs (e.g., 5′-upstream, 3′-untranslated regions, intronic) and their possible functional effects, such as amino acid changes in protein structure, transcription factor binding sites in promoter or intronic enhancer regions, and alternative splicing regulation by disrupting exonic splicing enhancers (*ESE*) or silencers [21,22].

2.6. Statistical Analysis

All statistical analysis in this study was performed using SPSS version 18.0 (SPSS, Chicago, Il). Data of continuous variables were expressed as median and percentiles (25th–75th), while data of discrete variables [e.g., frequency (n, %)] were analyzed using Chi-squared or Fisher's exact tests. We used logistic regression tests to associate the SNPs with ACS under five inheritance models [16]. The correction of the p-values (pC) was performed with the Bonferroni test. Using the HAPLOVIEW version 4.1 software (Cambridge, MA, USA), we performed the haplotypes construction and linkage disequilibrium analysis (LD, D″). We tested whether our study population was in Hardy–Weinberg equilibrium (HWE) with a Chi-square test. Furthermore, we used the QUANTO software [http://biostats.usc.edu/software] to calculate the statistical power of our study and found it was 0.80. Using the Student's t-test, we analyzed the contribution of the genotypes on the P-selectin plasma levels. The values were expressed as means ± SD. The level of significance was set at $p < 0.05$.

3. Results

3.1. Characteristics of the Study Population

Clinical and biochemical characteristics of the ACS patients and healthy controls are shown in Table 1. There were significant differences between the ACS patients and healthy controls. Compared to healthy controls, the ACS patients had a higher frequency of T2DM, hypertension, dyslipidemia, and smoking habit. Conversely, the total cholesterol, triglycerides, and LDL-C levels in ACS patients were lower than those in the control group; this effect may be due to their treatment with statins.

Table 1. Clinical characteristics and biochemical parameters of the study individuals.

		ACS (*n* = 625)	**Healthy Controls** (*n* = 700)	***p*-Value**
		Median (percentile 25–75)	Median (percentile 25–75)	
Age (years)		57.72 (51–65)	54.39 (49–59)	<0.001
BMI (kg/m^2)		27.3 (25–29)	28.3 (26–31)	0.001
Blood pressure (mmHg)	Systolic	130.61 (114–144)	117.32 (106–126)	<0.001
	Diastolic	80.1 (70–90)	72.47 (66–77)	<0.001
Glucose (mg/dl)		158.51 (102–188)	98.73 (84–99)	<0.001
Total cholesterol (mg/dl)		164.22 (128–198)	190.4 (164–210)	<0.001
HDL-C (mg/dl)		38.32 (32–44)	44.6 (35–53)	<0.001
LDL-C (mg/dl)		106.4 (76–133)	115.8 (94–134)	<0.001
Triglycerides (mg/dl)		169.2 (109–201)	175.1 (112–208)	0.218
Gender n (%)	Male	510 (82)	463 (66)	<0.001
	Female	115 (18)	237 (34)	
Smoking n (%)	Yes	225 (35)	155 (22)	<0.001
Hypertension	Yes	355 (57)	206 (29)	<0.001
Diabetes mellitus	Yes	218 (35)	68 (10)	<0.001
Dyslipidemia n (%)	Yes	534 (85)	501 (71)	<0.001

Data are expressed as median and percentiles (25th–75th). *p*-values were estimated using Mann–Whitney U test for continuous variables and chi-square test for categorical values. ACS: acute coronary syndrome patients.

3.2. Allele and Genotype Frequencies

Genotype frequencies of the SNPs were in HWE. The frequencies of the *SELP Leu599Val* SNP was similar in ACS patients and healthy controls. Nonetheless, the SNPs [*SELP* Ser290Asn, and *SELP* Thr715Pro] were associated with a lower risk of ACS (Table 2). Under co-dominant, dominant, over-dominant, and additive models, the *A* (290Asn) allele of the *SELP* Ser290Asn SNP was associated with a lower risk of ACS (OR = 0.59, $pC_{Co\text{-}Dom} = 0.047$; OR = 0.59, $pC_{Dom} = 0.014$; OR = 0.58, $pC_{Over\text{-}Dom} = 0.061$, and OR = 0.62, $pC_{Add} = 0.015$, respectively). In the same way, under dominant, over-dominant, and additive models, the *C* (715Pro) allele of the *SELP* Thr715Pro SNP was associated with a lower risk of ACS (OR = 0.61, $pC_{Dom} = 0.028$; OR = 0.63, $pC_{Over\text{-}Dom} = 0.044$, and OR = 0.62, $pC_{Add} = 0.023$, respectively). All models were adjusted for gender, age, blood pressure, BMI, glucose, total cholesterol, HDL-C, LDL-C, triglycerides, and smoking habit.

Table 2. Distribution of *SEL-P* polymorphisms in ACS patients and healthy controls.

				MAF	Model	OR (95%CI)	*pC*
			***SELP G1057A* Ser290Asn (rs6131)**				
	GG	GA	AA				
Control (n = 691)	569 (0.823)	115 (0.166)	7 (0.010)	0.09	Co-dominant Dominant Recessive	0.59 (0.38–0.92) 0.59 (0.39–0.90) 0.58 (0.12–2.83)	0.047 0.014 0.49
ACS (n = 617)	541 (0.877)	73 (0.118)	3 (0.005)	0.06	Over-dominant Additive	0.61 (0.39–0.92) 0.62 (0.42–0.92)	0.019 0.015
			***SELP G1980T* Leu599Val (rs6133)**				
	GG	GT	TT				
Control (n = 682)	563 (0.825)	114 (0.167)	5 (0.007)	0.09	Co-dominant Dominant Recessive	0.28 (0.02–3.32) 1.07 (0.73–1.58) 0.27 (0.02–3.26)	0.46 0.73 0.26
ACS (n = 611)	505 (0.827)	105 (0.172)	1 (0.002)	0.09	Over-dominant Additive	1.12 (0.75–1.66) 1.02 (0.71–1.49)	0.57 0.90
			***SELP A2331C Thr715Pro* (rs6136)**				
	AA	AC	CC				
Control (n = 685)	580 (0.847)	97 (0.141)	8 (0.012)	0.08	Co-dominant Dominant Recessive	0.63 (0.40–0.99) 0.61 (0.39–0.95) 0.36 (0.04–2.95)	0.075 0.028 0.32
ACS (n = 607)	537 (0.884)	67 (0.110)	3 (0.005)	0.06	Over-dominant Additive	0.63 (0.40–0.99) 0.62 (0.41–0.94)	0.044 0.023

ACS, acute coronary syndrome, MAF, minor allele frequency, OR, odds ratio, CI, confidence interval, *pC*, *p*-value corrected. The p-values were calculated by the logistic regression analysis, and the ORs were adjusted for gender, age, blood pressure, BMI, glucose, total cholesterol, HDL-C, LDL-C, triglycerides, and smoking habit.

Considering that the prevalence of T2DM (35%) and hypertension (57%) are highest in ACS patients versus healthy controls (10% and 29%, respectively), we performed a sub-analysis of the polymorphisms associated with a low risk of ACS (*SELP* Ser290Asn and *SELP* Thr715Pro). This analysis was made comparing individuals with and without T2DM and the other hand, individuals with and without hypertension. The results show that both polymorphisms were not associated with T2DM or with hypertension (Supplementary Tables S1 and S2). Therefore, this analysis corroborates that the genetic variation of these polymorphisms of the *SELP* gene are associated to the ACS, and not comes of the T2DM or hypertension.

3.3. Linkage Disequilibrium Analysis

We used the Haploview version 4.1 program for the analysis of the linkage disequilibrium and construction of haplotypes. In this analysis, the *SELP* Thr715Pro and *SELP* Leu599Val SNPs showed a strong linkage disequilibrium (D′ = 0.95). In addition, Haploview revealed strong evidence of recombination of the polymorphisms *SELP* Thr715Pro versus *SELP* Ser290Asn and *SELP Leu599Val* versus *SELP* Ser290Asn (D '= 0.17 and D' = 0.28, respectively; data not shown). This analysis marked three haplotypes with different distributions in ACS patients and healthy controls (Table 3). The "Thr-Leu-Ser" haplotype was associated with a higher risk of developing ACS (OR = 1.28, 95% CI: 1.05–1.54, pC = 0.006), while the "Pro-Leu-Ser" and "Thr-Leu-Asn" haplotypes were associated with a lower risk of developing ACS (OR = 0.72, 95% CI: 0.52-0.99, pC = 0.022, and OR = 0.71, 95% CI: 0.51–1.00, pC = 0.027, respectively).

Table 3. Haplotype frequencies (Hf) of *SEL-P* haplotypes in ACS patients and healthy controls.

Haplotypes	Thr715Pro	Leu599Val	Ser290Asn	ACS (n = 605)	Controls (n = 676)	OR	95%CI	P
				Hf	Hf			
H1	Thr	Leu	Ser	0.804	0.763	1.28	1.05–1.54	0.006
H2	Thr	Val	Ser	0.073	0.067	1.08	0.80–1.47	0.32
H3	Pro	Leu	Ser	0.057	0.077	0.72	0.52–0.99	0.022
H4	Thr	Leu	Asn	0.049	0.066	0.71	0.51–1.00	0.027
H5	Pro	Val	Asn	0.014	0.022	0.62	0.33–1.13	0.063

Abbreviations: Hf, Haplotype frequency; *P*, *p*-value; OR, odds ratio; 95% CI, confidential interval. The order of the polymorphisms in the haplotypes is according to the positions in the chromosome (*SELP A2331C Thr715Pro* (rs6136), *SELP G1980T* Leu599Val (rs6133), and *SELP G1057A* Ser290Asn (rs6131). Bold numbers indicate significant associations.

3.4. Association of Polymorphisms with Plasma P-Selectin Levels

In order to define the functional effect of the *SELP* Ser290Asn and *SELP* Thr715Pro SNPs associated with a lower risk of ACS, we determined the plasma levels of P-selectin in individuals with different genotypes of these two polymorphisms. For this analysis, we included a subgroup of 30 healthy controls for *SELP* Ser290Asn (7 *AA*, 11 *GA* and 12 *GG*) and a subgroup of 30 healthy controls for the *SELP* Thr715Pro SNP (8 *CC*, 11 *AC* and 11 *AA*). In this study, we did not include the analysis of plasma P-selectin levels in patients with ACS, due to the fact that in the setting of the coronary syndrome, the comorbidities, such as insulin resistance/T2DM, hypertension, and inflammatory processes, as well as the use of the anti-dyslipidemic and/or anti-hypertensive drugs, may have altered the inflammatory markers levels, such as inflammatory cytokines, adhesion molecules, and C-reactive protein, masking the real impact of *SELP* polymorphisms on plasma P-selectin levels [23–25]. In this context, subjects carrying the *AA* (Ans/Ans*)* genotype of the *SELP* Ser290Asn SNP had a lower P-selectin plasma concentration (33.93 ± 9.79 ng/mL) than carriers of the *GG* (Ser/Ser*)* (44.76 ± 6.54 ng/mL, *p* =0.032) or GA (Ser/Ans*)* genotypes (48.04 ± 16.57 ng/mL, *p* = 0.049) (Figure 1A). On the other hand, the analysis of the *SELP* Thr715Pro polymorphism showed that individuals with the *CC* (Pro/Pro) genotype had a lower concentration of P-selectin (26.44 ± 10.77 ng/mL) than *AA* (Thr/Thr) carriers (55.35 ± 14.05 ng/dl, *p* = 0.001). In addition, the individuals with the *AC* (Thr/Pro*)* genotype had lower P-selectin levels than *AA* (Thr/Thr) carriers (34.91 ± 14.46 ng/dl, *p* = 0.005) (Figure 1B).

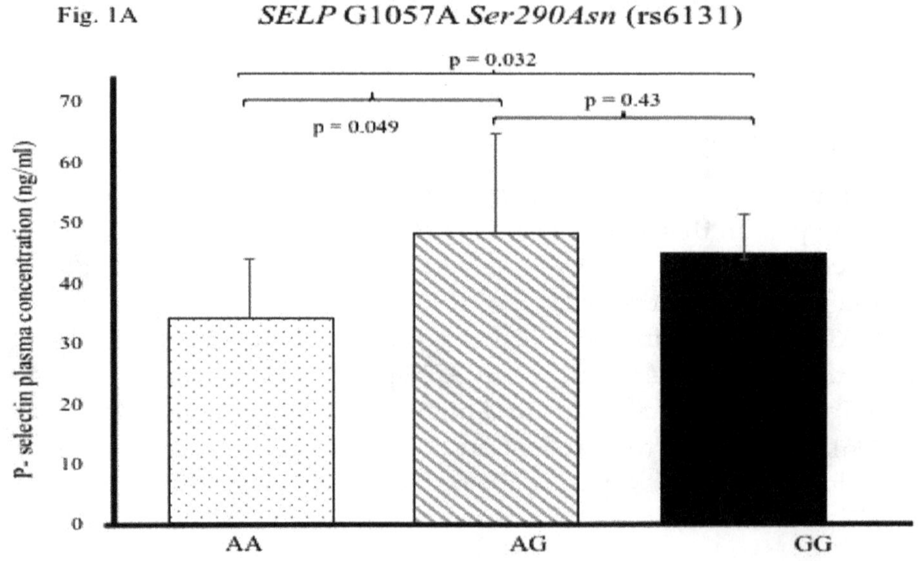

Figure 1. *Cont.*

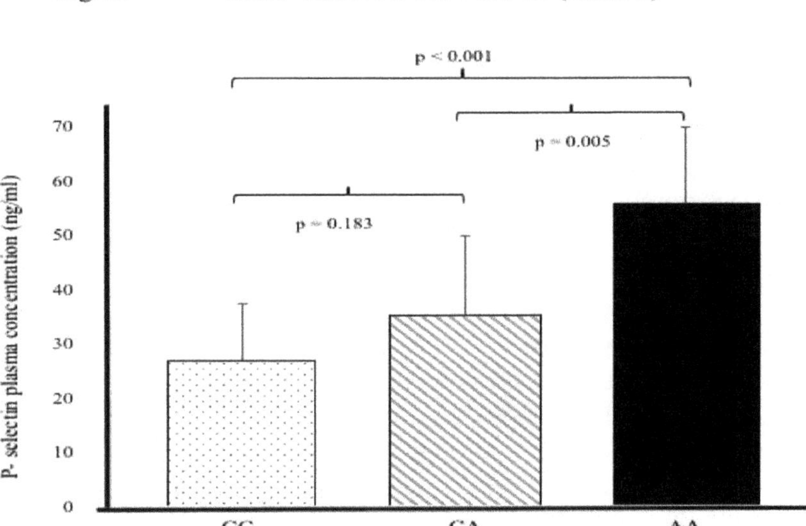

Figure 1. Genetic contribution of the *SELP G1057A* and *SELP A2331C* polymorphisms on P-selectin levels. (**A**) P-selectin plasma levels in individuals with different genotypes of the *SELP G1057A* polymorphism. (**B**) P-selectin plasma levels in individuals with different genotypes of the *SELP A2331C* polymorphism.

3.5. Functional Prediction

The functional prediction analysis showed that the presence of the *A* (Asn) allele of the *SELP* Ser290Asn polymorphism potentially produces a binding motif for Srp40 protein. In contrast, no evidence of potentially functional motifs was found for the *SELP* Thr715Pro polymorphism.

4. Discussion

In this study, we analyzed three relevant polymorphisms (Ser290Asn, Leu599Val, and Thr715Pro, respectively) of the *SELP* gene. The association of these SNPs with several inflammatory diseases in different populations is controversial, with positive and negative results [8–15]. In our study, the distribution of the *SELP* Leu599Val SNP was similar in both ACS patients and healthy controls. Nonetheless, the presence of the 290*Asn* and 715*Pro* alleles (*SELP* Ser290Asn and *SELP* Thr715Pro polymorphisms, respectively) was associated with a lower risk of developing ACS. In the same way, Reiner et al. reported in the CARDIA study that the *SELP* Ser290Asn and *SELP* Thr715Pro SNPs are associated with carotid intima-media thickness in young adults; however, these associations are different in European-American and African-American individuals [9]. In line with these data, Nasibullin et al. reported that the 290*Ans* allele of the *SELP* Ser290Asn SNP is associated with a lower risk of MI in a Russian population [13]. Similarly, the study of the risk of atherosclerosis in communities (ARIC), as well as the study of the Framingham heart (FHS) have shown that the genotype Pro715Pro is associated with a decreased risk of atherosclerosis in American and European populations [26,27]. In contrast with these data, in the ARIC study, Volcik et al. reported that the 290*Ans* and 715*Pro* alleles (*SELP* Ser290Asn and *SELP* Thr715Pro SNPs, respectively) were associated with the development of coronary heart disease in white but not in African Americans [11]. Similarly, Timasheva et al. reported that the *290*Ans allele of the *SELP* Ser290Asn SNP is associated with the development of hypertension in ethnic Tatars originating from the Republic of Bashkortostan (Russian Federation) [12]. By the same token, Kou et al. reported that *Thr715Pro* or *Pro715Pro* genotypes of the *SELP* Thr715Pro polymorphism increased the risk of developing cardiovascular diseases (CVD) in a Chinese Han population [28]. Additionally, we found that the H3 (Pro-Leu-Ser) and H4 (Thr-Leu-Asn) haplotypes were associated with a lower risk of developing ACS, whereas H1 (Thr-Leu-Ser) was associated with a higher risk. As can be seen, the haplotypic combinations between *SELP* Thr715Pro and *SELP* Ser290Asn polymorphisms were not in linkage disequilibrium. Nonetheless, the protection haplotypes carry *715Pro* and 290*Ans* alleles, and both of them were associated independently with a lower risk of cardiovascular diseases and other inflammatory diseases. This finding corroborated the role of these two alleles with the presence of ACS, whether they were analyzed independently or as haplotypes.

It is important to note that ACS patients and the healthy donors have much greater variation in blood glucose (102-188 versus 84-99) and diabetes mellitus (35% versus 10%). Considering these data, it is important to establish whether the polymorphisms are associated with T2DM or hypertension. In a sub-analysis, we showed that both polymorphisms were not associated with T2DM or with hypertension.

As can be seen, the associations of the *SELP* Ser290Asn and *SELP* Thr715Pro polymorphisms with ACS are contradictory in different study populations. We suggest that these discrepancies could be due to the classical cardiovascular risk factors and the environmental factors, such as diet, exercise, and lifestyle, which have an important role in the development of inflammatory diseases [29,30]. Another reason may be the fact that the allelic distribution of these polymorphisms varies according to the ethnic origin of the study populations. According to data obtained from the National Center for Biotechnology Information, populations from European, Asian, and African ancestry in Southwest US present a higher frequency of the *A* allele of the *SELP G1057A* Ser290Asn (rs6131) polymorphism (21.7%, 20.2% and 32.9%, respectively) when compared to Mexican mestizos and white American populations with a lower frequency of the *A* allele (9% and 14%, respectively). Concerning the *SELP A2331C* Thr715Pro (rs6136) SNP, Mexican mestizos, Europeans, and white Americans present a higher frequency of the *C* allele (8%, 8.8%, and 8.2%, respectively) than populations with Asian and African ancestry (0.2% and 2.5%, respectively) (https://www.ncbi.nlm.nih.gov/variation/tools/1000genomes/), (https://www.ensembl.org/index.html).

We further determined the effect of the *SELP* gene polymorphisms on plasma P-selectin levels using genotype groups. We found that the *AA* (290 Asn/Asn) and *CC* (715 Pro/Pro) genotypes were associated with low P-selectin levels. As far as we know, this is the first study that showed the association of the *SELP* Ser290Asn and *SELP* Thr715Pro polymorphisms in P-selectin levels in individuals without the use of the anti-dyslipidemic or anti-hypertensive drugs. These drugs may modify the levels of the inflammatory markers, such as pro-inflammatory cytokines, adhesion molecules and C-reactive protein, masking the real impact of *SELP* gene polymorphisms on plasma P-selectin [23–25]. Nonetheless, the results concerning the association between P-selectin plasma levels and heart diseases are still contradictory. For example, Reiner et al. reported in the CARDIA study that the *A* (290Asn) and *C* (715Pro) alleles are associated with decreased plasma P-selectin levels and with the risk of developing atherosclerosis [9]. By the same token, Volcik et al. documented that the 715Pro allele is associated with lower P-selectin levels in the Atherosclerosis Risk in Communities (ARIC) study [27]. Similarly, Lee et al. determined that the lower serum levels of P-selectin decreased the risk of atherosclerosis [26]. At the same time, other reports have shown that the 715Pro *(C)* allele increased the expression of SELP mRNA, as well as the concentration of P-selectin levels in other inflammatory diseases, such as rheumatoid arthritis and T2DM [8,31]. As far as we know, the precise mechanism by which low and/or high P-selectin levels are associated with ACS remains to be elucidated. Nonetheless, recent data provide evidence that P-selectin upregulation on the endothelial cell surface mediates the effects of angiotensin II (Ang II), which has an important role in the development atherosclerosis [32]. In addition, Ang II stimulates not only the production of several molecules (adhesion molecules, chemokines, and cytokines) but also the oxidation and uptake of LDL, which promotes endothelial dysfunction [6,32]. On the other hand, Ang II triggers the synthesis of matrix metalloproteinases, the plasminogen activator inhibitor-1, and the proliferation of vascular smooth cells; this effect leads to the destabilization of atherosclerotic plaques [6]. Furthermore, using bioinformatics tools, we determined the potential effect of the *SELP* gene polymorphisms associated with ACS. The analysis of the *SELP* Thr715Pro polymorphism did not provide evidence of potential functional motifs. Nonetheless, the analysis of the *SELP* Ser290Asn polymorphism showed that the 290 Asn (*A)* allele generates a binding site for the Srp40 proteins. These proteins have multiple functions in the pre-mRNA splicing process, as well as in the regulation of alternative splicing, which leads to the production of protein isoforms [33,34]. In this context, we think that future investigations are warranted to understand the effect of these polymorphisms on P-selectin levels.

Some limitations should be considered. The P-selectin levels were only measured in a small sample of control individuals and experiments on RNA transcription or protein stability were not made. Considering these limitations, the effect of the SNPs on P-selectin plasma levels should be taken with care and studies in a large number of individuals are necessary to corroborate this association. In the same way, in our study it was not possible to determine the expression levels of P-selectin on the leukocyte's surface to confirm the data obtained in plasma.

In summary, this study demonstrated that the *SELP* Ser290Asn and *SELP* Thr715Pro polymorphisms are associated with a lower risk of developing ACS in a Mexican population. It was possible to distinguish two haplotypes (Pro-Leu-Ser and Thr-Leu-Asn) associated with a lower risk of developing ACS. On the other hand, both polymorphisms were associated with lower P-selectin levels in plasma. Lastly, due to the specific genetic characteristics of the Mexican population, we consider that additional studies will need to be undertaken in a larger number of individuals and in populations with different ethnic origins; these studies could help define the true role of these polymorphisms as markers of risk or protection from developing ACS and other cardiovascular events.

Author Contributions: Conceptualization, G.H.-M., G.V.-A., O.P.-M. and J.M.F.; Data curation, O.P.-M., T.J.-C. and A.V.-M.; Formal analysis, G.H.-M., R.P.-S., F.M., T.J.-C., G.E., A.V.-M. and J.M.F.; Investigation, G.V.-A., O.P.-M. and J.M.F.; Methodology, O.P.-M., R.P.-S., F.M., G.E. and A.V.-M.; Resources, G.H.-M., O.P.-M., T.J.-C. and G.E.; Software, G.H.-M., R.P.-S., F.M., T.J.-C., G.E. and A.V.-M.; Supervision, J.M.F.; Validation, A.V.-M.; Writing – original draft, J.M.F.; Writing – review & editing, G.V.-A. and J.M.F. All authors have read and agreed to the published version of the manuscript.

Acknowledgments: This work was submitted in fulfilment of the requirements to obtaining the Doctoral degree of Gabriel Herrera-Maya in the PhD program of Biological Sciences of the Universidad Nacional Autónoma de Mexico (UNAM). Gabriel Herrera-Maya was supported by a fellowship from the *Consejo Nacional de Ciencia y Tecnología* (*CONACyT*) Mexico City, Mexico with **CVU number 545322**. The authors are grateful to the study participants. Institutional Review Board approval was obtained for all sample collections. The authors would like to thank the technicians Silvestre Ramirez-Fuentes and Marva Arellano-Gonzalez for their participation in sample collection and DNA extraction.

Abbreviations

HDL-C	High-density lipoprotein–cholesterol
LDL	Low-density lipoprotein–cholesterol
SELP	P-selectin gene
T2DM	Type 2 diabetes mellitus
SNP	Single nucleotide polymorphism
ACS	Acute coronary syndrome

References

1. Libby, P. Inflammation and Atherosclerosis. *Nature* **2002**, *420*, 868–874. [CrossRef]
2. Virmani, R.; Kolodgie, F.D.; Burke, A.P.; Finn, A.V.; Gold, H.K.; Tulenko, T.N.; Wrenn, S.P.; Narula, J. Atherosclerotic plaque progression and vulnerability to rupture: angiogenesis as a source of intraplaque hemorrhage. *Arterioscler. Thromb. Vasc. Biol.* **2005**, *25*, 2054–2061. [CrossRef] [PubMed]

3. Achar, S.A.; Kundu, S.; Norcross, W.A. Diagnosis of acute coronary syndrome. *Am. Fam. Physician.* **2005**, *72*, 119–126. [PubMed]
4. Braunersreuther, V.; Mach, F.; Steffens, S. The specific role of chemokines in atherosclerosis. *Thromb. Haemost* **2007**, *97*, 714–721. [CrossRef]
5. Aukrust, P.; Halvorsen, B.; Yndestad, A.; Ueland, T.; Oie, E.; Otterdal, K.; Gullestad, L.; Damås, J.K. Chemokines and cardiovascular risk. *Arterioscler. Thromb. Vasc. Biol.* **2008**, *28*, 1909–1919. [CrossRef]
6. Montezano, A.C.; Nguyen Dinh Cat, A.; Rios, F.J.; Touyz, R.M. Angiotensin II and Vascular Injury. *Curr. Hypertens Rep.* **2014**, *16*, 431. [CrossRef]
7. Bland, A.D.; Nadar, S.K.; Lip, G.Y.H. The adhesion molecule P-selectin and cardiovascular disease. *Eur. Heart J.* **2003**, *24*, 2166–2179. [CrossRef]
8. Kaur, R.; Singh, J.; Kapoor, R.; Kaur, M. Association of SELP polymorphisms with soluble P-selectin levels and vascular risk in patients with type 2 diabetes mellitus: a case-control study. *Biochem. Genet.* **2019**, *57*, 73–97. [CrossRef]
9. Reiner, A.P.; Carlson, C.S.; Thyagarajan, B.; Reider, M.J.; Polak, J.F.; Siscovick, D.S.; Nickerson, D.A.; Jacobs, D.R., Jr.; Gross, M.D. Soluble P-selectin, SELP polymorphisms, and atherosclerotic risk European-American and African-African young adults: the coronary artery risk development in young adults (CARDIA) study. *Arterioscler. Thromb. Vasc. Biol.* **2008**, *28*, 1549–1555. [CrossRef]
10. Morris, D.L.; Graham, R.R.; Erwig, L.P.; Gaffney, P.M.; Moser, K.L.; Behrens, T.W.; Vyse, T.J.; Graham, D.C. Variation in the upstream region of P-selectin (SELP) is a risk factor for SLE. *Genes Immun.* **2009**, *10*, 404–413. [CrossRef] [PubMed]
11. Volcik, K.A.; Ballantyne, C.M.; Coresh, J.; Folsom, A.R.; Boerwinkle, E. Specific P-selectin and P-selectin glycoprotein ligand-1 genotypes/haplotypes are associated with risk of incidence CHD and ischemic stroke: the atherosclerosis risk in communities (ARIC) study. *Atherosclerosis* **2007**, *195*, e76–e82. [CrossRef] [PubMed]
12. Timasheva, Y.R.; Nasibullin, T.R.; Imaeva, E.B.; Erdman, V.; Kruzliak, P.; Tuktarova, I.A.; Nikolaeva, I.E.; Mustafina, O.E. Polymorphisms of inflammatory markers and risk of essential hypertension in Tartars from Russia. *Clin. Exp. Hypertens.* **2015**, *37*, 398–403. [CrossRef] [PubMed]
13. Nasibullin, T.R.; Timasheva, Y.R.; Sadikova, R.I.; Tuktarova, I.A.; Erdman, V.V.; Nikolaeva, I.E.; Sabo, J.; Kruzliak, P.; Mustafina, O.E. Genotype/allelic combinations as potential predictors of myocardial infarction. *Mol. Bio. Rep.* **2016**, *43*, 11–16. [CrossRef] [PubMed]
14. Kolahdouz, P.; Yazd, E.F.; Tajamolian, M.; Manaviat, M.R.; Sheikhha, M.H. The rs3917779 polymorphism of P-selectin significant association with proliferative diabetic retinopathy in Yazd, Iran. *Graefes Arch. Clin. Exp. Ophthalmol.* **2015**, *253*, 1967–1972. [CrossRef] [PubMed]
15. Fenoglio, C.; Scalabrini, D.; Piccio, L.; de Ris, M.; Venturelli, E.; Cortini, F.; Villa, C.; Serpente, M.; Parks, B.; Rinker, J.; et al. Candidate gene analysis of selectin cluster in patients with multiple sclerosis. *J. Neurol.* **2009**, *256*, 832–833. [CrossRef] [PubMed]
16. Cannon, C.P.; Battler, A.; Brindis, R.G.; Cox, J.L.; Ellis, S.G.; Every, N.R.; Flaherty, J.T.; Harrington, R.A.; Krumholz, H.M.; Simoons, M.L.; et al. American College of Cardiology key data elements and definitions for measuring the clinical management and outcomes of patients with acute coronary syndromes. A report of the American College of Cardiology Task Force on Clinical Data Standards (Acute Coronary Syndromes Writing Committee). *J. Am. Coll. Cardiol.* **2001**, *38*, 2114–2130.
17. Hamm, C.W.; Bassand, J.P.; Agewall, S.; Bax, J.; Boersma, E.; Bueno, H.; Caso, P.; Dudek, D.; Gielen, S.; Huber, K. ESC Guidelines for the management of acute coronary syndromes in patients presenting without persistent ST-segment elevation: The Task Force for the management of acute coronary syndromes (ACS) in patients presenting without persistent ST-segment elevation of the European Society of Cardiology (ESC). *Eur. Heart J.* **2011**, *32*, 2999–3054.
18. Posadas-Sanchez, R.; Perez-Hernandez, N.; Angeles-Martinez, J.; Lopez-Bautista, F.; Villarreal-Molina, T.; Rodríguez-Perez, J.M.; Fragoso, J.M.; Posadas-Romero, C.; Vargas-Alarcón, G. Interleukin 35 Polymorphisms Are Associated with Decreased Risk of Premature Coronary Artery Disease, Metabolic Parameters, and IL-35 Levels: The Genetics of Atherosclerotic Disease (GEA) Study. *Mediators Inflamm.* **2017**, *2017*, 6012795. [CrossRef]
19. DeLong, D.M.; DeLong, E.R.; Wood, P.D.; Lippel, K.; Rifkind, B.M. A comparison of methods for the estimation of plasma low- and very low-density lipoprotein cholesterol. The Lipid Research Clinics Prevalence Study. *JAMA.* **1986**, *256*, 2372–2377. [CrossRef]

20. Lahiri, D.K.; Nurnberger, J.I., Jr. A rapid non-enzymatic method for the preparation HMW DNA from blood for RFLP studies. *Nucleic Acids Res.* **1991**, *19*, 5444. [CrossRef]
21. Smith, P.J.; Zhang, C.; Wang, J.; Chew, S.L.; Zhang, M.Q.; Krainer, A.R. An increased specificity score matrix for the prediction of SF2/ASF-specific exonic splicing enhancers. *Hum. Mol. Genet.* **2006**, *15*, 2490–2508. [CrossRef] [PubMed]
22. Xu, Z.; Taylor, J.A. SNPinfo: integrating GWAS and candidate gene information into functional SNP selection for genetic association studies. *Nucleic Acids Res.* **2009**, *37*, W600–W605. [CrossRef] [PubMed]
23. Agabiti Rosei, E.; Morelli, P.; Rizzoni, D. Effects of nifedipine GITS 20 mg or enalapril 20 mg on blood pressure and inflammatory markers in patients with mild-moderate hypertension. *Blood Press Suppl.* **2005**, *1*, 14–22. [CrossRef] [PubMed]
24. Golia, E.; Limongelli, G.; Natale, F.; Fimiani, F.; Maddaloni, V.; Pariggiano, I.; Bianchi, R.; Crisci, M.; Giordano, R.; Di Palma, G.; et al. Inflamation and cardiuovascular disease: From pathogenesis and therapeutic target. *Curr. Atheroscler. Rep.* **2014**, *16*, 435. [CrossRef]
25. Ruszkowski, P.; Masajtis-Zagajewska, A.; Nowicki, M. Effects of combined statin and ACE inhibitor therapy on endothelial function and blood pressure in essential hypertension-a radomised double-blind, placebo controlled crossover study. *J. Renin. Angiotensin Aldosterone Syst.* **2019**, *20*, 1–9. [CrossRef]
26. Lee, D.S.; Larson, M.G.; Lunetta, K.L.; Dupuis, J.; Rong, J.; Keaney, J.F., Jr.; Lipinska, I.; Baldwin, C.T.; Vasan, R.S.; Benjamin, E.J. Clinical and genetic correlates of soluble P-selectin in the community. *J. Thromb. Haemost.* **2008**, *6*, 20–31. [CrossRef]
27. Volcik, K.A.; Catellier, D.; Folson, A.R.; Matijevic, N.; Wasserman, B.; Boerwinkle, E. SELP and SELPG genetic variation is associated with cell surface measures of SELp and SELPG: the atherosclerosis risk in communities (ARIC) study. *Clin. Chem.* **2009**, *55*, 1076–1082. [CrossRef]
28. Kuo, L.; Yang, N.; Dong, B.; Li, Y.; Tang, J.; Qin, Q. Interaction between SELP genetic polymorphisms with inflammatory cytokine interleukin-6 (IL_6) gene variants on cardiovascular disease in Chinese Han population. *Mamm. Genome* **2017**, *28*, 436–442.
29. Bielinski, S.J.; Berardi, C.; Decker, P.A.; Kirsch, P.S.; Larson, N.B.; Pankow, J.S.; Sale, M.; De Andrade, M.; Sicotte, H.; Tang, W.; et al. P-selectin and subclinical and clinical atherosclerosis: the multi-ethnic study of atherosclerosis (MESA). *Atherosclerosis* **2015**, *240*, 3–9. [CrossRef]
30. Nettleton, J.A.; Matijevic, N.; Follis, J.L.; Folsom, A.R.; Boerwinkle, E. Associations between dietary patterns and flow cytometry-measured biomarkers of inflammation and cellular activation in the Atherosclerosis Risk in Communities (ARIC) Carotid Artery MRI Study. *Atherosclerosis* **2010**, *212*, 260–267. [CrossRef]
31. Burkhardt, J.; Blume, M.; Petit-Teixeira, E.; Hugo Teixeira, V.; Steiner, A.; Quente, E.; Wolfram, G.; Scholz, M.; Pierlot, C.; Migliorini, P.; et al. Cellular Adhesion Gene SELP Is Associated with Rheumatoid Arthritis and Displays Differential Allelic Expression. *PLoS ONE* **2014**, *9*, e103872. [CrossRef] [PubMed]
32. Piqueras, L.; Kubes, P.; Alvarez, A.; O'Connor, E.; Issekutz, A.C.; Esplugues, J.V.; Sanz, M.J. Angiotensin II Induces leukocyte–endothelial cell interactions in vivo via AT1 and AT2 receptor-mediated P-selectin upregulation. *Circulation* **2000**, *102*, 2118–2123. [CrossRef] [PubMed]
33. Tardos, J.G.; Eisenreich, A.; Deikus, G.; Bechhofer, D.H.; Chandradas, S.; Zafar, U.; Rauch, U.; Bogdanov, V.Y. SR proteins ASF/SF2 and SRp55 participoate in tissue factor biosynthesis in human monocyte cells. *J. Thromb. Haemost.* **2008**, *6*, 877–884. [CrossRef] [PubMed]
34. Graveley, B.R. Sorting out the complexity of SR protein functions. *RNA* **2000**, *6*, 1197–1211. [CrossRef] [PubMed]

12

Ceruloplasmin, NT-proBNP and Clinical Data as Risk Factors of Death or Heart Transplantation in a 1-Year Follow-Up of Heart Failure Patients

Ewa Romuk [1,*], Wojciech Jacheć [2], Ewa Zbrojkiewicz [3], Alina Mroczek [3], Jacek Niedziela [4], Mariusz Gąsior [4], Piotr Rozentryt [3,4] and Celina Wojciechowska [2]

1 Department of Biochemistry, Faculty of Medical Sciences in Zabrze, Medical University of Silesia, 40-055 Katowice, Poland
2 Second Department of Cardiology, Faculty of Medical Sciences in Zabrze, Medical University of Silesia, 40-055 Katowice, Poland; wjachec@interia.pl (W.J.); wojciechowskac@wp.pl (C.W.)
3 Department of Toxicology and Health Protection, Faculty of Health Sciences in Bytom, Medical University of Silesia, 40-055 Katowice, Poland; ezbrojkiewicz@op.pl (E.Z.); alina.mroczek@wp.pl (A.M.); prozentryt@sum.edu.pl (P.R.)
4 3rd Department of Cardiology, Faculty of Medical Sciences in Zabrze, Medical University of Silesia, Silesian Centre for Heart Disease, 41-800 Zabrze, Poland; jacek.niedziela@gmail.com (J.N.); m.gasior@op.pl (M.G.)
* Correspondence: eromuk@gmail.com

Abstract: We investigated whether the additional determination of ceruloplasmin (Cp) levels could improve the prognostic value of N-terminal pro-B-type natriuretic peptide (NT-proBNP) in heart failure (HF) patients in a 1-year follow-up. Cp and NT-proBNP levels and clinical and laboratory parameters were assessed simultaneously at baseline in 741 HF patients considered as possible heart transplant recipients. The primary endpoint (EP) was a composite of all-cause death (non-transplant patients) or heart transplantation during one year of follow-up. Using a cut-off value of 35.9 mg/dL for Cp and 3155 pg/mL for NT-proBNP (top interquartile range), a univariate Cox regression analysis showed that Cp (hazard ratio (HR) = 2.086; 95% confidence interval (95% CI, 1.462–2.975)), NT-proBNP (HR = 3.221; 95% CI (2.277–4.556)), and the top quartile of both Cp and NT-proBNP (HR = 4.253; 95% CI (2.795–6.471)) were all risk factors of the primary EP. The prognostic value of these biomarkers was demonstrated in a multivariate Cox regression model using the top Cp and NT-proBNP concentration quartiles combined (HR = 2.120; 95% CI (1.233–3.646)). Lower left ventricular ejection fraction, VO_2max, lack of angiotensin-converting enzyme inhibitor or angiotensin receptor blocker therapy, and nonimplantation of an implantable cardioverter-defibrillator were also independent risk factors of a poor outcome. The combined evaluation of Cp and NT-proBNP had advantages over separate NT-proBNP and Cp assessment in selecting a group with a high 1-year risk. Thus multi-biomarker assessment can improve risk stratification in HF patients.

Keywords: ceruloplasmin; NT-proBNP; heart failure

---

1. Introduction

Systolic heart failure (HF) is a complex disease caused by reduced ejection fraction of the left ventricle, often leading to the worsening of symptoms and poor quality of life, despite proper diagnosis and treatment according to current guidelines. All-cause mortality in these patients remains high and heart transplantation is a therapeutic option in end-stage HF. Adverse outcomes for HF patients are associated with many contributing factors. Stratification of risk factors is a great challenge in out-patient clinic cohorts, in which patients still undergo significant mortality and morbidity, despite stable HF. Different clinical and laboratory parameters can be helpful to identify patients at higher risk of adverse outcomes. Biological markers reflecting several pathophysiological abnormalities of HF have become powerful and convenient noninvasive tools for the stratification of HF patients [1–3]. Brain natriuretic peptide (BNP) and N-terminal pro-BNP (NT-proBNP) are secreted by cardiomyocytes in response to hemodynamic overload or neurohormonal disturbances. In clinical practice, NT-proBNP is recommended as a marker over BNP, because of its longer plasma half-life and lower levels of biological variation. NT-proBNP is the best-known diagnostic biomarker [4]. The usefulness of NT-proBNP for risk stratification varies depending on the stage of HF, time of assessment (onset of hospitalization, pre-discharge, or out-patient clinic evaluation), and duration of follow-up. However, there is no conclusive evidence that plasma NT-proBNP concentration is a guide for more effective therapy [5–8]. Ceruloplasmin (Cp) is an acute-phase reactant that is synthesized and secreted by the liver and monocyte/macrophages. It is elevated in conditions of acute inflammation. Cp contains seven copper atoms per molecule, participates in copper transport and metabolism, and has ferroxidase activity [9,10]. Furthermore, Cp is involved in the modulation of coagulation and angiogenesis and the inactivation of biogenic amines [11,12]. It is possible that increased levels of Cp may decrease available plasma NO, thus increasing reactive oxygen species formation and oxidative cell injury [13]. Several recent reports have indicated that Cp levels are elevated in patients with heart failure, regardless of its etiology [14–16].

Different pathobiological processes are involved in heart failure; thus, it is not surprising that single biomarkers, even natriuretic peptides, fail to predict all risks associated with HF.

The aim of this study was to examine the prognostic value of clinical factors, with special consideration of Cp, in a large cohort of HF patients and to investigate whether the combination of Cp and NT-proBNP could provide additional prognostic information in HF patients in a 1-year follow-up.

2. Materials and Methods

2.1. Clinical Assessment

We analyzed data in a subgroup of patients included in the Prospective Registry of Heart Failure (PR-HF) and Studies Investigating Co-morbidities Aggravating Heart Failure (SICA-HF) studies described elsewhere [17]. A cohort of patients with chronic systolic HF were prospectively recruited from patients referred to our inpatients clinic as potential candidates for heart transplantation. The main inclusion criteria were reduced left ventricular ejection fraction (LVEF $\leq$ 40%) and symptomatic HF, despite pharmacological treatment according to the current published ESC guidelines, at least 3 months before inclusion. The exclusion criteria included acute myocardial infarction; pulmonary thromboembolism; constrictive pericarditis; infectious pericarditis; prior heart transplantation; noncardiac conditions resulting in an expected mortality of less than 12 months, as judged by the treating physician; and a history of alcohol abuse or known antioxidant supplementation. These criteria were fulfilled in the 1216 PR-HF and SICA-HF studies. We analyzed data from 741 participants (aged 48–59 years) who had completed clinical and laboratory assessments.

A detailed description of the clinical echocardiographic evaluation of patients included in the study has been presented elsewhere [18].

The primary outcome was a composite of death from all causes (nontransplant patients) or heart transplantation. In the case of heart transplantation, the endpoint was reached and the patient was not followed up further. Patients were followed for a year via direct or phone contact. In some cases, the exact data regarding patient death were obtained from family members or the national identification number database by dedicated research personnel. Prior to enrolment in the study, all participants provided written informed consent. The local ethics committee of Silesian Medical University approved the study protocol (NN-6501-12/I/04). All procedures were performed in accordance with the 1975 Declaration of Helsinki and its revision in 2008.

2.2. Biochemical Methods

Venous blood samples obtained at enrollment were processed, separated by centrifugation at 1500× g for 10 min, frozen at −70 °C, and partially stored at −70 °C until assayed. Serum protein, albumin, fibrinogen, CRP, alanine aminotransferase, aspartate aminotransferase, gamma-glutamyl-transferase (GGTP), alkaline phosphatase, bilirubin, and lipid parameters and serum iron, sodium, creatinine, glucose, and uric acid concentrations were measured by colorimetric methods (Cobas 6000 e501; Roche, Basel, Switzerland). Hemoglobin, leukocytes, and platelets were measured using a MEDONIC M32C analyzer (Alpha Diagnostics, Warsaw, Poland). NT-proBNP was measured using a chemiluminescence method (Cobas 6000 e501).

Serum Cp concentration was determined spectrophotometrically, according to the Richterich reaction with p-phenyl-diamine [19]. Cp catalyzes the oxidation of colorless p-phenylenediamine, resulting in a blue-violet dye. Twenty microliters of serum was added to the test sample, while 20 µL of serum and 200 µL of sodium azide solution were added to the control sample to stop the reaction. Then, 1 mL of p-phenylenediamine dihydrochloride in acetate buffer was added to both test and control samples. After a 15-min incubation, 200 µL of sodium azide was added to the test sample. Finally, after a 15-min incubation, the absorbance of test and control samples was measured at 560 nm using a PerkinElmer VICTOR-X3 plate reader. The samples were not previously thawed before Cp assays. The intra-assay coefficient of variation was 3.7% and the intra-assay precision was 4%.

2.3. Statistical Analysis

Study participants were divided into subgroups based on Cp concentration quartiles (Table 1). Moreover, two subgroups, firstly, both Cp and NT-proBNP in the top quartile and, secondly, remaining patients (Cp or NT-proBNP in I–III quartiles including patients with Cp in I–III quartiles and NT-proBNP in I–IV quartiles or NT-proBNP in I–III quartiles and Cp in I–IV quartiles), were also compared (Table 2). The Shapiro–Wilk test was used to evaluate the distribution of all continuous variables. Continuous data are presented as the median, with the first and fourth quartiles (because of non-normal distribution of the data). Categorical data are presented as absolute numbers and percentages. The Kruskal-Wallis ANOVA test was used to compare both continuous and categorical data.

Estimations of risk were performed using a Cox proportional hazards model. Only complete data were analyzed. All demographic; clinical; echocardiography; laboratory; medication; and Cp and NT-proBNP data, expressed as the top quartiles individually or as the combined top quartiles of Cp and NT-proBNP concentration, were included in a univariate Cox analysis. Variables with a value of $p \leq 0.05$ in the univariate analysis were included in the multivariate analysis. Two multivariate analysis models were built. The first model was based on the top Cp and NT-proBNP concentration quartiles separately and the second model was based on the combined top quartiles of Cp and NT-proBNP concentrations.

The results of the Cox analysis are presented as relative risks, with 95% confidence intervals (CIs). Cumulative survival curves for all-cause death or heart transplantation were constructed as the time to endpoint occurrence, using the Kaplan–Meier method. Survival curves were compared among groups according to quartiles of Cp, quartiles of NT-proBNP and between groups presented in Table 2, using the log-rank test, as appropriate.

The odds ratio (OR) of achieving the endpoint for the top quartiles of Cp and NT-proBNP concentrations were calculated. The same calculations were performed for the combined top quartiles of Cp and NT-proBNP concentrations. The predictive value of these parameters was then compared.

Statistical significance was set at $p < 0.05$. Statistical analyses were performed using STATISTICA 13.1 PL software (StatSoft, Cracow, Poland).

3. Results

3.1. *Baseline Characteristics of the Entire Study Population and Subgroups in Relation to Ceruloplasmin Concentration*

The study group included 741 systolic HF patients, with a median Cp concentration of 28.7 mg% (range, 23.7–35.8). The cohort was divided into quartiles of serum Cp concentration as follows: group I, 184 (24.8%) patients with a Cp concentration range of 8.0–23.6 mg/dL; group II, 184 (24.8%) patients with 23.7–28.6 mg/dL Cp; group III, 187 (25.2%) patients with 28.7–35.8 mg/dL Cp; and group IV, 186 (25.1%) patients with the highest Cp concentration quartile of 35.9–81.0 mg/dL. One hundred and twenty-eight (17.42%) patients reached the combined endpoint (101 deaths, 27 heart transplantations). The overall mortality rate during the 1-year follow-up period was 13.76% and the heart transplantation rate was 3.64%. The demographic, clinical, and laboratory parameters of all patient groups and subgroups, divided according to quartiles of serum Cp concentration, are presented in Table 1.

Table 1. Characteristic of the examined group with division according to ceruloplasmin concentration quartiles.

Ceruloplasmin Quartiles (mg/dL)	All Group	I Quartile 8.0–23.6	II Quartile 23.7–28.6	III Quartile 28.7–35.8	IV Quartile 35.9–81.0	
Number	$N = 741$	$N = 184$	$N = 184$	$N = 187$	$N = 186$	
	Demographic and clinical parameters					ANOVA
Deaths (n)/HT (n) All n (%)	101/27 128 (17.27)	16/4 20 (10.87)	24/5 29 (15.76)	23/6 29 (15.51)	38/12 50 (26.88)	$p < 0.001$
Female n (%)	105 (14.17)	18 (9.78)	25 (13.59)	28 (14.97)	34 (18.28)	NS
Age (years)	54.00 (48.0–59.0)	54.00 (48.00–58.00)	55.00 (49.00–60.00)	54.00 (48.00–59.00)	55.00 (49.00–60.00)	NS
BMI (kg/m^2)	26.29 (23.50–29.32)	26.49 (24.04–29.06)	26.66 (23.58–29.70)	26.15 (23.36–29.69)	25.96 (22.50–28.89)	NS
Duration of symptoms before inclusion (months)	33.83 (13.07–69.67)	29.82 (13.40–58.47)	33.60 (12.80–69.02)	31.83 (12.90–68.70)	43.77 (14.13–79.93)	NS
	Exercise, capacity, echocardiography					
NYHA class III–IV n (%)	417 (56.28)	77 (41.85)	99 (53.80)	119 (63.64)	122 (65.59)	$p < 0.001$
VO_2max (mL/min/kg b.w.)	14.35 (11.70–17.60)	15.30 (12.30–19.50)	14.70 (12.00–17.70)	14.20 (11.40–17.10)	13.40 (10.75–16.55)	$p < 0.001$
LVEF (%)	24.00 (20.00–30.00)	25.00 (20.50–32.50)	24.00 (20.00–30.00)	24.00 22.00–28.00)	22.00 (19.00–28.00)	$p < 0.01$
	Laboratory parameters					
NT-proBNP (pg/mL) /100	13.92 (6.44–31.55)	9.30 (5.00–20.09)	14.82 (6.64–34.77)	15.48 (6.55–31.95)	18.42 (8.97–37.96)	$p < 0.001$
Ceruloplasmin (mg/dL)	28.70 (23.70–35.80)	20.75 (18.20–22.40)	26.25 (24.90–27.50)	31.90 (30.00–33.50)	42.35 (38.10–49.30)	$p < 0.001$
Hemoglobin (g/dL)	14.02 (13.05–14.99)	14.02 (13.05–14.83)	14.02 (12.89–14.99)	14.02 (13.22–15.15)	14.18 (13.05–15.15)	NS
Leukocytes (10^9/L)	6.94 (5.82–8.27)	6.83 (5.53–8.26)	6.77 (5.55–8.27)	7.23 (5.88–8.65)	6.92 (6.07–7.84)	0.060
Blood platelets (10^9/L)	185.00 (152.00-223.00)	183.00 (148.00-218.50)	185.00 (156.50-220.50)	197.00 (160.00-238.00)	174.00 (150.00-218.00)	$p < 0.05$
Sodium (mmol/L)	136.00 (134.00–139.00)	137.00 (135.00–139.00)	137.00 (134.50–138.00)	135.00 (133.00–138.00)	136.00 (134.00–138.00)	$p < 0.001$
Creatinine clearance (mL/min)	95.11 (69.98–119.44)	101.49 (80.86–125.04)	93.51 (70.86–117.35)	88.85 (70.07–116.43)	93.27 (61.00–117.28)	$p < 0.01$
Uric acid (μmol/L)/10	40.90 (33.00–50.60)	37.85 (33.05–45.00)	41.10 (32.95–50.15)	41.50 (33.10–50.80)	43.25 (32.90–55.60)	$p < 0.001$

Table 1. *Cont.*

Ceruloplasmin Quartiles (mg/dL)	All Group	I Quartile 8.0–23.6	II Quartile 23.7–28.6	III Quartile 28.7–35.8	IV Quartile 35.9–81.0	
Number	**N = 741**	**N = 184**	**N = 184**	**N = 187**	**N = 186**	
			Laboratory parameters			
Serum protein (g/L)	71.00 (67.00–75.00)	70.00 (66.00–73.50)	70.00 (66.00–74.00)	72.00 (67.00–76.00)	73.00 (69.00–77.00)	$p < 0.001$
Albumin (g/l)	42.00 (39.00–44.00)	42.00 (39.00–44.00)	41.00 (39.00–43.50)	41.00 (38.00–44.00)	43.00 (40.00–45.00)	$p < 0.05$
Fibrinogen (mg/dL)	397.00 (338.00–462.00)	367.00 (320.50–433.50)	395.50 (340.00–454.50)	425.00 (367.00–495.00)	409.50 (343.00–491.00)	$p < 0.001$
C-reactive protein (mg/dL)	2.94 (1.34–6.67)	1.97 (0.91–4.55)	2.65 (1.27–6.04)	4.11 (1.82–7.35)	3.83 (1.86–8.90)	$p <0.001$
Iron concentration (μmol/L)	17.10 (12.00–22.20)	16.91 (13.00–20.25)	17.10 (11.14–21.40)	16.90 (11.80–22.40)	17.60 (12.00–23.92)	NS
Bilirubin (μmol/L)	13.70 (9.70–20.50)	12.00 (8.45–16.15)	13.65 (10.00–18.35)	14.70 (9.30–21.10)	16.55 (11.00–26.60)	$p < 0.001$
Aspartate transaminase (IU/L)	23.0 (19.0–30.9)	23.0 (18.0–29.0)	23 (19.0–28.6)	24 (18.0–310)	24 (20.0–33.0)	NS
Alanine transaminase (IU/L)	24 (17.0–36.0)	23 (17.5–35.5)	24 (17.0–36.0)	24 (17.0–34.0)	25 (18.0–38.0)	NS
γ-glutamyl transpeptidase (IU/L)	49 (27.0–100.0)	39 (24.5–75.5)	45.5 (27.0–79.0)	54 (27.0–112.0)	67.5 (33.0–152.0)	$p < 0.001$
Alkaline phosphatase (IU/L)	68.0 (56.0–90.0)	65.0 (52.0–80.4)	65.0 (54.0–84.0)	72.0 (58.0–94.0)	78.0 (61.0–108.0)	$p < 0.001$
Fasting glucose (mmol/L)	5.50 (5.00–6.20)	5.50 (5.00–6.20)	5.45 (4.85–6.20)	5.60 (5.10–6.70)	5.50 (4.90–6.10)	NS
Total Cholesterol (mmol/L)	4.29 (3.64–5.22)	4.30 (3.60–5.10)	4.25 (3.65–5.19)	4.25 (3.62–5.34)	4.41 (3.67–5.21)	NS
Triglycerides (mmol/L)	1.20 (0.89–1.73)	1.17 (0.83–1.73)	1.22 (0.89–1.93)	1.23 (0.97–1.69)	1.20 (0.85–1.74)	NS
Cholesterol HDL (mmol/L)	1.14 (0.94–1.40)	1.19 (0.98–1.43)	1.14 (0.92–1.39)	1.13 (0.94–1.32)	1.13 (0.88–1.42)	NS
Cholesterol LDL (mmol/L)	2.45 (1.90–3.16)	2.46 (1.89–3.08)	2.39 (1.88–3.20)	2.38 (1.85–3.25)	2.54 (2.00–3.16)	NS
			Comorbidities			
Non ischemic DCM; *n* (%)	280 (37.79)	58 (31.52)	77 (41.85)	78 (41.71)	67 (36.02)	NS
Diabetes; *n* (%)	211 (28.48)	43 (23.37)	53 (28.80)	61 (32.62)	54 (29.03)	NS
Arterial hypertension; *n* (%)	408 (55.06)	100 (54.35)	104 (56.52)	91 (48.66)	113 (60.75)	NS
Permanent atrial fibrillation; *n* (%)	176 (23.75)	24 (13.04)	42 (22.83)	48 (25.67)	62 (33.33)	$p < 0.001$
ICD presence; *n* (%)	207 (27.94)	50 (27.17)	63 (34.24)	52 (27.81)	42 (22.58)	NS
Smoker; *n* (%)	257 (34.68)	64 (34.78)	78 (42.39)	72 (38.50)	43 (23.12)	$p < 0.001$
			Pharmacotherapy			
Beta-blockers; *n* (%)	726 (97.98)	182 (98.91)	181 (98.37)	180 (96.26)	183 (98.39)	NS
ACE–inhibitors; *n* (%)	641 (86.50)	166 (90.22)	161 (87.50)	159 (85.03)	155 (83.33)	NS
Angiotensin-2 receptor blockers; *n* (%)	76 (10.26)	17 (9.24)	20 (10.87)	24 (12.83)	15 (8.06)	NS

Table 1. *Cont.*

Ceruloplasmin Quartiles (mg/dL)	All Group	I Quartile 8.0–23.6	II Quartile 23.7–28.6	III Quartile 28.7–35.8	IV Quartile 35.9–81.0	
Number	$N = 741$	$N = 184$	$N = 184$	$N = 187$	$N = 186$	
		Pharmacotherapy				
ACE–inhibitor or/and * ARB; *n* (%)	693 (93.52)	178 (96.74)	174 (94,57)	174 (93,05)	167 (89,78)	$p < 0.05$
Loop diuretic; *n* (%)	647 (87.31)	145 (78.80)	168 (91.30)	169 (90.37)	165 (88.71)	$p < 0.001$
Thiazide diuretics; *n* (%)	93 (12.55)	14 (7.61)	19 (10.33)	34 (18.18)	26 (13.98)	$p < 0.05$
Aldosterone receptor antagonist; *n* (%)	683 (92.19)	163 (88.65)	171 (92.93)	177 (94.65)	172 (92.47)	NS
Statins; *n* (%)	487 (65.72)	128 (69.57)	127 (69.02)	124 (66.31)	108 (58.06)	NS
Digitalis; *n* (%)	339 (45.75)	57 (30.98)	82 (44.57)	102 54.55	98 (52.69)	$p < 0.001$

HT: Heart Transplantation; BMI: body mass index; NYHA: New York Heart Association functional class; VO_2max: maximum oxygen output; LVEF: left ventricle ejection fraction; NT-proBNP: N-terminal pro-B-type natriuretic peptide; HDL: high density lipoproteins; LDL: low density lipoproteins; ICD: Implantable Cardioverter Defibrillator; ACE-inhibitor: angiotensin-converting-enzyme inhibitor; ARB: angiotensin-2 receptor blockers; * (24 patients received ACE-I and ARB simultaneously).

Neither age, sex, BMI, nor duration of symptoms before enrollment differed between groups. LVEF was reduced to a greater extent in group IV. The percentage of patients with atrial fibrillation was higher in group IV, but the frequencies of coronary artery disease, hypertension, diabetes mellitus, and implantable cardioverter-defibrillators (ICDs) were similar between groups. Pharmacological treatments were comparable between groups in terms of the use of angiotensin-converting enzyme inhibitors (ACE-Is), angiotensin receptor blockers (ARBs), beta-blockers, mineralocorticoid receptor antagonists (MRAs), and statins, but loop and thiazide diuretics and digitalis were more frequently used by group III patients. If ACE-I or ARB treatment was analyzed, their use was the lowest in patients in the 4th Cp quartile.

The following laboratory parameters, assessed in serum samples, were different among groups: NT-proBNP, Cp, sodium, creatinine clearance, protein, fasting glucose, lipid parameters, uric acid, bilirubin, aspartate transaminase, alanine transaminase, alkaline phosphatase, and GGTP (Table 1). Characteristic of examined group with division according to ceruloplasmin and NT-proBNP concentration quartiles are presented in Table 2

Table 2. Characteristic of examined group with division according to ceruloplasmin and N-terminal pro-B-type natriuretic peptide (NT-proBNP) concentration quartiles.

Ceruloplasmin/NT-pro-BNP Quartiles (mg/dL)	I–III Quartile	IV–IV Quartiles	ANOVA
Number	$N = 683$	$N = 58$	
Demographic and clinical parameters			
Deaths (*n*)/HT (*n*) All *n* (%)	79/21 100 (14.64)	23/5 28 (48.28)	$p < 0.001$
Female *n* (%)	96 (14.06)	9 (15.52)	NS
Age (years)	54.00 (49.00–59.00)	56,50 (45,00–61,00)	NS
BMI (kg/m^2)	26.44 (23.74–29.41)	23.55 (19,86–26.76)	$p < 0.001$
Duration of symptoms before inclusion (months)	33.53 (12.93–68.70)	43.12 (14.3–92.20)	NS

Table 2. *Cont.*

Ceruloplasmin/NT-pro-BNP Quartiles (mg/dL)	I–III Quartile	IV–IV Quartiles	ANOVA
Number	*N* = 683	*N* = 58	
Exercise, capacity, echocardiography			
NYHA class III-IV *n* (%)	369 (54.03)	48 (82.76)	$p < 0.001$
VO_2max (mL/min/kg b.w.)	14.50 (11.70–18.00)	12.30 (9.20–14.50)	$p < 0.001$
LVEF (%)	24.00 (20.00-30.00)	20.00 (17.00-24.00)	$p < 0.001$
Laboratory parameters			
NT-proBNP (pg/mL) /100	12.78 (5.97–25.70)	52.34 (41.31–78.06)	$p < 0.001$
Ceruloplasmin (mg/dL)	28.00 (23.40–33.70)	46.30 (38.10–54.30)	$p < 0.001$
Hemoglobin (g/dL)	14.02 (13.05–14.99)	13.62 (12.73–15.15)	NS
Leukocytes (10^9/L)	6.94 (5.79–8.31)	7.01 (6.17–8.19)	NS
Blood platelets (10^9/L)	185.00 (152.00–224.00)	185.00 (152.00–219.00)	NS
Sodium (mmol/L)	137.00 (134.00–139.00)	134.00 (132.00–137.00)	$p < 0.001$
Creatinine clearance (mL/min)	96.93 (73.45–120.64)	66.41 (50.32–103.34)	$p < 0.001$
Uric acid (μmol/L)/10	40.80 (32.90–49.50)	44.40 (33.70–69.00)	$p < 0.01$
Serum protein (g/L)	71.00 (67.00–75.00)	71.50 (67.00–77.00)	NS
Albumin (g/L)	42.00 (39.00–44.00)	40.00 (38.00–44.00)	$p < 0.05$
Fibrinogen (ug/mL)	396.00 (337.00–458.00)	434.00 (360.00–536.00)	$p < 0.01$
C-reactive protein (mg/dL)	2.80 (1.27–6.12)	7.18 (2.67–14.75)	$p < 0.001$
Iron concentration (μmol/L)	17.20 (12.10–22.20)	16.15 (10.50–21.30)	NS
Bilirubin (μmol/L)	13.40 (9.50–19.30)	22.90 (13.80–32.50)	$p < 0.001$
Aspartate transaminase (IU/L)	23.00 (18.00–30.00)	27.00 (21.00–37.00)	$p < 0.01$
Alanine transaminase (IU/L)	24.00 (17.00–36.00)	25.00 (18.00–41.00)	NS
γ-glutamyl transpeptidase (IU/L)	47.00 (27.00–92.00)	133.50 (49.00–218.00)	$p < 0.001$
Alkaline phosphatase (IU/L)	67.00 (55.00–88.00)	99.50 (73.00–143.00)	$p < 0.001$
Fasting glucose (mmol/L)	5.50 (5.00–6.30)	5.20 (4.70–5.90)	$p < 0.05$
Total Cholesterol (mmol/L)	4.31 (3.66–5.27)	3.97 (3.33–3.86)	NS
Triglycerides (mmol/L)	1.22 (0.89–1.75)	1.07 (0.78–1.36)	$p < 0.05$
Cholesterol HDL (mmol/L)	1.15 (0.95–1.40)	1.05 (0.79–1.29)	$p < 0.05$
Cholesterol LDL (mmol/L)	2.46 (1.91–3.19)	2.29 (1.85–3.00)	NS

Table 2. *Cont.*

Ceruloplasmin/NT-pro-BNP Quartiles (mg/dL)	I–III Quartile	IV–IV Quartiles	ANOVA
Number	$N = 683$	$N = 58$	
Comorbidities			
Non ischemic DCM; *n* (%)	252 (36.90)	28 (48.27)	NS
Diabetes; *n* (%)	190 (27.82)	21 (36.21)	NS
Arterial hypertension; *n* (%)	382 (56.93)	20 (34.48)	$p < 0.01$
Permanent atrial fibrillation; *n* (%)	155 (22.69)	21 (36.21)	$p < 0.05$
ICD presence; *n* (%)	192 (28.11)	15 (25.86)	NS
Smoker; *n* (%)	241 (35.29)	16 27.59)	NS
Pharmacotherapy			
Beta-blockers; *n* (%)	668 (97,80)	58 (100,00)	NS
ACE–inhibitors; *n* (%)	595 (87,12)	46 (79.310	NS
Angiotensin-2 receptor blockers; *n* (%)	71 (10,40)	5 (79,31)	NS
ACE–inhibitors or/and ARB; *n* (%)	643 (94.14)	50 (86,21)	$p < 0.05$
Loop diuretic; *n* (%)	590 (86.38)	57 (98.28)	$p < 0.05$
Thiazide diuretics; *n* (%)	79 (11.57)	14 (24.14)	$p < 05$
Aldosterone receptor antagonist; *n* (%)	628 (91,95)	54 (93,10)	NS
Statins; *n* (%)	457 (66.91)	30 (51.72)	$p < 0.05$
Digitalis; *n* (%)	305 (44.66)	34 (58.62)	NS

HT: Heart Transplantation; BMI: body mass index; NYHA: New York Heart Association functional class; VO_2max: maximum oxygen output; LVEF: left ventricle ejection fraction; NT-proBNP: N-terminal pro-B-type natriuretic peptide; HDL: high density lipoproteins; LDL: low density lipoproteins; ICD: Implantable Cardioverter Defibrillator; ACE-inhibitors: angiotensin-converting-enzyme inhibitor; ARB: angiotensin -2 receptor blockers.

3.2. Ceruloplasmin, NT-proBNP and Prognosis

3.2.1. Univariate Cox Regression Analysis

All demographic, clinical, exercise capacity, echocardiography, laboratory parameter, comorbidity, and pharmacotherapy data presented in Table 1 were assessed as risk factors for all-cause death or heart transplantation in a 1-year follow-up.

In univariate Cox regression analyses, among others, the top quartiles of NT-proBNP concentration (hazard ratio (HR) = 3.221, 95% CI (2.277–4.556)), Cp concentration (HR = 2.086, 95% CI (1.462–2.975)), and combined Cp and NT-proBNP concentration (HR = 4.253, 95% CI (2.795–6.471) were associated with a higher risk of death or heart transplantation.

All variables that reached $p < 0.05$ in a univariate Cox regression analysis are presented in Table 3.

3.2.2. Multivariate Cox Regression Analysis

In the first multivariate Cox regression model, after adjusting for other clinical and pharmacotherapeutic predictors, neither the top Cp concentration quartile nor the top NT-proBNP concentration quartile were significant predictors of unfavorable outcomes (Cp, HR = 1.511, 95% CI (0.980–2.330); NT-proBNP, HR = 1.287, 95% CI (0.815–2.033))

The results of the second multivariate Cox regression model, in which the top individual Cp and NT-proBNP concentration quartiles were replaced with the combined top quartiles of Cp and NT-proBNP concentrations, are presented in Table 3. In this model, an LVEF lower by 1 % (HR = 1.069, 95% CI (1.032–1.106)), a maximum measured VO_2 lower by 1 mL/min/kg b.m. (HR = 1.113, 95% CI (1.048–1.181)), absence of an ICD (HR = 7.575, 95% CI (3.278–17.502)), and lack of ACE-I and/or ARB therapy (HR = 2.195, 95% CI (1.234–3.906)) remained significant predictors of unfavorable outcomes. Among the laboratory parameters measured, only the combined top quartiles of Cp and NT-proBNP concentrations was associated with a higher risk of all-cause death and HT in a 1-year follow-up (HR = 2.120, 95% CI (1.233–3.646)).

Table 3. Predictors of death or heart transplantation in one-year follow-up. The results of uni- and multivariable Cox regression analysis, model-2.

	Univariable Cox Regression			**Multivariable Cox Regression**		
	HR	**95%CI**	***P***	**HR**	**95%CI**	***P***
General characteristics						
BMI ↑ (1 kg/m²)	0.945	0.908–0.985	$p < 0.01$	0.966	0.912–1.022	NS
Duration of symptoms before inclusion ↑ (1month)	1.004	1.000–1.007	$p < 0.05$	1.000	0.996–1.004	NS
NYHA class ↑ (1 class)	2.936	2.280–3.779	$p < 0.001$	1.099	0.759–1.592	NS
VO_2max ↓ (1 mL/min/kg b.m.)	1.198	1.142–1.256	$p < 0.001$	1.113	1.048–1.181	$p < 0.001$
LVEF ↓ (1 %p)	1.091	1.059–1.122	$p < 0.001$	1.069	1.032–1.106	$p < 0.001$
Basic biochemistry						
Sodium ↓ (1 mmol/L)	1.111	1.070–1.155	$p < 0.001$	1.039	0.990–1.092	NS
Creatinine clearance ↓ (1 mL/min)	1.014	1.008–1.019	$p < 0.001$	1.001	0.993–1.008	NS
Albumin ↓ (1 g/L)	1.068	1.026–1.114	$p < 0.01$	1.023	0.966–1.083	NS
Cholesterol HDL ↓ (1 mmol/L)	1.805	1.121–2.907	$p < 0.05$	0.954	0.591–1.593	NS
Cp and NT-proBNP "both in top quartile" (yes/no)	4.253	2.795–6.471	$p < 0.001$	2.120	1.233–3.646	$p < 0.01$
Fibrinogen ↑ (1 mg/dL)	1.003	1.001–1.004	$p < 0.001$	1.001	1.000–1.003	NS
Uric acid ↑ (10 μmol/L)	1.030	1.018–1.041	$p < 0.001$	1.012	0.999–1.026	NS
Bilirubin ↑ (1 μmoL/L)	1.028	1.018–1.039	$p < 0.001$	0.994	0.976–1.012	NS
Alkaline phosphatase ↑ (1 U/L)	1.006	1.004–1.009	$p < 0.001$	1.000	0.995–1.006	NS
γ-Glutamyl trans peptidase ↑ (1 U/L)	1.001	1.000–1.002	$p < 0.05$	1.000	0.998–1.002	NS
Comorbidities						
Diabetes t.2 (yes/no)	1.604	1.123–2.291	$p < 0.01$	1.450	0.949–2.217	NS
ICD absence (yes/no)	9.929	3.922–20.000	$p < 0.001$	7.575	3.278–17.502	$p < 0.001$
Pharmacotherapy						
Lack of ACE - I or/and ARB (yes/no)	3.428	2.126–5.256	$p < 0.001$	2.195	1.234–3.906	$p < 0.01$
Loop diuretics (yes/no)	4.895	1.809–13.248	$p < 0.01$	1.735	0.525–5.730	NS
Thiazide diuretics (yes/no)	2.296	1.518–3.473	$p < 0.001$	1.317	0.781–2.221	NS
Statins (yes/no)	0.699	0.492–0.993	$p < 0.05$	1.294	0.825–2.032	NS
Digitalis (yes/no)	1.439	1.016–2.036	$p < 0.05$	0.833	0.547–1.267	NS

BMI: body mass index; NYHA: New York Heart Association functional class; VO_2max: maximum oxygen output; LVEF: left ventricle ejection fraction; NT-proBNP: N-terminal pro-B-type natriuretic peptide; Cp: ceruloplasmin, ICD: Implantable Cardioverter Defibrillator; ACE-I: angiotensin-converting-enzyme inhibitor; ARB: Angiotensin-2 receptor blocker.

3.2.3. Kaplan–Meier Survival Analysis and Endpoint Odds Ratios

There were 128 endpoints in groups I (20, 10.9%), II (29, 15.8%), III (29, 15.5%), and IV (50, 26.9%). Kaplan–Meier survival curves for the four groups according to Cp and NT-proBNP quartiles are presented in Figures 1 and 2. Patients with both Cp and NT-proBNP concentrations in the top quartile were compared with the remaining patients (quartile I–III of Cp or NT-proBNP concentration), as shown in Figure 3.

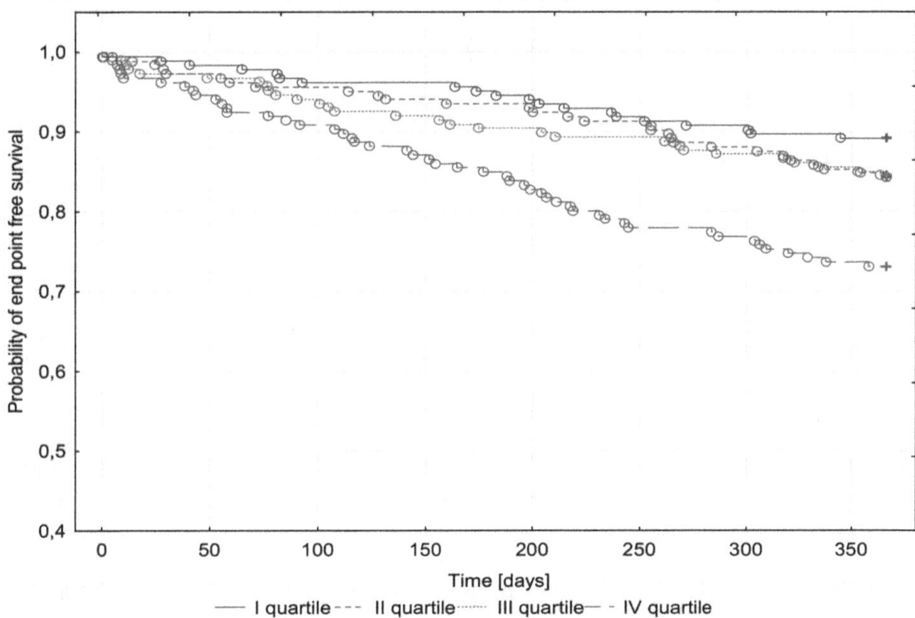

Figure 1. Probability of survival of time free of death or heart transplantation depending on quartiles of ceruloplasmin concentration in 1-year follow-up, $p < 0.001$.

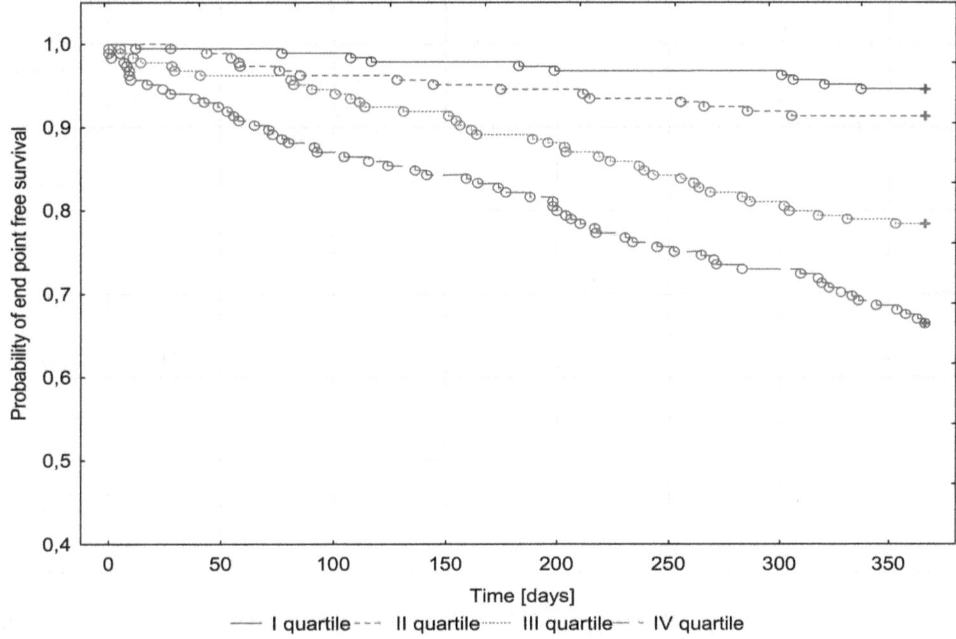

Figure 2. Probability of survival of time free of death or heart transplantation depending on quartiles of NT-proBNP concentrations in 1-year follow-up, $p < 0.001$.

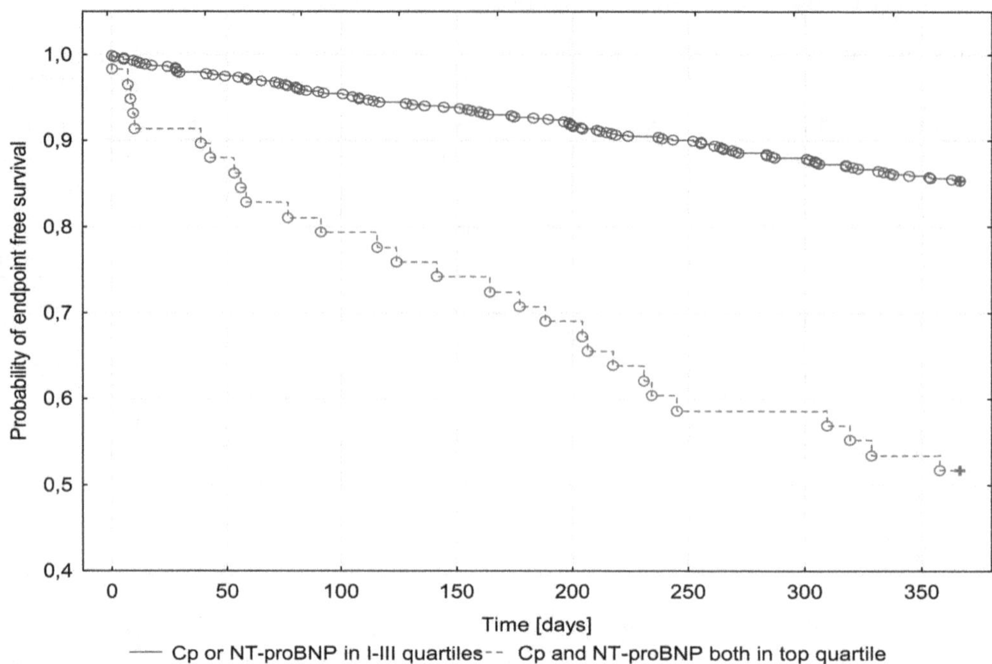

Figure 3. Probability of endpoint free survival in 1-year follow-up. Patients with Ceruloplasmin or NT-proBNP concentrations in I–III quartiles vs. both Cp and NT-proBNP in the top quartile, log rank $p < 0.001$.

A log-rank analysis revealed a significantly different probability of all-cause death or heart transplantation over time in patients stratified by quartiles of Cp or NT-proBNP concentration in the 1-year follow-up period ($p < 0.001$). After the stratification of patients based on the combination of CP and NT-proBNP concentration, patients with both Cp and NT-proBNP in the upper quartile had the highest probability of an endpoint occurrence (Table 4).

Table 4. Probability of death or heart transplantation occurrence in 1-year follow-up.

	I-III Quartiles of Cp (mg%) (8.0–35.8)	Top Quartile of Cp (mg%) (35.9–81.0)	I-III Quartiles of NT-proBNP (pg/mL) (122.9–3155.0)	Top Quartile of NTpro-BNP (pg/mL) (3156.0–22378.0)	I-III Quartiles of Cp or NT-proBNP	Cp and NT-proBNP Both in Top Quartile
End point (+) (*n*)	78	50	66	62	100	28
End point (−) (*n*)	477	136	490	123	583	30
Probability of end point (%) with confidence intervals	14.054 (11.159–16.941)	26.881 (20.508–33.251)	11.871 (9.182–14.558)	33.513 (26.708–40.312)	14.641 (11.989–17.291)	48.276 (35.416–61.136)
Odds ratio	2.248 95%CI (1.503–3.364) $p < 0.001$		3.742 95%CI (2.511–5.578) $p < 0.001$		5.441 95%CI (3.117–9.498) $p < 0.001$	
Sensitivity (%)	26.88		33.51		48.28	
Specificity (%)	77.81		79.93		95.10	

Cp—ceruloplasmin; NT-proBNP—N-terminal Type B pro peptide.

Detailed results for the top quartiles of Cp and NT-proBNP concentration, as well as the combination of the top quartiles of Cp and NT-proBNP concentrations, with the sensitivity and specificity of their predictive values, are presented in Table 4. For patients with a Cp concentration in the top quartile, the risk of death or heart transplantation was two-fold higher than in patients with Cp concentrations in quartiles I–III. Similarly, NT-proBNP concentration in the top quartile indicated approximately a 4-fold increase in the probability of an endpoint occurrence. The predictive values of Cp and NT-proBNP concentrations did not differ significantly (NT-proBNP vs. Cp, OR = 1.371, 95% CI (0.878–2.140)). The greatest prognostic value was seen for the combination of Cp and NT-proBNP concentrations in the top quartile, which was associated with more than a five-fold increased risk. Cp and NT-proBNP concentrations (both in the top quartile) showed a significantly higher predictive value than the top quartile of Cp (OR = 2.539; 95% CI (1.381–4.666)) or NT-proBNP (OR = 1.852; 95% CI (1.018–3.370)) concentrations individually (Table 4).

4. Discussion

There are many papers documenting the association between Cp and cardiovascular disease in clinical and experimental studies [20–22]. However, data confirming the effect of Cp concentration on prognosis in patients with HF are limited. This study intended to determine the clinical utility of a single baseline Cp measurement and other common risk factors as prognostic markers of all-cause mortality or heart transplantation in HF patients. We showed a significantly higher risk of all-cause death or heart transplantation in a 1-year follow-up of patients with Cp concentration in the top quartile. Similarly, patients with NT-proBNP concentration in the top quartile had a higher risk of endpoint occurrence. However, after adjustment for known clinical and laboratory parameters and treatments, neither NT-proBNP nor Cp remained significant predictors. Interestingly, the combination of elevated Cp and NT-proBNP concentrations (both in the top quartile) had greater specificity and sensitivity for endpoint prediction than CP or NT-proBNP concentrations alone. Other independent endpoint predictors were LVEF, peak VO_2, ACE-I/ARB therapy, and prior ICD implantation. Although clinical assessment had a strong prognostic role, it is worth highlighting that peak oxygen consumption (peak VO_2) rather than New York Heart Association class, should be used to estimate functional capacity. The utility of peak VO_2 and other parameters of the Heart Failure Survival Score (ischemic heart disease, mean blood pressure, LVEF, heart rate, serum sodium, intraventricular conduction defect) for predicting prognosis and assessing candidacy for heart transplantation, have been documented across races and genders [23].

Recently, Paolillo et al. showed that the cut-off values of peak VO_2 able to identify a 10% or 20% risk (in 10 years of follow-up) of unfavorable outcomes decreased over 20 years up to 2010, with similar cut-off values observed over this time period [24]. As a possible explanation, they suggested that the most effective treatment options were introduced to the guidelines by 2010, such that a similar risk level was observed in patients enrolled after 2010. In our study, patients were enrolled before 2010 and a decrease in peak VO_2 by 1 mL/min/kg was associated with an 11% increase in the risk of endpoints in a 1-year follow-up. Lower values of the main echocardiographic parameter, LVEF, were associated with increased mortality or heart transplantation rate.

On the contrary, Lai et al. showed that, at initial presentation, LVEF did not have outcome-predictive power Additionally, they showed that the 12-month mortality risk in patients with LVEF $\geq$ 50% was similar to those with LVEF < 40% [7]. However, in this study, patients were hospitalized with acute HF, and therefore, LVEF data may reflect exacerbated heart function, rather than a chronic stable status.

Referring to guideline-based therapy, patient treatment in our study was considered to be optimized by the physicians [25]. Although we did not analyze the reasons for not using this treatment, in most cases there were contraindications to the use of this therapy. Moreover, we did not analyze the ACE-I/ARB dose, since even low-dose ACE-I/ARB therapy is superior to no one treatment as it decreases 1-year mortality rates [26]. Patient treatment may be a limitation of the study (see study limitation section). Beta-blockers were used in the majority of patients (97%). Notably, the percentage of patients with ICDs in our study was rather low (approximately 27%). The lack of ICD implantation was an independent risk factor of all-cause mortality (not only sudden cardiac death) and heart transplantation. Improved survival of patients with implanted ICDs has previously been observed in clinical trials [27]. ICD implantation was different between groups according to Cp concentration quartiles. In the highest

Cp quartile the percentage of patients who did not receive ACE-I and /or ARB was the lowest. In our study, many of the analyzed laboratory parameters were risk factors of unfavorable outcomes only in univariable analyses. However, none of them were shown to affect mortality or heart transplantation after adjusting for other predictive factors. Only the combination of the top quartiles of NT-proBNP and Cp concentrations was useful for the prediction of unfavorable outcomes.

Previously, some investigations with various study designs have demonstrated the prognostic power of natriuretic peptide concentration [28–30]. Lai et al. reported that increased plasma NT-pro BNP level (≥11755 ng/L) was an independent predictor of 1- and 3-month mortality, but not of mortality in more extended follow-up [7]. Bettencourt and colleagues showed that an NT-proBNP concentration > 6779 pg/mL at admission was a weaker predictor of readmission or death than a post-treatment NT-proBNP concentration of 4137 pg/mL, with an 8% increase in the probability of death or readmission over 6 months per 1000 pg/mL of NT-proBNP [31]. Finally, the current ACC/AHA/HFSA Guideline for the Management of Heart Failure recommends the assessment of natriuretic peptide biomarkers on admission in acutely decompensated HF patients and before discharge, to establish a prognosis [32].

We evaluated NT-proBNP concentrations in stable, nonhospitalized patients and found that an NT-proBNP concentration > 3155pg/mL (upper quartile) did not have significant predictive value in a multivariate analysis in a 1-year follow-up. A comparison of our results with other studies is difficult because of different follow-up periods, endpoint definitions, and types of cohorts. Bayes-Genis et al. performed a serial assessment of NT-proBNP concentration in an outpatient group (patient decompensated, but not requiring emergency hospital admission) with reduced LVEF (27 +/− 9%). The percentage reduction in NT-proBNP concentration in the first four weeks (not baseline concentration) was a predictor of death and hospitalization during three months of follow-up [33].

Multiple biomarker strategies, involving a combination of NPs with other biomarkers, have been proposed to create more accurate predictive scores in HF [34]. Multimarker approaches combining NT-pro-BNP and Cp have been used to assess the risk of HF incidence and mortality in patients in the Atherosclerosis Risk in Communities (ARIC) study. In this population, the strongest associations of Cp were observed with HF and all-cause mortality. These associations persisted after adjusting for biomarkers known to have a role in HF prediction, such as NT-proBNP, troponin, and CRP [35]. Engstrom et al. also reported Cp as a risk factor for HF incidence in Caucasian men with a high risk of cardiovascular disease [36].

Elevated Cp levels have been shown in many cardiovascular disorders, including coronary heart disease, myocardial infarction, and arteriosclerosis. The oxidative effects of Cp on serum lipids, in combination with decreased antioxidant protection, can predominate in CAD patients. Ceruloplasmin has diverse functions. It is involved in iron homeostasis and angiogenesis. It is the major source of serum ferroxidase activity and can act as a pro- or antioxidant molecule [37–39]. Many previous studies have reported an elevated Cp concentration during HF [40,41]. Some study demonstrated that the Cp can be a significant marker of heart failure in patients with ST segment elevated myocardial infarction [42]. A possible association between ceruloplasmin and progression of HF was study by Cabassi et al. [43].

To the best of our knowledge, only one previous study has evaluated the prognostic value of the simultaneous assessment of Cp and BNP in stable HF patients undergoing elective cardiac evaluation, including coronary angiography. In that study, Hammadah et al. reported that elevated Cp levels increase the risk of 5-year all-cause mortality. Even after adjusting for a large panel of other risk factors and medications, Cp concentration in the third or fourth quartile (> 25.6 mg/dL) remained a significant predictor of increased 5-year mortality. Further analysis, with additional adjustment for heart rate, QRS duration and ICD placement, revealed that a Cp concentration in the upper quartile (> 30.2 mg/dL) remained predictive. Additionally, within each group of defined BNP concentration range, higher Cp levels were associated with poorer outcomes. Similar to our study, the authors shown that the combined use of biomarkers can help identify patients with the highest probability of death [44].

The reasons for the increased Cp concentration in HF are not well understood, but it is possible that the measurement of Cp (in combination with NT-proBNP) can help identify patients with the highest long-term mortality risk.

5. Conclusions

The determination of Cp concentration is cost-effective and relatively easy. Data from the present study confirmed the association between Cp concentration and the severity of HF. The combined measurement of Cp and NT-proBNP concentrations has an advantage over measuring NT-proBNP concentration alone in selecting a group of high-risk HF patients in a 1-year follow-up.

Study Limitations

Our study has several limitations. Firstly, these results may not be applicable to the general population, since the age range of patients in this study was 48–59 years. Secondly, it was a single-center study of stable outpatients considered as potential recipients of the heart. Thirdly, ARNI and SGLT2 were not used, since patient enrollment occurred before 2010. Fourthly, low percentage of patients with implanted ICD.

Author Contributions: Conceptualization, E.R., C.W., and W.J.; Methodology, C.W., E.R., and W.J.; Software, W.J.; Validation, E.R., C.W., and W.J.; Formal Analysis, E.R., C.W., and W.J.; Investigation, E.R., C.W., and W.J.; Resources, M.G., E.Z., and P.R.; Data Curation, A.M., E.Z.; Writing—Original Draft Preparation, E.R., C.W., and W.J.; Writing—Review & Editing, E.R., C.W., and W.J.; Visualization, J.N., A.M., and W.J.; Supervision, M.G., P.R.; Project Administration, E.R., C.W., and W.J. All authors have read and agreed to the published version of the manuscript.

References

1. Seino, Y.; Ogawa, A.; Yamashita, T.; Fukushima, M.; Ogata, K.; Fukumoto, H.; Takan, T. Application of NT-proBNP and BNP measurements in cardiac care: A more discerning marker for the detection and evaluation of heart failure. *Eur. J. Heart Fail.* **2004**, *6*, 295–300. [CrossRef] [PubMed]
2. Anker, S.; Doehner, W.; Rauchhaus, M.; Sharma, R.; Francis, D.; Knosalla, C.; Davos, C.H.; Cicoira, M.; Shamim, W.; Kemp, M.; et al. Uric Acid and Survival in Chronic Heart Failure Validation and Application in Metabolic, Functional, and Hemodynamic Staging. *Circulation* **2003**, *107*, 1991–1997. [CrossRef] [PubMed]
3. Yin, W.H.; Chen, J.W.; Jen, L.H.; Chiang, M.C.; Huang, W.P.; Feng, A.N.; Young, M.S.; Lin, S.J. Independent prognostic value of elevated high-sensitivity C-reactive protein in chronic heart failure. *Am. Heart J.* **2004**, *147*, 931–938. [CrossRef] [PubMed]
4. Ponikowski, P.; Voors, A.A.; Anker, S.D.; Bueno, H.; Cleland, J.G.F.; Coats, A.J.S.; Falk, V.; González-Juanatey, J.R.; Harjola, V.P.; Jankowska, E.A.; et al. 2016 ESC Guidelines for the diagnosis and treatment of acute and chronic heart failure: The Task Force for the diagnosis and treatment of acute and chronic heart failure of the European Society of Cardiology (ESC). Developed with the special contribution of the Heart Failure Association (HFA) of the ESC. *Eur. Heart J.* **2016**, *37*, 2129–2200. [CrossRef]
5. Neuhold, S.; Huelsmann, M.; Strunk, G.; Stoiser, B.; Struck, J.; Morgenthaler, N.G.; Bergmann, A.; Moertl, D.; Berger, R.; Pacher, R. Comparison of copeptin, B-type natriuretic peptide, and amino-terminal pro-B-type natriuretic peptide in patients with chronic heart failure: Prediction of death at different stages of the disease. *J. Am. Coll. Cardiol.* **2008**, *52*, 266–272. [CrossRef]
6. Chow, S.L.; Chow, S.L.; Maisel, A.S.; Anand, I.; Bozkurt, B.; de Boer, R.A.; Felker, G.M.; Fonarow, G.C.; Greenberg, B.; Januzzi, J.L., Jr.; et al. Role of biomarkers for the prevention, assessment, and management of heart failure a scientific statement from the American Heart Association. *Circulation* **2017**, *135*, 1054–1091. [CrossRef]
7. Lai, M.Y.; Kan, W.C.; Huang, Y.T.; Chen, J.; Shiao, C.C. The Predictivity of N-Terminal Pro b-Type Natriuretic Peptide for All-Cause Mortality in Various Follow-Up Periods among Heart Failure Patients. *J. Clin. Med.* **2019**, *13*, 357. [CrossRef]

8. Januzzi, J.L.; Rehman, S.U.; Mohammed, A.A.; Bhardwaj, A.; Barajas, L.; Barajas, J.; Kim, H.N.; Baggish, A.L.; Weiner, R.B.; Chen-Tournoux, A.; et al. Use of amino-terminal pro-B type natriuretic peptide to guide outpatient therapy of patients with chronic left ventricular systolic dysfunction. *J. Am. Coll. Cardiol.* **2011**, *58*, 1881–1889. [CrossRef]
9. Floris, G.; Medda, R.; Padiglia, A.; Musci, G. The physiopathological significance of caeruloplasmin. *Biochem. Pharmacol.* **2000**, *60*, 1735–1741. [CrossRef]
10. Harris, E.D. A requirement for copper in angiogenesis. *Nutr. Rev.* **2004**, *62*, 60–64. [CrossRef]
11. Hannan, G.N.; McAuslen, B.R. Modulation of synthesis of specific proteins in endothelial cells by copper, cadmium, and disulfiram: An early response to an angiogenic inducer of cell migration. *J. Cell. Physiol.* **1982**, *111*, 207–212. [CrossRef] [PubMed]
12. Shukla, N.; Maher, J.; Masters, J.; Angelini, G.D.; Jeremy, J.Y. Does oxidative stress change ceruloplasmin from a protective to a vasculopathic factor. *Atherosclerosis* **2006**, *187*, 238–250. [CrossRef] [PubMed]
13. Shiva, S.; Wang, X.; Ringwood, L.A.; Xu, X.; Yuditskaya, S.; Annavajjhala, V.; Miyajima, H.; Hogg, N.; Harris, Z.L.; Gladwin, M.T. Ceruloplasmin is a NO oxidase and nitrite synthase that determines endocrine NO homeostasis. *Nat. Chem. Biol.* **2006**, *2*, 486–493. [CrossRef] [PubMed]
14. Xu, Y.; Lin, H.; Zhou, Y.; Cheng, G.; Xu, G. Ceruloplasmin and the extent of heart failure in ischemic and nonischemic cardiomyopathy patients. *Mediat. Inflamm.* **2013**, *2013*, 348145. [CrossRef] [PubMed]
15. Kaya, Z.; Kaya, B.; Sezen, H.; Bilinc, H.; Asoglu, R.; Yildiz, A.; Taskin, A.; Yalcin, S.; Sezen, Y.; Aksoy, N. Serum ceruloplasmin levels in acute decompensated heart failure. *Clin. Ter.* **2013**, *164*, 87–91.
16. Ahmed, M.S.; Jadhav, A.B.; Hassan, A.; Meng, Q.H. Acute Phase Reactants as Novel Predictors of Cardiovascular Disease. *ISRN Inflamm.* **2012**. [CrossRef]
17. Studies Investigating Co-Morbidities Aggravating Heart Failure (SICA-HF). 2016. Available online: https://clinicaltrials.gov/ (accessed on 18 November 2019).
18. Romuk, E.; Wojciechowska, C.; Jacheć, W.; Nowak, J.; Niedziela, J.; Malinowska-Borowska, J.; Głogowska-Gruszka, A.; Birkner, E.; Rozentryt, P. Comparison of Oxidative Stress Parameters in Heart Failure Patients Depending on Ischaemic or Nonischaemic Aetiology. *Oxid. Med. Cell. Longev.* **2019**, *2019*, 13. [CrossRef]
19. Richterich, R.; Gautier, E.; Stillharth, H.; Rossi, E. Serum ceruloplasmin concentration was determined spectrophotometrically according to Richterich reaction with p-phenyl-diamine. The heterogeneity of caeruloplasmin nd the enzymatic defect in Wilson's disease. *Helv. Paediatr. Acta* **1960**, *15*, 424–436.
20. Singh, T.K. Serum ceruloplasmin in acute myocardial infarction. *Acta Cardiol.* **1992**, *47*, 321–329.
21. Manttari, M.; Manninen, V.; Huttunen, J.K.; Palosuo, T.; Ehnholm, C.; Heinonen, O.P.; Frick, M.H. Serum ferritin and ceruloplasmin as coronary risk factors. *Eur. Heart J.* **1994**, *15*, 1599–1603. [CrossRef]
22. Atanasiu, R.; Dumoulin, M.J.; Chahine, R.; Mateescu, M.A.; Nadeau, R. Antiarrhythmic effects of ceruloplasmin during reperfusion in the ischemic isolated rat heart. *Can. J. Physiol. Pharmacol.* **1995**, *73*, 1253–1261. [CrossRef]
23. Goda, A.; Lund, L.H.; Mancini, D.M. Comparison across races of peak oxygen consumption and heart failure survival score for selection for cardiac transplantation. *Am. J. Cardiol.* **2010**, *15*, 1439–1444. [CrossRef]
24. Paolillo, S.; Veglia, F.; Salvioni, E.; Corrà, U.; Piepoli, M.; Lagioia, R.; Limongelli, G.; Sinagra, G.; Cattadori, G.; Scardovi, A.B.; et al. Heart failure prognosis over time: How the prognostic role of oxygen consumption and ventilatory efficiency during exercise has changed in the last 20 years. *Eur J. Heart Fail.* **2019**, *21*, 208–217. [CrossRef]
25. Tai, C.; Gan, T.; Zou, L.; Sun, Y.; Zhang, Y.; Chen, W.; Li, J.; Zhang, J.; Xu, Y.; Lu, H.; et al. Effect of angiotensin-converting enzyme inhibitors and angiotensin II receptor blockers on cardiovascular events in patients with heart failure: A meta-analysis of randomized controlled trials. *BMC Cardiovasc. Disord.* **2017**, *17*, 257. [CrossRef]
26. Rochon, P.A.; Sykora, K.; Bronskill, S.E.; Mamdani, M.; Anderson, G.M.; Gurwitz, J.H.; Gill, S.; Tu, J.V.; Laupacis, A. Use of angiotensin-converting enzyme inhibitor therapy and dose-related outcomes in older adults with new heart failure in the community. *J. Gen. Intern. Med.* **2004**, *19*, 676–683. [CrossRef]
27. Al-Khatib, S.M.; Hellkamp, A.; Bardy, G.H.; Hammill, S.; Hall, W.J.; Mark, D.B.; Anstrom, K.J.; Curtis, J.; Al-Khalidi, H.; Curtis, L.H.; et al. Survival of patients receiving a primary prevention implantable cardioverter-defibrillator in clinical practice vs clinical trials. *JAMA* **2013**, *309*, 55–62. [CrossRef]

28. Kociol, R.D.; Horton, J.R.; Fonarow, G.C.; Reyes, E.M.; Shaw, L.K.; O'Connor, C.M.; Felker, G.M.; Hernandez, A.F. Admission, discharge, or change in B-type natriuretic peptide and long-term outcomes: Data from Organized Program to Initiate Lifesaving Treatment in Hospitalized Patients with Heart Failure (OPTIMIZE-HF) linked to Medicare claims. *Circ. Heart Fail.* **2011**, *4*, 628–636. [CrossRef]
29. Khanam, S.S.; Son, J.W.; Lee, J.W.; Youn, Y.J.; Yoon, J.; Lee, S.H.; Kim, J.Y.; Ahn, S.G.; Ahn, M.S.; Yoo, B.S. Prognostic value of short-term follow-up BNP in hospitalized patients with heart failure. *BMC Cardiovasc. Disord.* **2017**, *17*, 215. [CrossRef]
30. Cheng, V.; Kazanagra, R.; Garcia, A.; Lenert, L.; Krishnaswamy, P.; Gardetto, N.; Clopton, P.; Maisel, A. A rapid bedside test for B-type peptide predicts treatment outcomes in patients admitted for decompensated heart failure: A pilot study. *J. Am. Coll. Cardiol.* **2001**, *37*, 386–391. [CrossRef]
31. Bettencourt, P.; Azevedo, A.; Pimenta, J.; Frioes, F.; Ferreira, S.; Ferreira, A. N-terminal-pro-brain natriuretic peptide predicts outcome after hospital discharge in heart failure patients. *Circulation* **2004**, *110*, 2168–2174. [CrossRef]
32. Yancy, C.W.; Jessup, M.; Bozkurt, B.; Butler, J.; Casey, D.E., Jr.; Colvin, M.M.; Drazner, M.H.; Filippatos, G.S.; Fonarow, G.C.; Givertz, M.M.; et al. 2017 ACC/AHA/HFSA Focused Update of the 2013 ACCF/AHA Guideline for the Management of Heart Failure. A Report of the American College of Cardiology/American Heart Association Task Force on Clinical Practice Guidelines and the Heart Failure Society of America. *Circulation* **2017**, *136*, 137–161. [CrossRef]
33. Bayes-Genis, A.; Pascual-Figal, D.; Fabregat, J.; Domingo, M.; Planas, F.; Casas, T.; Ordonez-Llanos, J.; Valdes, M.; Cinca, J. Serial NT-proBNP monitoring and outcomes in outpatients with decompensation of heart failure. *Int. J. Cardiol.* **2007**, *120*, 338–343. [CrossRef]
34. Bayes-Genis, A.; Ordonez-Llanos, J. Multiple biomarker strategies for risk stratification in heart failure. *Clin. Chim. Acta* **2015**, *443*, 120–125. [CrossRef]
35. Dadu, R.T.; Dodge, R.; Nambi, V.; Virani, S.S.; Hoogeveen, R.C.; Smith, N.L.; Chen, F.; Pankow, J.S.; Guild, C.; Tang, W.H.W.; et al. Ceruloplasmin and heart failure in the Atherosclerosis Risk in Communities study. *Circ. Heart Fail.* **2013**, *6*, 936–943. [CrossRef]
36. Engström, G.; Hedblad, B.; Tydén, P.; Lindgärde, F. Inflammation-sensitive plasma proteins are associated with increased incidence of heart failure: A population-based cohort study. *Atherosclerosis* **2009**, *202*, 617–622. [CrossRef]
37. Bustamante, J.B.; Mateo, M.C.; Fernandez, J.; de Quiros, B.; Manchado, O.O. Zinc, copper and ceruloplasmin in arteriosclerosis. *Biomed. Express* **1976**, *25*, 244–245.
38. Reunanen, A.; Knekt, P.; Aaran, R.K. Serumceruloplasmin level and the risk ofmyocardial infarction and stroke. *Am. J. Epidemiol.* **1992**, *136*, 1082–1090. [CrossRef]
39. Göçmen, A.Y.; Sahin, E.; Semiz, E.; Gümuşlü, S. Is elevated serum ceruloplasmin level associated with increased risk of coronary artery disease? *Can. J. Cardiol.* **2008**, *24*, 209–212. [CrossRef]
40. Sezen, H.; Sezen, Y. How to Change Ceruloplasmin Levels in Heart Disease? *Koşuyolu Heart J.* **2018**, *21*, 61–64. [CrossRef]
41. Cao, D.J.; Hill, J.A. Copper Futures: Ceruloplasmin and Heart Failure. *Circ. Res.* **2014**, *114*, 1678–1680. [CrossRef]
42. Correale, M.; Brunetti, M.D.; de Gennaro, L.; di Biase, M. Acute phase proteins in atherosclerosis (Acute Coronary Syndrome). *Cardiovasc. Hematol. Agents Med. Chem.* **2008**, *6*, 272–277. [CrossRef]
43. Cabassi, A.; Binno, S.M.; Tedeschi, S.; Ruzicka, V.; Dancelli, S.; Rocco, R.; Vicini, V.; Coghi, P.; Regolisti, G.; Montanari, A.; et al. Low Serum Ferroxidase I Activity Is Associated With Mortality in Heart Failure and Related to Both Peroxynitrite-Induced Cysteine Oxidation and Tyrosine Nitration of Ceruloplasmin. *Circ. Res.* **2014**, *114*, 1723–1732. [CrossRef]
44. Hammadah, M.; Fan, Y.; Wu, Y.; Hazern, S.L.; Wilson Tang, W.H. Prognostic Value of Elevated Serum Ceruloplasmin Levels in Patients with Heart Failure. *J. Card. Fail.* **2014**, *20*, 946–952. [CrossRef]

13

Diagnosis of Non-Alcoholic Fatty Liver Disease (NAFLD) is Independently Associated with Cardiovascular Risk in a Large Austrian Screening Cohort

David Niederseer [1,*,†], Sarah Wernly [2,†], Sebastian Bachmayer [2], Bernhard Wernly [3], Adam Bakula [1], Ursula Huber-Schönauer [2], Georg Semmler [2], Christian Schmied [1], Elmar Aigner [4] and Christian Datz [2]

1 Department of Cardiology, University Heart Center Zurich, University of Zurich, University Hospital Zurich, 8091 Zurich, Switzerland; adam.bakula@usz.ch (A.B.); christian.schmied@usz.ch (C.S.)

2 Department of Internal Medicine, General Hospital Oberndorf, Teaching Hospital of the Paracelsus Medical University Salzburg, 5110 Oberndorf, Austria; sarah_wernly@airpost.net (S.W.); S.Bachmayer@kh-oberndorf.at (S.B.); huber.schoenauer@gmail.com (U.H.-S.); georg.semmler@hotmail.com (G.S.); c.datz@kh-oberndorf.at (C.D.)

3 Department of Internal Medicine II, Paracelsus Medical University Salzburg, 5020 Salzburg, Austria; bernhard@wernly.net

4 Department of Internal Medicine I, Paracelsus Medical University Salzburg, 5020 Salzburg, Austria; e.aigner@salk.at

* Correspondence: david.niederseer@usz.ch

† These authors contributed equally to this work.

Abstract: Background: Many patients with non-alcoholic fatty liver disease (NAFLD) simultaneously suffer from cardiovascular (CV) disease and often carry multiple CV risk factors. Several CV risk factors are known to drive the progression of fibrosis in patients with NAFLD. Objectives: To investigate whether an established CV risk score, the Framingham risk score (FRS), is associated with the diagnosis of NAFLD and the degree of fibrosis in an Austrian screening cohort for colorectal cancer. Material and Methods: In total, 1965 asymptomatic subjects (59 ± 10 years, 52% females, BMI 27.2 ± 4.9 kg/m^2) were included in this study. The diagnosis of NAFLD was present if (1) significantly increased echogenicity in relation to the renal parenchyma was present in ultrasound and (2) viral, autoimmune or hereditary liver disease and excess alcohol consumption were excluded. The FRS (ten-year risk of coronary heart disease) and NAFLD Fibrosis Score (NFS) were calculated for all patients. High CV risk was defined as the highest FRS quartile (>10%). Both univariable and multivariable logistic regression models were used to calculate associations of FRS with NAFLD and NFS. Results: Compared to patients without NAFLD (n = 990), patients with NAFLD (n = 975) were older (60 ± 9 vs. 58 ± 10 years; $p < 0.001$), had higher BMI (29.6 ± 4.9 vs. 24.9 ± 3.6 kg/m^2; $p < 0.001$) and suffered from metabolic syndrome more frequently (33% vs. 7%; $p < 0.001$). Cardiovascular risk as assessed by FRS was higher in the NAFLD-group (8.7 ± 6.4 vs. 5.4 ± 5.2%; $p < 0.001$). A one-percentage-point increase of FRS was independently associated with NAFLD (OR 1.04, 95%CI 1.02–1.07; $p < 0.001$) after correction for relevant confounders in multivariable logistic regression. In patients with NAFLD, NFS correlated with FRS ($r = 0.29$; $p < 0.001$), and FRS was highest in patients with significant fibrosis (F3-4; 11.7 ± 5.4) compared to patients with intermediate results (10.9 ± 6.3) and those in which advanced fibrosis could be ruled-out (F0-2, 7.8 ± 5.9, $p < 0.001$). A one-point-increase of NFS was an independent predictor of high-risk FRS after correction for sex, age, and concomitant diagnosis of metabolic syndrome (OR 1.30, 95%CI 1.09–1.54; $p = 0.003$). Conclusion: The presence of NAFLD might independently improve prediction of long-term risk for CV disease and the diagnosis of NAFLD might be a clinically relevant piece in the puzzle of predicting long-term CV outcomes. Due to the significant overlap of advanced NAFLD and high CV risk, aggressive treatment of established CV risk factors could improve prognosis in these patients.

Keywords: NAFLD; cardiovascular risk; Framingham risk score; CVD; risk prediction; secondary prevention; primary prevention; metabolic syndrome; NAFLD fibrosis score

---

1. Introduction

With a constant increase in the incidence of metabolic syndrome, the prevalence of non-alcoholic fatty liver disease (NAFLD) is estimated to be around 25% in Europe. A steep rise in the prevalence of NAFLD from 15% in 2005 to 25% in 2010 has been observed [1]. This increase mirrors obesity rates, which nearly tripled since 1975 and reached epidemic levels [2]. Components of the metabolic syndrome such as hypertension, dyslipidemia, dysglycemia, and abdominal obesity are established risk factors for NAFLD [3]. Since they have also been established as risk factors for CVD, patients frequently suffer from both conditions.

CVD is a leading cause of death worldwide both in the general population and patients with NAFLD [4–6]. NAFLD is independently associated with several markers of subclinical atherosclerosis such as coronary artery calcification, impaired flow-mediated vasodilation, arterial stiffness, carotid artery inflammation and thickening of carotid intima-media as well as left ventricular hypertrophy and diastolic dysfunction [7,8]. Importantly, some of these studies suggest an association of these two disease entities independent from traditional risk factors. Several lines of evidence suggest that NAFLD may be causally and independently involved in CVD pathogenesis [9,10].

Different possible pathophysiological pathways link NAFLD with CVD [11]. Markers of inflammation such as cytokines, CRP, or interleukin-6 are overexpressed in these patients and also correlate with a higher degree of liver fibrosis [12]. Furthermore, patients with hepatic steatosis show elevated levels of pro-coagulant factors such as fibrinogen, von Willebrand factor and plasminogen activator inhibitor-1 [13]. Additionally, hepatic insulin resistance and atherogenic dyslipidemia seem to contribute to the development of CVD [14]. These mechanisms are possible explanations for the fact that the severity of NAFLD, especially if progressed to non-alcoholic steatohepatitis (NASH) with fibrosis, additionally contributes to CV risk [15].

In our study, we examined the prevalence of NAFLD in an Austrian screening cohort for colorectal cancer (SAKKOPI). An established non-invasive estimate of fibrosis severity i.e., the NAFLD fibrosis score (NFS) was calculated and the relation of fibrosis with CV risk as assessed by the Framingham Risk Score (FRS) evaluated.

2. Methods

2.1. Study Subjects

The study cohort consisted of 1965 Caucasians undergoing routine screening colonoscopy at a single center in Austria. All Patients were recruited between 2010 and 2014. Informed consent was obtained, and the study was approved by the local ethics committee (Ethikkommission des Landes Salzburg, approval no. 415-E/1262/2-2010).

2.2. Assessment

As previously described, participants were examined on two consecutive days [16]. On the day of admission, venous blood was drawn after an overnight fast. A whole blood count, kidney and liver tests, lipids, CRP, as well as hemoglobin A1c, an oral glucose tolerance test, and insulin levels were measured. The participants completed a detailed questionnaire including past medical history, current medical regimen, family history, smoking history ("never smokers", "former smokers", or "current smokers") dietary habits and physical activity. A standard physical examination including blood pressure, height, weight, and waist circumference) was performed. Importantly, all patients underwent abdominal ultrasonography. The liver was considered normal if echogenicity was similar to the renal parenchyma. If areas showed a significantly increased echogenicity compared to the renal parenchyma, the liver was considered steatotic. On the second day, all subjects underwent complete colonoscopy.

2.3. Definitions

The diagnosis of NAFLD was made after exclusion of viral, autoimmune and hereditary liver diseases (Wilson disease, hereditary haemochromatosis, alpha-1 antitrypsin deficiency) and excess daily alcohol consumption ≥30 g for men and ≥20 g for women according to the European clinical practice guidelines for the management of NAFLD [17]. NAFLD fibrosis score (NFS) was calculated as previously described [18]. Briefly, NFS (age, body mass index (BMI), presence of impaired fasting glucose or diabetes, aspartate-aminotransferase (AST), alanine-aminotransferase (AST), platelets and albumin) was used to stratify patients according to their risk of significant fibrosis. Specifically, patients with a NFS < -1.455 were graded as F0-2, those with NFS > 0.676 as "F3-4", and patients with a NFS between -1.455 and 0.676 as "intermediate".

Metabolic syndrome was diagnosed when three or more of the following criteria were met [19]: fasting blood glucose level ≥100 mg/dL or antidiabetic therapy, waist circumference >102 cm in males and >88 cm in females, blood pressure ≥130/85 mmHg or current antihypertensive treatment, plasma triglycerides ≥150 mg/dL, and plasma HDL <40 mg/dL in males and <50 mg/dL in females.

2.4. Cardiovascular Risk Assessment

We evaluated patients for cardiovascular disease applying the Framingham Risk Score (FRS) [20]. Although the FRS is not validated in subjects with diabetes (T2DM), we did include subjects with T2DM in our analysis and performed a separate analysis, excluding all subjects with T2DM. Since results were not changed when subjects with T2DM were excluded, we report the results including T2DM to allow for greater generalizability of our results.

2.5. Statistical Analysis

Continuous variables are expressed as mean (±standard deviation) and compared using *t*-test or ANOVA. Categorical data are expressed as numbers (percentage). Chi-square test was applied to calculate differences between groups. Both univariable and multivariable logistic regression was used to evaluate associations of FRS with NAFLD and NFS with CV risk. For multivariable logistic regression, elimination criteria was a p-value of < 0.10 following backward elimination. Variables were included in the multivariable model based on literature. All variables included in the multivariable models evidenced a univariable association at a p-value of $p < 0.05$. A p-value of < 0.05 was considered statistically significant. SPSS version 22.0 (IBM, USA) was used for statistical analyses.

3. Results

3.1. Analysis of the Total Study Cohort, NAFLD versus Non-NAFLD Patients

Overall, 49.6% ($n = 975$) of patients had NAFLD as defined by hepatic steatosis in ultrasound, while 990 patients (50.4%) did not have NAFLD. NAFLD patients were older (60 ± 9 vs. 58 ± 10 years; $p < 0.001$), evidenced higher BMI (29.6 ± 4.9 vs. 24.9 ± 3.6 kg/m^2; $p < 0.001$) and more frequently fulfilled criteria for metabolic syndrome (33% vs. 7%; $p < 0.001$). Characteristics of NAFLD versus non-NAFLD patients are shown in Table 1.

Table 1. Baseline characteristics of patients without ($n = 990$) and with ($n = 975$) non-alcoholic fatty liver disease (NAFLD).

	No NAFLD	NAFLD	Total Cohort	p-Value
	$n = 990$	$n = 975$	$n = 1965$	
Female	61%	43%	52%	<0.001
Age (years)	58 (10)	60 (9)	59 (10)	<0.001
Systolic RR (mmHg)	128 (18)	135 (19)	131 (18)	<0.001
Diastolic RR (mmhg)	79 (10)	83 (11)	81 (10)	<0.001
BMI (kg/m^2)	25 (4)	26 (5)	27 (4)	<0.001
Waist circumference (cm)	90 (11)	105 (12)	97 (11)	<0.001
Waist to hip ratio	1 (0.1)	1 (0.1)	1 (0.1)	<0.001
Bilirubine (mg/dL)	0.72 (0.4)	0.73 (0.4)	0.72 (0.4)	0.4
GGT (U/L)	31 (46)	48 (71)	40 (46)	<0.001
AST (U/L)	22 (12)	26 (18)	24 (12)	<0.001
INR	1.0 (0.1)	1.0 (0.1)	1.0 (0.1)	0.24
Total cholesterol (mg/dL)	219 (40)	217 (44)	218 (40)	0.25
HDL (mg/dL)	67 (18)	56 (16)	62 (18)	<0.001
LDL (mg/dL)	137 (36)	142 (39)	139 (36)	0.02
Triglycerices (mg/dL)	101 (51)	145 (85)	123 (51)	<0.001
Thrombocytes (G/L)	236 (66)	227 (65)	232 (66)	0.001
Fasting glucose (mg/dL)	97 (15)	109 (30)	103 (15)	<0.001
HbA1c (%)	5.6 (0.5)	5.9 (0.8)	5.8 (0.5)	<0.001
Metabolic syndrome	7%	33%	20%	<0.001
T2DM	9%	24%	16%	<0.001
Current smoker	19%	17%	20%	0.48
		Medication		
ASS	11%	17%	14%	0.001
Statin	15%	23%	19%	<0.001
ACE-I/ARB	13%	27%	20%	<0.001
Metformin	2%	8%	5%	<0.001
		CV risk score		
FRS	5.41 (5.20)	8.71 (6.38)	7.05 (5.20)	<0.001
FRS 0-2%	41%	19%	30%	<0.001
FRS >2–5%	21%	19%	20%	
FRS >5–10%	22%	30%	25%	
FRS >10%	16%	33%	24%	

NAFLD: Non-alcoholic fatty liver disease; NFS: NAFLD fibrosis score; FRS: Framingham Risk Score; RR: blood pressure; GGT: gamma-glutamyl-transferase; AST: Aspartate transaminase; INR: International normalized ratio; HDL: High-density lipoprotein; LDL: Low-density lipoprotein; HbA1c: Glycated hemoglobin; T2DM: type 2 diabetes mellitus; ASS: acetylsalicylic acid; CV: cardiovascular; OR: odds ratio.

CV risk assessed by FRS was higher in the NAFLD-group (8.7 ± 6.4 vs. 5.4 ± 5.2%; $p < 0.001$). After allocation of subjects to FRS into risk quartiles (Q1: FRS 0%–2%; Q2: FRS 2%–5%; Q3: FRS 5%–10%, Q4: FRS > 10%), patients with NAFLD more often were in the Q4-FRS group (33% vs. 16%; $p < 0.001$) compared to non-NAFLD patients.

In univariable logistic regression, this relationship corresponded to an increase of OR of 1.11, (95%CI 1.09–1.13; $p < 0.001$) in the likelihood for NAFLD per one-percentage-point increase of FRS. This association remained significant after correction for age, sex and metabolic syndrome (OR, 1.04 95%CI 1.02–1.07; $p < 0.001$) in a multivariable model (Table 2). In an additional sensitivity analysis, a one-percentage-point increase of FRS remained associated with an increased likelihood for NAFLD both in males (OR 1.08, 95%CI 1.06–1.11; $p < 0.001$) and females (OR 1.13, 95%CI 1.09–1.18; $p < 0.001$).

Table 2. Univariable and multivariable associations with the presence of NAFLD.

	Univariable			Multivariable		
	OR	95%CI	*p*-Value	OR	95%CI	*p*-Value
Age	1.03	1.02–1.04	<0.001	1.010	0.998–1.023	0.11
Female gender	0.48	0.40–0.58	<0.001	0.68	0.54–0.86	0.001
Metabolic syndrome	6.08	4.63–7.99	<0.001	5.02	3.77–6.70	<0.001
FRS	1.11	1.09–1.13	<0.001	1.06	1.04–1.08	<0.001

3.2. Analysis of Patients with NAFLD

Patients with NAFLD were grouped according to their NFS into F0-F2 ($n = 604$), intermediate ($n = 138$) and F3-4 ($n = 10$). The characteristics of patients according to their NFS are shown in Table 3. Over the whole NAFLD cohort, NFS correlated with FRS ($r = 0.29$; $p < 0.001$), and FRS was highest in the F3-4 group (11.7 ± 5.4%; $p < 0.001$ vs. F0-F2) compared to the intermediate (10.9 ± 6.3%) and the F0-F2 group (7.8 ± 5.9%). When grouping intermediate and F3-4 into an "at-risk" group (due to small sample size in F3-4), the significant differences between F0-2 essentially persisted (Table 4).

In univariable logistic regression, a one-point increase of NFS was associated with a higher likelihood of high-risk FRS (OR 1.60, 95%CI 1.41–1.83; $p < 0.001$). NFS remained an independent predictor of Q4-FRS after correction for sex, age, and concomitant diagnosis of metabolic syndrome (OR 1.30, 95%CI 1.09–1.54; $p = 0.003$). In a sensitivity analysis in both males (OR 1.84, 95%CI 1.54–2.20; $p < 0.001$) and females (OR 2.06, 95%CI 1.52–2.78; $p < 0.001$) a one-point increase of NFS remained associated with high-quartile FRS. Univariable and multivariable significant associations of age, female gender, metabolic syndrome, and FRS with the presence of high risk NFS are depicted in Table 5.

Table 3. Baseline characteristics of patients according to their NAFLD Fibrosis Score (NFS) score: F0-F2 ($n = 604$), intermediate ($n = 138$) and F3-F4 ($n = 10$).

	F0-F2		Intermediate		F3-F4		
	n = 604		*n* = 138		*n* = 10		
	Mean	SD	Mean	SD	Mean	SD	*p*-Value
Female	36%		43%		50%		0.80
Age (years)	59	9	66	8	67	9	<0.001
Systolic RR (mmHg)	134	18	139	19	148	26	<0.001
Diastolic RR (mmhg)	82	11	85	12	85	12	0.07
BMI (kg/m^2)	29	4	33	6	35	4	<0.001
Waist circumference (cm)	103	11	111	12	115	14	<0.001
Waist to hip ratio	0.96	0	0.97	0	0.97	0	0.23
Bilirubine (mg/dL)	0.70	0	0.80	1	1.57	1	<0.001
GGT (U/L)	48	76	53	70	115	145	0.02
AST (U/L)	25	15	30	24	55	61	<0.001
INR	0.99	0	1.02	0	1.17	0	<0.001
Total cholesterol (mg/dL)	221	44	202	42	221	52	<0.001
HDL (mg/dL	57	16	53	13	57	13	0.03
LDL (mg/dL)	145	40	130	37	142	41	<0.001
Triglycerices (mg/dL)	145	84	147	101	142	68	0.97
Thrombocytes (G/L)	243	62	176	52	128	88	<0.001
Fasting glucose (mg/dL)	107	28	115	28	97	16	0.01
HbA1c (%)	5.9	1	6.0	1	5.6	0	0.08
Metabolic syndrome	30%		43%		40%		0.01
T2DM	20%		44%		20%		<0.001
Current Smoker	19%		6%		0%		0.02
Medication							
ASS	24%		31%		13%		0.21
Statin	24%		31%		13%		0.21
ACE-I/ARB	22%		38%		20%		0.02
Metformin	8%		10%		0%		0.42
FRS	7.83	5.92	10.87	6.29	11.70	5.44	<0.001

Table 4. Baseline characteristics of patients according to their NFS score: F0-F2 (n = 604), and intermediate or F3-F4 (n = 148).

	F0-F2	Intermediate or F3-F4	*p*-Value
	n = 604	n = 148	
Female	41%	43%	0.64
Age (years)	59 (9)	66 (9)	<0.001
Systolic RR (mmHg)	134 (18)	140 (18)	<0.001
Diastolic RR (mmhg)	82 (11)	85 (11)	0.02
BMI (kg/m^2)	29 (4)	33 (4)	<0.001
Waist circumference (cm)	103 (11)	111 (11)	<0.001
Waist to hip ratio	1 (0)	1 (0)	0.09
Bilirubine (mg/dL)	1 (0)	1 (0)	<0.001
GGT (U/L)	48 (76)	57 (76)	0.16
AST (U/L)	25 (15)	32 (15)	<0.001
INR	0.99 (0.07)	1.03 (0.07)	<0.001
Total cholesterol (mg/dL)	221 (44)	203 (44)	<0.001
HDL (mg/dL	57 (16)	53 (16)	0.01
LDL (mg/dL)	145 (40)	131 (40)	<0.001
Triglycerices (mg/dL)	145 (84)	147 (84)	0.87
Thrombocytes (G/L)	243 (62)	173 (62)	<0.001
Fasting glucose (mg/dL)	107 (28)	113 (28)	0.01
HbA1c (%)	5.9 (0.7)	6.0 (0.7)	0.12
Metabolic syndrome	30%	43%	0.003
T2DM	20%	40%	<0.001
Current Smoker	19%	6%	0.003
Medication			
ASS	16%	21%	0.11
Statin	24%	30%	0.20
ACE-I/ARB	22%	37%	0.01
Metformin	8%	10%	0.39
FRS	7.83 (5.92)	10.92 (5.92)	<0.001

Table 5. Univariable and multivariable associations with the presence of high risk NFS score.

	Univariable			Multivariable		
	OR	95%CI	*p*-Value	OR	95%CI	*p*-Value
Age	1.11	1.09–1.13	<0.001	1.17	1.14–1.21	<0.001
Female gender	0.15	0.10–0.21	<0.001	0.02	0.01–0.04	<0.001
Metabolic syndrome	2.46	1.86–3.26	<0.001	4.15	2.64–6.55	<0.001
FRS	1.60	1.41–1.83	<0.001	1.30	1.09–1.54	0.003

4. Discussion

Our study confirms that there is a "silent epidemic" of NAFLD. In the present cohort of asymptomatic individuals undergoing colonoscopy screening between 50 and 75 years of age, around 50% were diagnosed with NAFLD. In total, 14.2% of the screened patients were categorized as being intermediate and 1% of patients were at high risk for advanced fibrosis by the NFS. Importantly, patients with NAFLD had higher CV risk as defined by the FRS compared to patients without NAFLD. Finally, the CV risk was highest in patients with highest NFS scores.

The NFS does not only predict the risk for advanced liver fibrosis, but also CV risk. Interestingly, in a post-hoc analysis of the IMPROVE-IT trial the NFS identified patients who were at the highest risk for recurrent cardiovascular events. The IMPROVE-IT compared statin therapy alone to the add-on of ezetimibe in post ACS patients [21]. In this trial, higher NFS identified patients more likely to benefit from aggressive lipid-lowering therapy. Thus, although the IMPROVE-IT trial was not designed to assess the link between NAFLD and ACS, it offers important data on the potential link between fatty liver severity and atherosclerosis [21].

The most obvious link between CV risk and NFS is the fact that this score is constituted of factors like age, BMI, ALT, AST, platelets, albumin, and the presence or absence of diabetes, all of which reflect metabolic and inflammatory processes. Of note, inflammation and fibrosis are hallmarks of both liver and cardiovascular disease [18] and may therefore indicate common systemic mechanisms.

In our analysis, NAFLD was an independent risk indicator for CV risk. This is in concordance with a meta-analysis of pooled studies from European, Asian, and American countries suggesting an independent association of NAFLD with CV risk [10]. However, a British study including 17.7 million patients found that the diagnosis of NAFLD was not associated with increased risk for acute myocardial infarction or stroke after adjustment for established CV risk factors [22]. Nevertheless, in another meta-analysis of Targher et al., patients with NAFLD evidenced an increased risk of fatal and non-fatal CV disease [23]. Although the link between NAFLD and CV risk seems intuitive, the effect on CV mortality or events has not been demonstrated. Also, a role for a specific medical treatment for NAFLD in preventing CV events and mortality beyond lifestyle advice and current CV guidelines is not established [24,25]. The data in this manuscript suggests an independent relationship of CV risk and NAFLD in an Austrian cohort. Specific management strategies may be considered based on this evidence to improve liver outcomes in CV patients and CV outcomes in liver patients.

4.1. CV Risk Assessment for NALFD Patients

Considering the Joint Clinical Practice Guidelines of EASL-EASD-EASO for the management of NAFLD patients [17], a non-invasive test should be used as the first screening tool to assess disease severity. Depending on the result, patients can be graded into low, intermediate and high risk with regard to advanced fibrosis. For patients in the low risk group, their individual cardiovascular risk should be assessed by risk scores as for example by the FRS. Target goals for risk factors, e.g., for blood pressure, LDL levels, body weight or blood glucose should be treated according to primary prevention guidelines [25].

Patients with intermediate and high risk for advanced fibrosis should be referred to a hepatologist. In patients with advanced fibrosis stage or even cirrhosis CV risk should be assessed by a cardiologist as described in by Choudhary and Duseja [26]. All other patients should be clinically assessed, stratified by a CV risk score and should be managed according to respective prevention guidelines [25] (Figure 1).

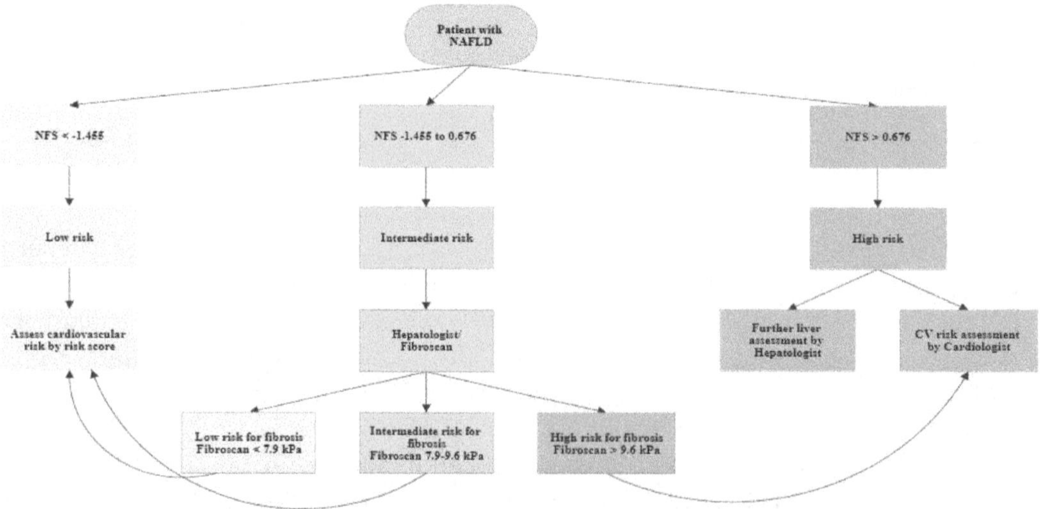

Figure 1. Cardiovascular (CV) assessment algorithm in patients with diagnosed NAFLD.

4.2. Screening for NAFLD in CV Patients

For patients after an CV event or at with a high CV risk we suggest the following approach to detect NAFLD. As a screening test the NFS could be calculated. For patients with low risk for advanced fibrosis, lifestyle modification changes could be recommended. Patients with an intermediate risk could be referred to a liver ultrasound exam and to a hepatologist with expertise in transient elastography. If these exams show no fibrosis or a low stage of fibrosis they should be managed as patients in the low risk group. For patients with intermediate risk in the NFS and advanced fibrosis or cirrhosis in the further exams as well as for patients with a high risk NFS score a hepatologist should be consulted. We are aware, that NFS was developed to estimate fibrosis in the presence of NAFLD. However, we here propose NFS as cheap and non-invasive "screening tool" for NAFLD in patients after an CV event or with a high CV risk. All patients should be treated according to the current guidelines of the European Society of Cardiology [24] (Figure 2).

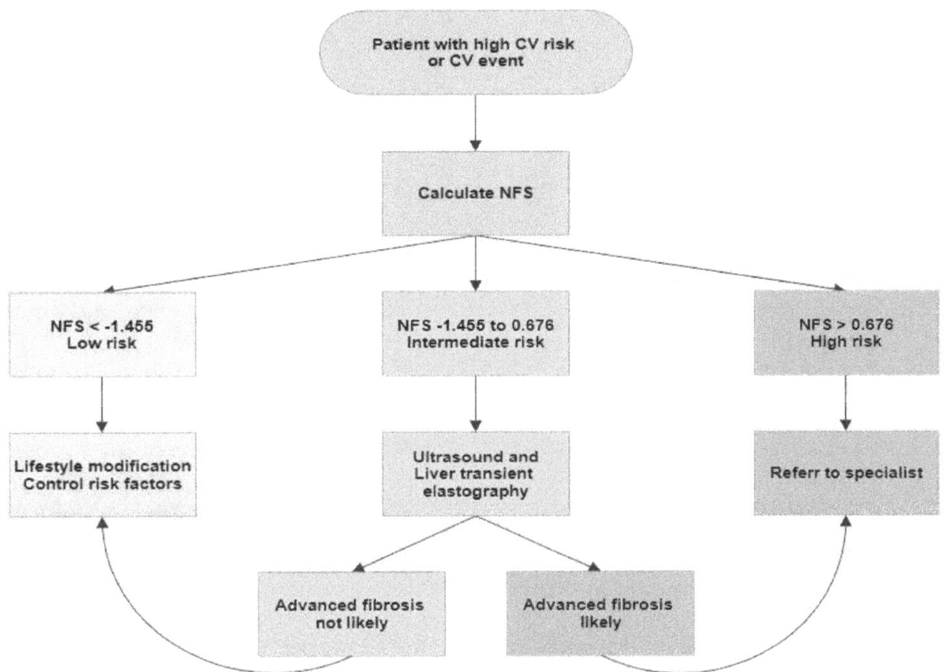

Figure 2. Liver assessment in patients with high cardiovascular risk or with a cardiovascular event in the past medical history.

5. Limitations

This study is a post-hoc analysis of a single-center prospective register and the results remain thesis-generating. However, these data mirror a real-world Austrian population and indicate a high prevalence of undetected NAFLD in the general population. Although this study cannot provide longitudinal CV outcome data, we provide data from a carefully characterized cohort in a cross-sectional study. Another limitation of this study is the linearity of the models especially in using a high number of contributing factors, an assumption that is implicit due to the design of the study.

Furthermore, ultrasound and not liver transient elastography was used to diagnose NAFLD. Finally, clinical data and established surrogate risk scores for calculation of the CV risk as well as the determination of the degree of liver fibrosis by non-invasive scores were used, even though there are other but more expensive and sometime even more invasive methods available to determine CV risk or liver fibroses such as magnetic resonance imaging, liver biopsy, liver transient elastography, vascular ultrasound, or coronary calcium scoring.

6. Conclusions

The presence of NAFLD might independently predict long-term risk for CV disease. Therefore, patients with high risk for or known CV events should be screened for the presence of NAFLD and risk scores should be routinely applied. Non-invasive risk scores for CV risk and fibrosis could help to facilitate and optimize management of patients with NAFLD with increased CV risk. The care for patients with both NAFLD and CV disease is challenging and due to the vast overlap of patients screening for liver disease in CV patients as well as screening for NAFLD in CV patients seems reasonable [26]. Cardiologists and hepatologists should team up in the treatment of their patients [27].

Author Contributions: D.N., C.D., B.W., S.W.: Conceptualization; D.N., S.W., B.W., U.H.-S., G.S., E.A., G.S., C.S., A.B.: Data curation; B.W., S.W.: Formal analysis; C.D.: Funding acquisition; D.N., C.D.: Methodology; D.N.: Project administration; D.N., C.D.: Supervision; B.W., S.W.: Visualization; D.N., S.W.: Writing—original draft; S.B., B.W., A.B., U.H.-S., G.S., C.S., E.A., C.D.: Writing—review & editing. All authors have read and agreed to the published version of the manuscript.

References

1. Younossi, Z.M.; Koenig, A.B.; Abdelatif, D.; Fazel, Y.; Henry, L.; Wymer, M. Global epidemiology of nonalcoholic fatty liver disease-Meta-analytic assessment of prevalence, incidence, and outcomes. *Hepatology* **2016**, *64*, 73–84. [CrossRef] [PubMed]
2. WHO Expert Consultation. Appropriate body-mass index for Asian populations and its implications for policy and intervention strategies. *Lancet* **2004**, *363*, 157–163. [CrossRef]
3. Expert Panel on Detection, Evaluation. Treatment of High Blood Cholesterol in, A. Executive Summary of The Third Report of The National Cholesterol Education Program (NCEP) Expert Panel on Detection, Evaluation, And Treatment of High Blood Cholesterol In Adults (Adult Treatment Panel III). *JAMA* **2001**, *285*, 2486–2497. [CrossRef]
4. Roth, G.A.; Johnson, C.; Abajobir, A.; Abd-Allah, F.; Abera, S.F.; Abyu, G.; Ahmed, M.; Aksut, B.; Alam, T.; Alam, K.; et al. Global, Regional, and National Burden of Cardiovascular Diseases for 10 Causes, 1990 to 2015. *J. Am. Coll. Cardiol.* **2017**, *70*, 1–25. [CrossRef]
5. Rafiq, N.; Bai, C.; Fang, Y.; Srishord, M.; McCullough, A.; Gramlich, T.; Younossi, Z.M. Long-term follow-up of patients with nonalcoholic fatty liver. *Clin. Gastroenterol. Hepatol.* **2009**, *7*, 234–238. [CrossRef]
6. Ong, J.P.; Pitts, A.; Younossi, Z.M. Increased overall mortality and liver-related mortality in non-alcoholic fatty liver disease. *J. Hepatol.* **2008**, *49*, 608–612. [CrossRef]
7. Oni, E.T.; Agatston, A.S.; Blaha, M.J.; Fialkow, J.; Cury, R.; Sposito, A.; Erbel, R.; Blankstein, R.; Feldman, T.; Al-Mallah, M.H.; et al. A systematic review: Burden and severity of subclinical cardiovascular disease among those with nonalcoholic fatty liver; should we care? *Atherosclerosis* **2013**, *230*, 258–267. [CrossRef]
8. Mantovani, A.; Pernigo, M.; Bergamini, C.; Bonapace, S.; Lipari, P.; Pichiri, I.; Bertolini, L.; Valbusa, F.; Barbieri, E.; Zoppini, G.; et al. Nonalcoholic Fatty Liver Disease Is Independently Associated with Early Left Ventricular Diastolic Dysfunction in Patients with Type 2 Diabetes. *PLoS ONE* **2015**, *10*, e0135329. [CrossRef]
9. Targher, G.; Day, C.P.; Bonora, E. Risk of cardiovascular disease in patients with nonalcoholic fatty liver disease. *N. Engl. J. Med.* **2010**, *363*, 1341–1350. [CrossRef]
10. Wu, S.; Wu, F.; Ding, Y.; Hou, J.; Bi, J.; Zhang, Z. Association of non-alcoholic fatty liver disease with major adverse cardiovascular events: A systematic review and meta-analysis. *Sci. Rep.* **2016**, *6*, 33386. [CrossRef]
11. Byrne, C.D.; Targher, G. NAFLD: A multisystem disease. *J. Hepatol.* **2015**, *62*, S47–S64. [CrossRef]
12. Wieckowska, A.; Papouchado, B.G.; Li, Z.; Lopez, R.; Zein, N.N.; Feldstein, A.E. Increased hepatic and circulating interleukin-6 levels in human nonalcoholic steatohepatitis. *Am. J. Gastroenterol.* **2008**, *103*, 1372–1379. [CrossRef] [PubMed]

13. Targher, G.; Bertolini, L.; Zoppini, G.; Zenari, L.; Falezza, G. Increased plasma markers of inflammation and endothelial dysfunction and their association with microvascular complications in Type 1 diabetic patients without clinically manifest macroangiopathy. *Diabet. Med.* **2005**, *22*, 999–1004. [CrossRef] [PubMed]
14. Howard, G.; O'Leary, D.H.; Zaccaro, D.; Haffner, S.; Rewers, M.; Hamman, R.; Selby, J.V.; Saad, M.F.; Savage, P.; Bergman, R. Insulin sensitivity and atherosclerosis. The Insulin Resistance Atherosclerosis Study (IRAS) Investigators. *Circulation* **1996**, *93*, 1809–1817. [CrossRef] [PubMed]
15. Ekstedt, M.; Hagstrom, H.; Nasr, P.; Fredrikson, M.; Stal, P.; Kechagias, S.; Hultcrantz, R. Fibrosis stage is the strongest predictor for disease-specific mortality in NAFLD after up to 33 years of follow-up. *Hepatology* **2015**, *61*, 1547–1554. [CrossRef] [PubMed]
16. Despotovic, D.; Niederseer, D.; Brunckhorst, C. CME-EKG 60: Akut auftretende Thoraxschmerzen und Dyspnoe: Das EKG als Schlussel zur Diagnose. *Praxis* **2018**, *107*, 223–224. [CrossRef]
17. European Association for the Study of the Liver (EASL); European Association for the Study of Diabetes (EASD); European Association for the Study of Obesity (EASO). EASL-EASD-EASO Clinical Practice Guidelines for the management of non-alcoholic fatty liver disease. *J. Hepatol.* **2016**, *64*, 1388–1402. [CrossRef]
18. Angulo, P.; Hui, J.M.; Marchesini, G.; Bugianesi, E.; George, J.; Farrell, G.C.; Enders, F.; Saksena, S.; Burt, A.D.; Bida, J.P.; et al. The NAFLD fibrosis score: A noninvasive system that identifies liver fibrosis in patients with NAFLD. *Hepatology* **2007**, *45*, 846–854. [CrossRef]
19. Grundy, S.M.; Cleeman, J.I.; Daniels, S.R.; Donato, K.A.; Eckel, R.H.; Franklin, B.A.; Gordon, D.J.; Krauss, R.M.; Savage, P.J.; Smith, S.C., Jr.; et al. Diagnosis and management of the metabolic syndrome: An American Heart Association/National Heart, Lung, and Blood Institute scientific statement: Executive Summary. *Crit. Pathw. Cardiol.* **2005**, *4*, 198–203. [CrossRef]
20. Wilson, P.W.; D'Agostino, R.B.; Levy, D.; Belanger, A.M.; Silbershatz, H.; Kannel, W.B. Prediction of coronary heart disease using risk factor categories. *Circulation* **1998**, *97*, 1837–1847. [CrossRef]
21. Simon, T.G.; Corey, K.E.; Cannon, C.P.; Blazing, M.; Park, J.G.; O'Donoghue, M.L.; Chung, R.T.; Giugliano, R.P. The nonalcoholic fatty liver disease (NAFLD) fibrosis score, cardiovascular risk stratification and a strategy for secondary prevention with ezetimibe. *Int. J. Cardiol.* **2018**, *270*, 245–252. [CrossRef] [PubMed]
22. Alexander, M.; Loomis, A.K.; Van der Lei, J.; Duarte-Salles, T.; Prieto-Alhambra, D.; Ansell, D.; Pasqua, A.; Lapi, F.; Rijnbeek, P.; Mosseveld, M.; et al. Non-alcoholic fatty liver disease and risk of incident acute myocardial infarction and stroke: Findings from matched cohort study of 18 million European adults. *BMJ* **2019**, *367*, l5367. [CrossRef] [PubMed]
23. Targher, G.; Byrne, C.D.; Lonardo, A.; Zoppini, G.; Barbui, C. Non-alcoholic fatty liver disease and risk of incident cardiovascular disease: A meta-analysis. *J. Hepatol.* **2016**, *65*, 589–600. [CrossRef] [PubMed]
24. Knuuti, J.; Wijns, W.; Saraste, A.; Capodanno, D.; Barbato, E.; Funck-Brentano, C.; Prescott, E.; Storey, R.F.; Deaton, C.; Cuisset, T.; et al. 2019 ESC Guidelines for the diagnosis and management of chronic coronary syndromes. *Eur. Heart J.* **2020**, *41*, 407–477. [CrossRef]
25. Piepoli, M.F.; Hoes, A.W.; Agewall, S.; Albus, C.; Brotons, C.; Catapano, A.L.; Cooney, M.T.; Corra, U.; Cosyns, B.; Deaton, C.; et al. 2016 European Guidelines on cardiovascular disease prevention in clinical practice: The Sixth Joint Task Force of the European Society of Cardiology and Other Societies on Cardiovascular Disease Prevention in Clinical Practice (constituted by representatives of 10 societies and by invited experts)Developed with the special contribution of the European Association for Cardiovascular Prevention & Rehabilitation (EACPR). *Eur. Heart J.* **2016**, *37*, 2315–2381. [CrossRef]
26. Choudhary, N.S.; Duseja, A. Screening of Cardiovascular Disease in Nonalcoholic Fatty Liver Disease: Whom and How? *J. Clin. Exp. Hepatol.* **2019**, *9*, 506–514. [CrossRef]
27. Wernly, B.; Wernly, S.; Niederseer, D.; Datz, C. Hepatitis C virus (HCV) infection and cardiovascular disease: Hepatologists and cardiologists need to talk! *Eur. J. Intern. Med.* **2020**, *71*, 87–88. [CrossRef]

14

Sarcomeric Gene Variants and Their Role with Left Ventricular Dysfunction in Background of Coronary Artery Disease

Surendra Kumar [1,†], Vijay Kumar [2,*,†] and Jong-Joo Kim [2,*]

1 Department of Anatomy, All India Institute of Medical Sciences, New Delhi 110029, India; surendrakhedarcbt@gmail.com
2 Department of Biotechnology, Yeungnam University, Gyeongsan, Gyeongbuk 38541, Korea
* Correspondence: vijaykumarcbt@gmail.com (V.K.); kimjj@ynu.ac.kr (J.-J.K.)

† These authors contributed equally to this work.

Abstract: Cardiovascular diseases are one of the leading causes of death in developing countries, generally originating as coronary artery disease (CAD) or hypertension. In later stages, many CAD patients develop left ventricle dysfunction (LVD). Left ventricular ejection fraction (LVEF) is the most prevalent prognostic factor in CAD patients. LVD is a complex multifactorial condition in which the left ventricle of the heart becomes functionally impaired. Various genetic studies have correlated LVD with dilated cardiomyopathy (DCM). In recent years, enormous progress has been made in identifying the genetic causes of cardiac diseases, which has further led to a greater understanding of molecular mechanisms underlying each disease. This progress has increased the probability of establishing a specific genetic diagnosis, and thus providing new opportunities for practitioners, patients, and families to utilize this genetic information. A large number of mutations in sarcomeric genes have been discovered in cardiomyopathies. In this review, we will explore the role of the sarcomeric genes in LVD in CAD patients, which is a major cause of cardiac failure and results in heart failure.

Keywords: sarcomere; dilated cardiomyopathy; left ventricle dysfunction; actin; myosin; troponin; tropomyosin

---

1. Introduction:

Cardiac diseases are one of the main causes of death these days, generally originating as coronary artery disease (CAD) or hypertension. In later stages, many patients may develop left ventricle dysfunction (LVD). Left ventricular ejection fraction (LVEF) is the most determining factor for the prognosis of CAD patients [1–3].

LVD is a complex multifactorial condition in which the left ventricle becomes functionally compromised. In the cardiovascular system, the left ventricle plays a central role in the maintenance of circulation because of its role as the major pump in the heart. In the case of LVD, the pumping function of the heart is reduced, leading to symptoms of congestive heart failure (CHF). CAD patients with severe LVD have a higher mortality than those with preserved LV function, and this mortality rate is proportional to the severity of LVD. The rising number of patients with ischemic LVD contributes significantly to the increased morbidity and mortality of cardiac arrests. Impaired pumping by the heart leads to other cardiovascular complications, such as heart failure, myocardial infarction, cardiomyopathies, etc. [3–6].

LVD includes two distinctive morphologies: hypertrophy and dilation. In LV hypertrophy, ventricular chamber volume remains the same, but the wall of the chamber is thickened. In LV dilation, the chamber volume of the left ventricle gets enlarged when the walls are either normal or thinned. These two conditions are associated with specific hemodynamic variations. In hypertrophic conditions, only diastolic relaxation is impaired, while in the dilated condition, systolic functions are diminished. This results in a change of heart shape from an elliptical to a more spherical form, which causes considerable mechanical inefficiency and deterioration, resulting in CHF [3,6]. Sarcomeric proteins are basic contractile units of the myocyte/myocardium. Several sarcomeric genes have been identified and associated with the pathogenesis of CHF.

This review will highlight the genetic basis of LVD in the background of CAD. We review the role of common sarcomeric genes (*MYBPC3, TNNT2, TTN, Myospryn*) and their genetic variants with LVD in CAD patients.

2. Common Sarcomeric Protein and Associated Gene Polymorphism

In recent years, remarkable developments have been made in identifying the genetic association of cardiac diseases, resulting in a better understanding of the underlying molecular mechanisms. Several genetic studies have found an association between LVD and dilated cardiomyopathy (DCM). Various sarcomeric protein-encoding genes such as cardiac myosin-binding protein C (MYBPC3), myosin heavy polypeptide, and cardiac troponin I gene mutations, as well as other gene mutations have been identified in DCM [7–13]. The common sarcomeric gene polymorphisms with their locations and functional roles are given in Table 1.

Table 1. Common sarcomeric gene polymorphism.

Genes	Location	Type of Polymorphism	Functional Role	Ref.
MYBPC3	11p11.2	25 bp Ins/del	*MYBPC3* gene mutation is associated with inherited cardiomyopathies and an increased heart failure risk	[14–18]
TNNT2	1q32	5 bp Ins/del	The 5 bp (CTTCT) deletion in intron 3 of the *TNNT2* gene at the polypyrimidine tract was found to affect the gene splicing and branch site selection	[10,19, 20]
TTN	2q31	18 bp Ins/del	This deletion is present within the PEVK region of *titin* gene that regulates the extensibility of the protein	[21,22]
Myospryn	5q14.1	K2906N	This polymorphism is associated with cardiac adaptation in response to pressure overload, left ventricular hypertrophy, and left ventricular diastolic dysfunction in hypertensive patients	[23]

3. Sarcomeric Proteins

A sarcomere is the functional unit of striated muscle tissue. Skeletal muscles are composed of myocytes formed during myogenesis. Muscle fibers are composed of numerous tubular myofibrils. These myofibrils are a bundle of sarcomeres with repeating units, which appear as alternating dark and light bands under a microscope. Sarcomeric proteins drive muscle contraction and relaxation as these protein filaments slide past each other during these processes. The main components of sarcomere myofilament are actin, myosin, tropomyosin (Tm), and troponin complex (TnT, TnC, and TnI). Myosin protein present in the center of the sarcomere in the form of a thick filament, while actin is thin myofilament and overlaps with myosin. Titin protein's C-terminus attaches to M-line, while N-terminus attaches to Z-disc. Titin is anchored to Z-disc by attaching both actin and myosin proteins [24–27]. During muscle contraction, a conformational rearrangement in the troponin complex is generated by binding calcium ions to TnC, resulting in the movement of Tm, which provides a space for myosin binding on actin, leading to a cross-bridge creation with the help of energy provided by ATP. The contractility of muscles is regulated by calcium ion, which acts on the thin filament's receptor molecule troponin. Calcium ion is bounded to TnC that successively binds to TnI, releasing it from its inhibitory site on actin [28–31]. The details are shown in Figure 1.

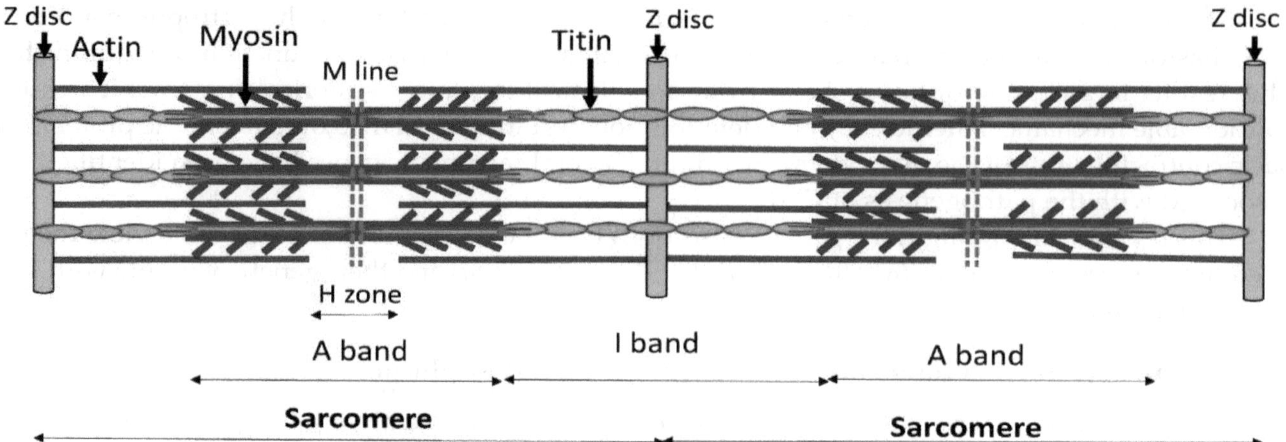

Figure 1. The location and arrangement of the thick and thin myofilament in the sarcomere.

3.1. *Myofilament Proteins*

Sarcomeres are in the form of thick and thin myofilament proteins. The thick filament is made up of C protein and myosin, while the thin filament is formed from actin, Tm, and troponin complex.

3.1.1. Myosin

Myosin is a motor molecule with actin myofilament, and generates force and motion. Myosin consists of two light chains (MLCs) and two heavy chains (MHCs) [32]. Cardiac MHCs have two isoforms in mammals (α and β-isoform) [33]. The α-isoform is related to better actomyosin ATPase activity than β-isoform. Thus, α-isoform has a fast-contractile velocity than β-isoform [34].

MHCs' isoform expression is sensitive to hormonal changes and cardiovascular stress [35,36]. Isoform shift was observed in human failing myocardium [37,38]. An increase in β-isoform was observed in cardiomyopathy, thyroid depletion, aging, and pressure overload condition [39]. In addition, mammalian myocardium normally primarily expresses α-isoform, but during experimental stimulation of heart failure, it shows upregulation of β-isoform and downregulation of α-isoform [40]. A localized shift of α and β isoforms is noticed in tissues of human ventricles. There is a higher expression of α-isoform in the sub-epicardial than in the sub-endocardial layer [40]. This localized shift of α and β isoforms is consistent with contraction duration and the shorter action potential in the sub-epicardium compared with sub-endocardium [41]. About 80% of atria tissues, present in human ventricular tissues, consist of α-isoform [42]. In atrial fibrillation, the β-isoform expression is approximately doubled [43], and in failing ventricles, α-isoform expression is decreased [42]. In sum, the MHC isoforms' transition may occur in human atrial and ventricular myocardial disease.

The β-myosin heavy chain (*MYH7*) gene is located on Chr. 14q11.2 and encodes the β isoform in the cardiac myosin heavy chain. Gene mutation in the *MYH7* gene leads to abnormal sarcomeric protein function. The deficiency or altered function of these proteins results in impaired muscle contraction, which results in heart failure [44,45].

3.1.2. Actin

Actin is essential for various cell functions. Actin isoforms in mammals are highly conserved. It consists of six isoforms encoded by six different genes. α-skeletal actin, α-cardiac actin, α-smooth actin, and γ-smooth actin are specific in their location and present in skeletal, cardiac, and smooth muscle, respectively. The other two isoforms, β -cyto actin and γ -cyto actin, are universally expressed in tissues [46]. The delicate variations in ratios of actin isoform may lead to alterations in contractility [46].

Additionally, evidence indicates that a reduction in cardiac contractility is associated with decreased expressions of α-cardiac isoform and aberrant expressions of γ-smooth isoform [47]. Humans generally have higher levels of α-skeletal isoform in the heart, compared to rats and mice [48].

3.1.3. Myospryn

In humans, myospryn protein is a large protein with 4069 amino acid residues (mol. wt. 449 kDa). The C-terminal portion of the protein is made up of approximately 570 amino acids and has tripartite motif (TRIM) proteins-like structure, while the rest of the protein consists of multiple glutamate-rich sequences. Based on this structure, myospryn has also been known as TRIM76 (HGNC Database 2008). Myospryn protein expression is restricted to cardiac and skeletal muscle only [49]. Myospryn protein is localized primarily in a Z-disc of sarcomere below the sarcolemma [50,51].

Myospryn gene is situated on Chr 5q14.1 and is related to Z-disc. The *Myospryn* gene is expressed in striated muscle cells, co-localized with the α-actinin sarcomeric protein. In the past, studies have reported an association of *Myospryn* K2906N (rs6859595) polymorphism with left ventricular hypertrophy, cardiac adaptation due to pressure overload [52], and LV diastolic dysfunction in hypertensive patients [23].

3.2. Regulatory Proteins

3.2.1. Tropomyosin (Tm)

Tropomyosin is a major regulatory protein, present in a supercoiled form by wrapping around each other—a dimer of two α-helical coil chains. In cells, Tm-isoforms collectively regulate the functional role of actin filaments. Tm-isoforms have two types—(a) muscle Tm-isoforms and (b) non-muscle Tm-isoforms [53]. The interactions between actin and myosin are controlled by these Tm-isoforms and play a pivotal role in controlling Ca^{++}sensitive regulation of contraction [54–56]. In humans, Tm-isoforms are encoded by four different genes (TPM1, TPM2, TPM3, and TPM4) [57]. α-Tm and κ-Tm from the *TPM1* gene, β-Tm from the *TPM2* gene, and γ-Tm transcribed from the *TPM3* gene are major Tm-isoforms present in human striated muscles. The ratio of β to α-Tm isomer varies from one species to another [58].

The Tm-isoform transition leads to cardiovascular disease. Purcell et al. reported that α-Tm isoform is exclusively expressed by failing heart ventricular muscles [59]. In the heart of chronic DCM patients was found increased expression of κ-Tm-isoform [60,61]. Tm-isoforms regulate cardiac contraction/relaxation, calcium sensitivity, and sarcomeric tension. Tm-isoform shifting potentially affects the overall cardiovascular system.

3.2.2. Troponins

The troponin complex controls the interaction of actin and myosin in striated muscle in response to calcium. This complex contains three regulatory subunits: Troponin-C (TnC; calcium-binding protein), Troponin-I (TnI; inhibitory protein), and Troponin-T (TnT; tropomyosin binding protein).

Troponin-C (TnC): Troponin-C is expressed in cardiac and skeletal muscle and has two isoforms, encoded by genes (*TNNC1* and *TNNC2*). The two isoforms are slow skeleton TnC isoform (ssTnC), encoded by the *TNNC1* gene and expressed in slow muscles and heart muscles; and the fast-skeletal isoform (fsTnC), encoded by the *TNNC2* gene. ssTnC is referred to as cTnC in the heart. The ssTnC/cTnC isoform has been expressed in both developing and adult hearts [55,62].

Troponin-I (TnI): Troponin-I has three isoforms: (a) ssTnI (slow skeletal muscle), (b) fsTnI (fast skeletal muscle), and (c) cTnI isoform (cardiac muscle), encoded by *TNNI1, TNNI2,* and *TNNI3* genes, respectively. During development, the ssTnI:cTnI ratio is continuously decreased, and the adult heart has mostly cTnI isoform [63,64]. As the developed heart only expresses cTnI, it does not go through isoform switching under pathological conditions such as DCM, ischemic, and heart failure [65]. In adult transgenic mice, due to increased calcium sensitivity, slow TnI overexpression may impair relaxation and diastolic cardiac function [66]. The cTnI knockout mice show developmental downregulation of ssTnI. TnI depletion changes the mechanical properties of the myocardium. Under relaxed conditions, the myocytes in ventricles show reduced sarcomeres, raised resting tension, and a decreased calcium sensitivity under activating conditions [67].

Troponin-T (TnT): The Tn-t protein is present in three isoforms: slow skeletal isoform (ssTnT), fast skeletal isoform (fsTnT), and cardiac isoform (cTnT), encoded by these genes: *TNNT1*, *TNNT3*, and *TNNT2*, respectively [68,69]. The human heart possesses four common isoforms of cardiac Tn-T (cTnT) i.e., (cTnT1, cTnT2, cTnT3, and cTnT4). A normal adult heart expresses only cTnT3 isoform, while the failing adult heart, as well as the fetal heart, expresses the cTnT4 isoform [70]. Unusual cTnT isoform expressions have been associated with heart ailments. An exon 4 skipped isoform was found highly expressed in failing human hearts [70], and familial HCM human hearts [71]. An over-expression of exon7-excluded cTnT isoform was observed by Craig et al. in a transgenic mouse heart leading to impaired systolic function [72]. The heterogeneous group of TnT isoforms or co-presence of multiple TnT isoforms desynchronize the calcium activation of thin filaments, resulting in cardiac performance reduction [73]. In comparison to wild–type controls, overexpression of one or more functionally different cardiac TnT isoforms in mice resulted in lower left ventricular pressure, declined stroke volume, and slower contractile and relaxation velocities. The author also suggests that co-expression of functionally distinct cTnT isoforms may impair cardiac function in adult ventricular muscle [73].

Troponin T (TNNT2) Gene: TNNT2 gene is located on Chr. 1q32. and encodes a tropomyosin-binding subunit of the troponin complex. This protein is situated on the thin filament of striated muscles and controls muscle contractility in response to Ca^{++} signals. Mutations in the *TNNT2* gene have been positively associated with DCM and familial HCM [20,74,75]. It has been reported that a 5-bp (CTTCT) I/ D polymorphism present in intron 3 of the *TNNT2* gene may impair the skipping of exon 4 and lead to LVD [10,19,20].

3.3. Sarcomeric Cytoskeletal Proteins

Cytoskeletal proteins provide mechanical resistance, morphological integrity, and play a major role in maintaining the cell shape of cardiomyocytes. Titin, α-actinin, myomesin, myosin-binding protein C (MyBP-C), and M-protein are the main constituent proteins of this group [76].

3.3.1. Titin Protein and Associated Gene Polymorphism

Titin is also known as connectin and encoded by the *TTN* gene, which is located on Chr. 2q31. It is a giant muscle protein of striated muscles that act as a molecular spring and are responsible for passive elasticity. Like a spring, it provides the force to control sarcomere contraction and signaling [22,77–79]. Titin is the third most abundant protein in cardiac muscle, after myosin and actin. It spans half of the sarcomere and connects M-line to Z-line. It is the key determinant of myocardial passive tension and plays an important role in the elasticity of cardiac myocytes. These proteins also contribute to the diastolic function of LV filling. Titin consists of two types of protein domains: 1) fibronectin type III domain and 2) immunoglobulin domain. The N-terminal of titin is located in the I-band and connected to Z-disc, and have elastic property. This I-band elastic region has a spring-like PEVK segment, rich in proline, glutamate, valine, and lysine [25–27,30,79].

A single gene encodes three major isoforms of titin through alternative splicing [21,79]. Change in ratios of cardiac titin isoforms has been associated with cardiovascular disease. Itoh-Satoh et al. found four possible DCM-associated mutations. The mutated gene expresses a non-functional titin protein that is unable to rotate half sarcomere and decreases binding affinities to Z-line proteins [80]. A familial DCM locus maps to Chr. 2q31 and causes early-onset congestive heart failure (CHF) [81]. RNA binding motif 20 (Rbm20) is a muscle-specific splicing factor, regulating alternative splicing of titin [82]. The Rbm20 knockout rats express a most compliant titin isoform that causes DCM [83,84]. This mutation is associated with the expression of a larger, compliant fetal cardiac titin isoform in severe DCM patients [82].

An 18 bp (TTTTCCTCTTCAGGAGCAA/T) I/D polymorphism falls within the PEVK region that controls the contractile nature of titin. It was previously reported that mutations in the *TTN* gene have been related to different forms of cardiomyopathy, including HCM, DCM, and arrhythmogenic right ventricular cardiomyopathy (ARVC) [9,21,22].

3.3.2. Myosin-Binding Protein C (Mybp-C) and Associated Gene Polymorphism

MyBP-C is a thick filament-associated striated muscle protein situated in the C zones cross-bridge of A-bands and binds to titin and myosin. MyBP-C and titin collectively form a firm ternary complex, where titin act as a molecular ruler and MyBP-C as a regulatory protein [85–87]. In the adult heart, MyBP-C is present in three isoforms in striated muscles, while skeletal muscle expresses only two isoforms. The fsMyBP-C is the fast-skeletal isoform encoded by the gene *MYBPC2* in humans. In humans, MYBPC1 encodes for ssMyBP-C, the slow form of skeletal muscle [88] while *MYBPC3* encodes for human cardiac MyBP-C (cMyBP-C) [89]. In the same sarcomere, fsMyBP-C and ssMyBP-C isoforms can be expressed simultaneously [90] and the diverse arrangements of the specific sarcomere bands are due to the co-existence of fsMyBP-C and ssMyBP-C in variable proportions [91]. The cMyBP-C isoform is found only in cardiac muscle and cannot be trans-complemented by skeletal MyBP-Cs [92].

The *MYBPC3* gene located on Chr. 11p11.2 and mutations in this gene were reported in HCM and DCM patients [17,93–95]. In 2–6% of Southeast Asian populations, *MYBPC3* 25 bp deletion, located in intron 32 at 3′ region of the gene is noted and associated with a high risk of LVD (left ventricular ejection fraction < 45). This 25-bp intronic deletion results in exon 33 skipping and incorporated missense amino acids at the C-terminal of the protein [14,18]. Incorporation of this mutated protein in myofibrils [14] may cause sarcomere breakdown. Moreover, authors have reported through a protein model that this deletion disrupts the α-helical stretch in the cMyBP-C and an additional α-helix and β-pleated sheets are incorporated in the mutated protein. As the cMyBP-C protein directly binds a subset of Ig domains with titin and myosin through its C8, C9, and C10 domains, any conformational changes in the mutated protein may cause alterations in conformation or direction of the C10 domain. Thus, the inability of myosin binding may have severe effects on sarcomeric organization, suggesting its involvement in the morphological and functional changes of cardiac muscle.

The pathophysiology of cardiac muscles due to truncated and missense MyBP-C has been explained by other mechanisms as well. Due to these mutations, MyBP-C3 mRNA may undergo nonsense-mediated mRNA decay (NMD), which disrupts its proteins through the UPS and may result in cardiac dysfunction [96]. UPS functions also decline with high oxidative stress and the age of an individual. Further, mutated protein may accumulate and disturb cellular homeostasis, and can initiate LVD [97,98]. This deletion polymorphism is also associated with other parameters of LV remodeling, i.e., LV dimensions (LV end-systolic and diastole dimension). This deletion may play an important role in conferring LVD risk in Southeast Asian populations and can be used as an early risk predictor [15].

The *MYBPC3* 25-bp deletion polymorphism is quite common with varied frequency in South Asian inhabitants. Studies have suggested that this deletion might have not been present in initial settlers who arrived 50000 to 20000 years ago from Africa, but might have surfaced later in India. The high frequency of this deleterious mutation is somewhat surprising. It has been suggested that with carrier frequency of 2–8% gradation from North to South India, this variation may contribute significantly to the burden of cardiac diseases in the subcontinent [14,99,100].

4. Common Sarcomeric Variants Reported with LVD

Studies have reported numerous genetic variants that play a vital role in the pathophysiology of left ventricular dysfunction [15,16,101]. Previously, the *TTN* and *TNNT2* gene variants were studied with various cardiac remodeling phenotypes. Mutation in the *TTN* and *TNNT2* genes were associated with different phenotypes of cardiac remodeling. In intron 3 of the *TNNT2* gene, a 5bp I/D polymorphism is associated with cardiac hypertrophy [20]. The DD genotype is associated with wall thickening of the ventricles and a greater LV mass in the hypertrophy population. Farza et al., however, observed no clinical importance of this variant in cardiac hypertrophy [102]. Rani et al. observed that 5bp deletion in this polymorphism leads to exon 4 skipping at the time of splicing, and is present in a significantly high concentration in HCM patients [19]. Nakagami et al. observed an association between cardiac hypertrophy and myospryn polymorphisms. Authors have reported that in the *Myospryn* gene, AA genotype of K2906N polymorphism plays a risk allele for left ventricular diastolic dysfunction in hypertensive patients [23]. Kumar et al. conducted a case-control study to explore the association of MYBPC3, titin, troponin T2, and myosporin gene deletion polymorphisms. A total of 988 angiographically proved CAD patients and 300 healthy controls were enrolled in this study. Of the 988 CAD patients, 253 were categorized as LVD with reduced left ventricular ejection fraction (LVEF ≤ 45%). The study concluded that there is a significant association of MYBPC3 25-bp deletion polymorphism with elevated risk of LVD (LVEF < 45) (healthy controls v/s LVD: OR = 3.85, p value < 0.001; and non-LVD v/s LVD: OR = 1.65, p value = 0.035), while the other three studied polymorphisms (Myosporin, TNNT2, TTN) do not seem to play a direct role in LVD as well as CAD risk in north Indians [15,16,103,104].

Several truncated and missense mutations were reported in MyBP-C, which generates poison peptides and haplo-insufficiency. Due to these mutations, MyBP-C3 mRNA may undergo nonsense-mediated mRNA decay (NMD), which disrupts its proteins through the UPS and may result in cardiac dysfunction [96]. UPS function also declines with high oxidative stress and age. Further, the mutated protein may accumulate and disturb cellular homeostasis and initiate LVD [97,98]. During adrenergic stimulation, cardiac contractility is regulated by MyBP-C. With the help of cyclic AMP-dependent protein kinase and calcium/calmodulin-dependent protein kinase II, MyBP-C goes through reversible phosphorylation [73,105]. A 25-bp deletion in the MyBP-C3 gene causes severe ischemic damage to the cardiac muscle and can develop severe LVD in CAD patients who carry this deletion [15]. In the South Asian population, this 25 bp deletion is relatively common. Analysis of this deletion in different subgroups based on LV ejection fraction (LVEF) shows a significant association of this polymorphism with severe LVD. Patients with LVEF (30–40%) and below 30% have a higher percentage of this deletion genotype. Additionally, this deletion polymorphism is also associated with echocardiogram results such as LV systolic and end-diastolic dimension. To rule out the possibilities of the development of LVD in CAD patients due to confounding factors such as diabetes, smoking, hypertension, and ST-elevation myocardial infarction, the authors performed a multivariate analysis, which shows that the above-stated association was only due to this 25 bp deletion only. This deletion may be responsible, for the development of LVD in CAD patients [15], alone or in combination with hypertension. Based on the above discussion, we proposed a model for left ventricular dysfunction (LVD)/heart failure (Figure 2).

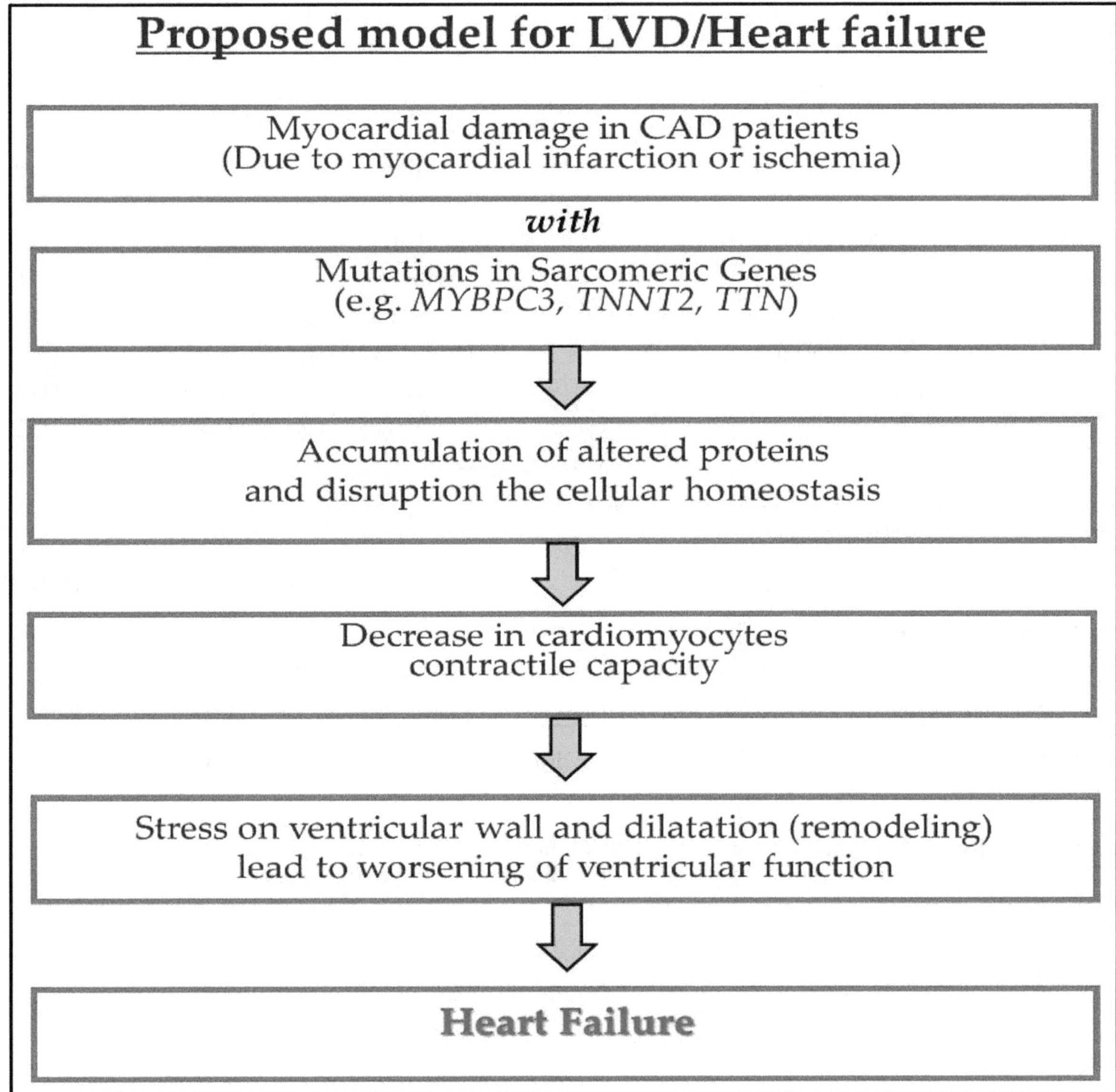

Figure 2. A model for left ventricular dysfunction (LVD)/heart failure. Coronary artery disease (CAD).

5. Conclusions

It is well established that left ventricular dysfunction is a complex condition, caused by numerous factors—mechanical, neurohormonal, and genetic. Some potential modifiers are shown in Table 2. Sarcomeric genes [15,16], matrix metalloproteinases (MMPs) [106], renin-angiotensin-aldosterone system (RAAS) [101], and inflammatory pathway genes [107] was previously associated with left ventricular dysfunction. In complex diseases, most genetic variants are known to exert minor, but significant effects on disease phenotype. It may be worthy to perform genome-wide association studies to identify novel loci, which may have a vital impact on the development of LVD. Moreover, it is suggested that large, well-designed association studies with functional studies for validation are conducted to establish the combined roles of SNPs in the predisposition and severity of the disease. Moreover, it is important to identify and validate novel mutations in sarcomeric genes using next-generation sequencing and microarrays methods for a complete analysis of genes involved in LVD.

Table 2. Potential modifier of Left Ventricular Dysfunction (LVD).

Common Factors	Effect	Ref.
Environmental Risk Factors		
Age	Higher in older patients	[108]
Gender	More in men	[109]
Ethnicity	High in African Athletes	[110]
Smoking status	Higher in smoker patients	[111]
Obesity	Higher in obese patients	[112]
Hypertension	Higher in hypertensive patients	[112]
Coronary artery disease	Higher in CAD patients	[112]
Renal disease	Higher in CKD patients	[112]
Genetic Risk Factors		
Sarcomeric gene mutations–*MYBPC3, TNNT2, TTN, MYH7, Myospryn*, etc.	↑ ventricular remodeling and LVD	[15,23]
Renin–Angiotensin–Aldosterone System (RAAS) pathway–*ACE* and *AT1* Gene	↑ ventricular remodeling and LVD	[101,113]
Matrix Metalloproteinase (MMPs)–*MMP2, MMP7* and *MMP9*	↑ LVD	[104,106]
Adrenergic pathway–*ADRB1, ADRA2A, ADRB3*	↑ ventricular remodeling and LVD	[103]
Inflammatory pathway–*NFKB1, IL6*, and *TNF-α*	↑ ventricular remodeling and LVD	[104,107]

Coronary artery disease (CAD); Chronic kidney disease (CKD); Left ventricle dysfunction (LVD).

Author Contributions: Conceptualization, S.K., V.K.; methodology, S.K., V.K.; writing—original draft preparation, S.K., V.K.; writing—review and editing J.-J.K., S.K., V.K. All authors have read and agreed to the published version of the manuscript.

References

1. Ghai, A.; Silversides, C.; Harris, L.; Webb, G.D.; Siu, S.C.; Therrien, J. Left ventricular dysfunction is a risk factor for sudden cardiac death in adults late after repair of tetralogy of Fallot. *J. Am. Coll. Cardiol.* **2002**, *40*, 1675–1680. [CrossRef]
2. McMurray, J.J.; Ezekowitz, J.A.; Lewis, B.S.; Gersh, B.J.; van Diepen, S.; Amerena, J.; Bartunek, J.; Commerford, P.; Oh, B.H.; Harjola, V.P.; et al. Left ventricular systolic dysfunction, heart failure, and the risk of stroke and systemic embolism in patients with atrial fibrillation: Insights from the ARISTOTLE trial. *Circ. Heart Fail.* **2013**, *6*, 451–460. [CrossRef] [PubMed]
3. Al-Khatib, S.M.; Stevenson, W.G.; Ackerman, M.J.; Bryant, W.J.; Callans, D.J.; Curtis, A.B.; Deal, B.J.; Dickfeld, T.; Field, M.E.; Fonarow, G.C.; et al. 2017 AHA/ACC/HRS Guideline for Management of Patients With Ventricular Arrhythmias and the Prevention of Sudden Cardiac Death. *Circulation* **2018**, *138*, e272–e391.
4. Stevens, S.M.; Reinier, K.; Chugh, S.S. Increased left ventricular mass as a predictor of sudden cardiac death: Is it time to put it to the test? *Circ. Arrhythm. Electrophysiol.* **2013**, *6*, 212–217. [CrossRef] [PubMed]
5. Chonchol, M.; Goldenberg, I.; Moss, A.J.; McNitt, S.; Cheung, A.K. Risk factors for sudden cardiac death in patients with chronic renal insufficiency and left ventricular dysfunction. *Am. J. Nephrol.* **2007**, *27*, 7–14. [CrossRef]
6. Benito, B.; Josephson, M.E. Ventricular tachycardia in coronary artery disease. *Rev. Esp. Cardiol.* **2012**, *65*, 939–955. [CrossRef] [PubMed]
7. Mestroni, L.; Brun, F.; Spezzacatene, A.; Sinagra, G.; Taylor, M.R. Genetic Causes of Dilated Cardiomyopathy. *Prog. Pediatr. Cardiol.* **2014**, *37*, 13–18. [CrossRef]

8. Favalli, V.; Serio, A.; Grasso, M.; Arbustini, E. Genetic causes of dilated cardiomyopathy. *Heart* **2016**, *102*, 2004–2014. [CrossRef]
9. McNally, E.M.; Mestroni, L. Dilated Cardiomyopathy: Genetic Determinants and Mechanisms. *Circ. Res.* **2017**, *121*, 731–748. [CrossRef]
10. Mattos, B.P.; Scolari, F.L.; Torres, M.A.; Simon, L.; Freitas, V.C.; Giugliani, R.; Matte, U. Prevalence and Phenotypic Expression of Mutations in the MYH7, MYBPC3 and TNNT2 Genes in Families with Hypertrophic Cardiomyopathy in the South of Brazil: A Cross-Sectional Study. *Arq. Bras. Cardiol.* **2016**, *107*, 257–265. [CrossRef]
11. Rafael, J.F.; Cruz, F.F.; Carvalho, A.C.C.; Gottlieb, I.; Cazelli, J.G.; Siciliano, A.P.; Dias, G.M. Myosin-binding Protein C Compound Heterozygous Variant Effect on the Phenotypic Expression of Hypertrophic Cardiomyopathy. *Arq. Bras. Cardiol.* **2017**, *108*, 354–360. [CrossRef] [PubMed]
12. Bienengraeber, M.; Olson, T.M.; Selivanov, V.A.; Kathmann, E.C.; O'Cochlain, F.; Gao, F.; Karger, A.B.; Ballew, J.D.; Hodgson, D.M.; Zingman, L.V.; et al. ABCC9 mutations identified in human dilated cardiomyopathy disrupt catalytic KATP channel gating. *Nat. Genet.* **2004**, *36*, 382–387. [CrossRef] [PubMed]
13. Kimura, A. Molecular basis of hereditary cardiomyopathy: Abnormalities in calcium sensitivity, stretch response, stress response and beyond. *J. Hum. Genet.* **2010**, *55*, 81–90. [CrossRef]
14. Dhandapany, P.S.; Sadayappan, S.; Xue, Y.; Powell, G.T.; Rani, D.S.; Nallari, P.; Rai, T.S.; Khullar, M.; Soares, P.; Bahl, A.; et al. A common MYBPC3 (cardiac myosin binding protein C) variant associated with cardiomyopathies in South Asia. *Nat. Genet.* **2009**, *41*, 187–191. [CrossRef] [PubMed]
15. Kumar, S.; Mishra, A.; Srivastava, A.; Bhatt, M.; Garg, N.; Agarwal, S.K.; Pande, S.; Mittal, B. Role of common sarcomeric gene polymorphisms in genetic susceptibility to left ventricular dysfunction. *J. Genet.* **2016**, *95*, 263–272. [CrossRef]
16. Srivastava, A.; Garg, N.; Mittal, T.; Khanna, R.; Gupta, S.; Seth, P.K.; Mittal, B. Association of 25 bp deletion in MYBPC3 gene with left ventricle dysfunction in coronary artery disease patients. *PLoS ONE* **2011**, *6*, e24123. [CrossRef]
17. Tanjore, R.R.; Rangaraju, A.; Kerkar, P.G.; Calambur, N.; Nallari, P. MYBPC3 gene variations in hypertrophic cardiomyopathy patients in India. *Can. J. Cardiol.* **2008**, *24*, 127–130. [CrossRef]
18. Waldmuller, S.; Sakthivel, S.; Saadi, A.V.; Selignow, C.; Rakesh, P.G.; Golubenko, M.; Joseph, P.K.; Padmakumar, R.; Richard, P.; Schwartz, K.; et al. Novel deletions in MYH7 and MYBPC3 identified in Indian families with familial hypertrophic cardiomyopathy. *J. Mol. Cell Cardiol.* **2003**, *35*, 623–636. [CrossRef]
19. Rani, D.S.; Nallari, P.; Dhandapany, P.S.; Tamilarasi, S.; Shah, A.; Archana, V.; AshokKumar, M.; Narasimhan, C.; Singh, L.; Thangaraj, K. Cardiac Troponin T (TNNT2) mutations are less prevalent in Indian hypertrophic cardiomyopathy patients. *DNA Cell Biol.* **2012**, *31*, 616–624. [CrossRef]
20. Komamura, K.; Iwai, N.; Kokame, K.; Yasumura, Y.; Kim, J.; Yamagishi, M.; Morisaki, T.; Kimura, A.; Tomoike, H.; Kitakaze, M.; et al. The role of a common TNNT2 polymorphism in cardiac hypertrophy. *J. Hum. Genet.* **2004**, *49*, 129–133. [CrossRef]
21. Bang, M.L.; Centner, T.; Fornoff, F.; Geach, A.J.; Gotthardt, M.; McNabb, M.; Witt, C.C.; Labeit, D.; Gregorio, C.C.; Granzier, H.; et al. The complete gene sequence of titin, expression of an unusual approximately 700-kDa titin isoform, and its interaction with obscurin identify a novel Z-line to I-band linking system. *Circ. Res.* **2001**, *89*, 1065–1072. [CrossRef]
22. Granzier, H.L.; Radke, M.H.; Peng, J.; Westermann, D.; Nelson, O.L.; Rost, K.; King, N.M.; Yu, Q.; Tschope, C.; McNabb, M.; et al. Truncation of titin's elastic PEVK region leads to cardiomyopathy with diastolic dysfunction. *Circ. Res.* **2009**, *105*, 557–564. [CrossRef] [PubMed]
23. Nakagami, H.; Kikuchi, Y.; Katsuya, T.; Morishita, R.; Akasaka, H.; Saitoh, S.; Rakugi, H.; Kaneda, Y.; Shimamoto, K.; Ogihara, T. Gene polymorphism of myospryn (cardiomyopathy-associated 5) is associated with left ventricular wall thickness in patients with hypertension. *Hypertens. Res.* **2007**, *30*, 1239–1246. [CrossRef] [PubMed]
24. Gregorio, C.C.; Trombitas, K.; Centner, T.; Kolmerer, B.; Stier, G.; Kunke, K.; Suzuki, K.; Obermayr, F.; Herrmann, B.; Granzier, H.; et al. The NH2 terminus of titin spans the Z-disc: Its interaction with a novel 19-kD ligand (T-cap) is required for sarcomeric integrity. *J. Cell Biol.* **1998**, *143*, 1013–1027. [CrossRef] [PubMed]

25. Guo, W.; Bharmal, S.J.; Esbona, K.; Greaser, M.L. Titin diversity–alternative splicing gone wild. *J. Biomed. Biotechnol.* **2010**, *2010*, 753675. [CrossRef]
26. Dos Remedios, C.; Gilmour, D. An historical perspective of the discovery of titin filaments. *Biophys. Rev.* **2017**, *9*, 179–188. [CrossRef]
27. Gonzalez-Morales, N.; Holenka, T.K.; Schock, F. Filamin actin-binding and titin-binding fulfill distinct functions in Z-disc cohesion. *PLoS Genet.* **2017**, *13*, e1006880. [CrossRef]
28. Gordon, A.M.; Homsher, E.; Regnier, M. Regulation of contraction in striated muscle. *Physiol. Rev.* **2000**, *80*, 853–924. [CrossRef]
29. Hamdani, N.; Kooij, V.; van Dijk, S.; Merkus, D.; Paulus, W.J.; Remedios, C.D.; Duncker, D.J.; Stienen, G.J.; van der Velden, J. Sarcomeric dysfunction in heart failure. *Cardiovasc. Res.* **2008**, *77*, 649–658. [CrossRef]
30. Tskhovrebova, L.; Trinick, J. Roles of titin in the structure and elasticity of the sarcomere. *J. Biomed. Biotechnol.* **2010**, *2010*, 612482. [CrossRef]
31. Rall, J.A. What makes skeletal muscle striated? Discoveries in the endosarcomeric and exosarcomeric cytoskeleton. *Adv. Physiol. Educ.* **2018**, *42*, 672–684. [CrossRef] [PubMed]
32. Rayment, I.; Holden, H.M.; Whittaker, M.; Yohn, C.B.; Lorenz, M.; Holmes, K.C.; Milligan, R.A. Structure of the actin-myosin complex and its implications for muscle contraction. *Science* **1993**, *261*, 58–65. [CrossRef] [PubMed]
33. Yamauchi-Takihara, K.; Sole, M.J.; Liew, J.; Ing, D.; Liew, C.C. Characterization of human cardiac myosin heavy chain genes. *Proc. Natl. Acad. Sci. USA* **1989**, *86*, 3504–3508. [CrossRef]
34. Holubarsch, C.; Goulette, R.P.; Litten, R.Z.; Martin, B.J.; Mulieri, L.A.; Alpert, N.R. The economy of isometric force development, myosin isoenzyme pattern and myofibrillar ATPase activity in normal and hypothyroid rat myocardium. *Circ. Res.* **1985**, *56*, 78–86. [CrossRef] [PubMed]
35. Allen, D.L.; Leinwand, L.A. Postnatal myosin heavy chain isoform expression in normal mice and mice null for IIb or IId myosin heavy chains. *Dev. Biol.* **2001**, *229*, 383–395. [CrossRef]
36. Lowes, B.D.; Minobe, W.; Abraham, W.T.; Rizeq, M.N.; Bohlmeyer, T.J.; Quaife, R.A.; Roden, R.L.; Dutcher, D.L.; Robertson, A.D.; Voelkel, N.F.; et al. Changes in gene expression in the intact human heart. Downregulation of alpha-myosin heavy chain in hypertrophied, failing ventricular myocardium. *J. Clin. Invest.* **1997**, *100*, 2315–2324. [CrossRef]
37. Miyata, S.; Minobe, W.; Bristow, M.R.; Leinwand, L.A. Myosin heavy chain isoform expression in the failing and nonfailing human heart. *Circ. Res.* **2000**, *86*, 386–390. [CrossRef]
38. Lompre, A.M.; Schwartz, K.; d'Albis, A.; Lacombe, G.; Van Thiem, N.; Swynghedauw, B. Myosin isoenzyme redistribution in chronic heart overload. *Nature* **1979**, *282*, 105–107. [CrossRef]
39. Swynghedauw, B. Developmental and functional adaptation of contractile proteins in cardiac and skeletal muscles. *Physiol. Rev.* **1986**, *66*, 710–771. [CrossRef]
40. Takahashi, T.; Schunkert, H.; Isoyama, S.; Wei, J.Y.; Nadal-Ginard, B.; Grossman, W.; Izumo, S. Age-related differences in the expression of proto-oncogene and contractile protein genes in response to pressure overload in the rat myocardium. *J. Clin. Invest.* **1992**, *89*, 939–946. [CrossRef]
41. Herron, T.J.; McDonald, K.S. Small amounts of alpha-myosin heavy chain isoform expression significantly increase power output of rat cardiac myocyte fragments. *Circ. Res.* **2002**, *90*, 1150–1152. [CrossRef]
42. Reiser, P.J.; Portman, M.A.; Ning, X.H.; Schomisch Moravec, C. Human cardiac myosin heavy chain isoforms in fetal and failing adult atria and ventricles. *Am. J. Physiol. Heart Circ. Physiol.* **2001**, *280*, H1814–H1820. [CrossRef]
43. Eiras, S.; Narolska, N.A.; van Loon, R.B.; Boontje, N.M.; Zaremba, R.; Jimenez, C.R.; Visser, F.C.; Stooker, W.; van der Velden, J.; Stienen, G.J. Alterations in contractile protein composition and function in human atrial dilatation and atrial fibrillation. *J. Mol. Cell Cardiol.* **2006**, *41*, 467–477. [CrossRef]
44. Meredith, C.; Herrmann, R.; Parry, C.; Liyanage, K.; Dye, D.E.; Durling, H.J.; Duff, R.M.; Beckman, K.; de Visser, M.; van der Graaff, M.M.; et al. Mutations in the slow skeletal muscle fiber myosin heavy chain gene (MYH7) cause laing early-onset distal myopathy (MPD1). *Am. J. Hum. Genet.* **2004**, *75*, 703–708. [CrossRef]
45. Darin, N.; Tajsharghi, H.; Ostman-Smith, I.; Gilljam, T.; Oldfors, A. New skeletal myopathy and cardiomyopathy associated with a missense mutation in MYH7. *Neurology* **2007**, *68*, 2041–2042. [CrossRef]
46. Suurmeijer, A.J.; Clement, S.; Francesconi, A.; Bocchi, L.; Angelini, A.; Van Veldhuisen, D.J.; Spagnoli, L.G.; Gabbiani, G.; Orlandi, A. Alpha-actin isoform distribution in normal and failing human heart: A morphological, morphometric, and biochemical study. *J. Pathol.* **2003**, *199*, 387–397. [CrossRef]

47. Kumar, A.; Crawford, K.; Flick, R.; Klevitsky, R.; Lorenz, J.N.; Bove, K.E.; Robbins, J.; Lessard, J.L. Transgenic overexpression of cardiac actin in the mouse heart suggests coregulation of cardiac, skeletal and vascular actin expression. *Transgenic Res.* **2004**, *13*, 531–540. [CrossRef]
48. Boheler, K.R.; Carrier, L.; de la Bastie, D.; Allen, P.D.; Komajda, M.; Mercadier, J.J.; Schwartz, K. Skeletal actin mRNA increases in the human heart during ontogenic development and is the major isoform of control and failing adult hearts. *J. Clin. Invest.* **1991**, *88*, 323–330. [CrossRef]
49. Benson, M.A.; Tinsley, C.L.; Blake, D.J. Myospryn is a novel binding partner for dysbindin in muscle. *J. Biol. Chem.* **2004**, *279*, 10450–10458. [CrossRef]
50. Durham, J.T.; Brand, O.M.; Arnold, M.; Reynolds, J.G.; Muthukumar, L.; Weiler, H.; Richardson, J.A.; Naya, F.J. Myospryn is a direct transcriptional target for MEF2A that encodes a striated muscle, alpha-actinin-interacting, costamere-localized protein. *J. Biol. Chem.* **2006**, *281*, 6841–6849. [CrossRef]
51. Kouloumenta, A.; Mavroidis, M.; Capetanaki, Y. Proper perinuclear localization of the TRIM-like protein myospryn requires its binding partner desmin. *J. Biol. Chem.* **2007**, *282*, 35211–35221. [CrossRef]
52. Kielbasa, O.M.; Reynolds, J.G.; Wu, C.L.; Snyder, C.M.; Cho, M.Y.; Weiler, H.; Kandarian, S.; Naya, F.J. Myospryn is a calcineurin-interacting protein that negatively modulates slow-fiber-type transformation and skeletal muscle regeneration. *FASEB J.* **2011**, *25*, 2276–2286. [CrossRef]
53. Pittenger, M.F.; Kazzaz, J.A.; Helfman, D.M. Functional properties of non-muscle tropomyosin isoforms. *Curr. Opin. Cell Biol.* **1994**, *6*, 96–104. [CrossRef]
54. Janco, M.; Suphamungmee, W.; Li, X.; Lehman, W.; Lehrer, S.S.; Geeves, M.A. Polymorphism in tropomyosin structure and function. *J. Muscle Res. Cell Motil.* **2013**, *34*, 177–187. [CrossRef]
55. Murakami, K.; Yumoto, F.; Ohki, S.Y.; Yasunaga, T.; Tanokura, M.; Wakabayashi, T. Structural basis for Ca2+-regulated muscle relaxation at interaction sites of troponin with actin and tropomyosin. *J. Mol. Biol.* **2005**, *352*, 178–201. [CrossRef]
56. Pathan-Chhatbar, S.; Taft, M.H.; Reindl, T.; Hundt, N.; Latham, S.L.; Manstein, D.J. Three mammalian tropomyosin isoforms have different regulatory effects on nonmuscle myosin-2B and filamentous beta-actin in vitro. *J. Biol. Chem.* **2018**, *293*, 863–875. [CrossRef]
57. Perry, S.V. Vertebrate tropomyosin: Distribution, properties and function. *J. Muscle Res. Cell Motil.* **2001**, *22*, 5–49. [CrossRef]
58. Denz, C.R.; Narshi, A.; Zajdel, R.W.; Dube, D.K. Expression of a novel cardiac-specific tropomyosin isoform in humans. *Biochem. Biophys. Res. Commun.* **2004**, *320*, 1291–1297. [CrossRef]
59. Purcell, I.F.; Bing, W.; Marston, S.B. Functional analysis of human cardiac troponin by the in vitro motility assay: Comparison of adult, foetal and failing hearts. *Cardiovasc. Res.* **1999**, *43*, 884–891. [CrossRef]
60. Karam, C.N.; Warren, C.M.; Rajan, S.; de Tombe, P.P.; Wieczorek, D.F.; Solaro, R.J. Expression of tropomyosin-kappa induces dilated cardiomyopathy and depresses cardiac myofilament tension by mechanisms involving cross-bridge dependent activation and altered tropomyosin phosphorylation. *J. Muscle Res. Cell Motil.* **2011**, *31*, 315–322. [CrossRef]
61. Rajan, S.; Jagatheesan, G.; Karam, C.N.; Alves, M.L.; Bodi, I.; Schwartz, A.; Bulcao, C.F.; D'Souza, K.M.; Akhter, S.A.; Boivin, G.P.; et al. Molecular and functional characterization of a novel cardiac-specific human tropomyosin isoform. *Circulation* **2010**, *121*, 410–418. [CrossRef]
62. Filatov, V.L.; Katrukha, A.G.; Bulargina, T.V.; Gusev, N.B. Troponin: Structure, properties, and mechanism of functioning. *Biochemistry* **1999**, *64*, 969–985. [PubMed]
63. Wilkinson, J.M.; Grand, R.J. Comparison of amino acid sequence of troponin I from different striated muscles. *Nature* **1978**, *271*, 31–35. [CrossRef]
64. Wade, R.; Eddy, R.; Shows, T.B.; Kedes, L. cDNA sequence, tissue-specific expression, and chromosomal mapping of the human slow-twitch skeletal muscle isoform of troponin I. *Genomics* **1990**, *7*, 346–357. [CrossRef]
65. Sasse, S.; Brand, N.J.; Kyprianou, P.; Dhoot, G.K.; Wade, R.; Arai, M.; Periasamy, M.; Yacoub, M.H.; Barton, P.J. Troponin I gene expression during human cardiac development and in end-stage heart failure. *Circ. Res.* **1993**, *72*, 932–938. [CrossRef]
66. Fentzke, R.C.; Buck, S.H.; Patel, J.R.; Lin, H.; Wolska, B.M.; Stojanovic, M.O.; Martin, A.F.; Solaro, R.J.; Moss, R.L.; Leiden, J.M. Impaired cardiomyocyte relaxation and diastolic function in transgenic mice expressing slow skeletal troponin I in the heart. *J. Physiol.* **1999**, *517*((Pt. 1)), 143–157. [CrossRef]

67. Huang, X.; Pi, Y.; Lee, K.J.; Henkel, A.S.; Gregg, R.G.; Powers, P.A.; Walker, J.W. Cardiac troponin I gene knockout: A mouse model of myocardial troponin I deficiency. *Circ. Res.* **1999**, *84*, 1–8. [CrossRef]
68. Sheng, J.J.; Jin, J.P. Gene regulation, alternative splicing, and posttranslational modification of troponin subunits in cardiac development and adaptation: A focused review. *Front. Physiol.* **2014**, *5*, 165. [CrossRef]
69. Samson, F.; Mesnard, L.; Mihovilovic, M.; Potter, T.G.; Mercadier, J.J.; Roses, A.D.; Gilbert, J.R. A new human slow skeletal troponin T (TnTs) mRNA isoform derived from alternative splicing of a single gene. *Biochem. Biophys. Res. Commun.* **1994**, *199*, 841–847. [CrossRef]
70. Anderson, P.A.; Malouf, N.N.; Oakeley, A.E.; Pagani, E.D.; Allen, P.D. Troponin T isoform expression in humans. A comparison among normal and failing adult heart, fetal heart, and adult and fetal skeletal muscle. *Circ. Res.* **1991**, *69*, 1226–1233. [CrossRef]
71. Thierfelder, L.; Watkins, H.; MacRae, C.; Lamas, R.; McKenna, W.; Vosberg, H.P.; Seidman, J.G.; Seidman, C.E. Alpha-tropomyosin and cardiac troponin T mutations cause familial hypertrophic cardiomyopathy: A disease of the sarcomere. *Cell* **1994**, *77*, 701–712. [CrossRef]
72. Craig, R.; Offer, G. The location of C-protein in rabbit skeletal muscle. *Proc. R Soc. Lond. B. Biol. Sci.* **1976**, *192*, 451–461. [PubMed]
73. Wakabayashi, T. Mechanism of the calcium-regulation of muscle contraction–in pursuit of its structural basis. *Proc. Jpn. Acad. Ser. B Phys. Biol. Sci.* **2015**, *91*, 321–350. [CrossRef] [PubMed]
74. Li, Y.D.; Ji, Y.T.; Zhou, X.H.; Li, H.L.; Zhang, H.T.; Xing, Q.; Hong, Y.F.; Tang, B.P. TNNT2 Gene Polymorphisms are Associated with Susceptibility to Idiopathic Dilated Cardiomyopathy in Kazak and Han Chinese. *Med. Sci. Monit.* **2015**, *21*, 3343–3347. [CrossRef]
75. Ripoll-Vera, T.; Gamez, J.M.; Govea, N.; Gomez, Y.; Nunez, J.; Socias, L.; Escandell, A.; Rosell, J. Clinical and Prognostic Profiles of Cardiomyopathies Caused by Mutations in the Troponin T Gene. *Rev. Esp. Cardiol.* **2016**, *69*, 149–158. [CrossRef]
76. Hein, S.; Kostin, S.; Heling, A.; Maeno, Y.; Schaper, J. The role of the cytoskeleton in heart failure. *Cardiovasc. Res.* **2000**, *45*, 273–278. [CrossRef]
77. Whiting, A.; Wardale, J.; Trinick, J. Does titin regulate the length of muscle thick filaments? *J. Mol. Biol.* **1989**, *205*, 263–268. [CrossRef]
78. Miller, M.K.; Granzier, H.; Ehler, E.; Gregorio, C.C. The sensitive giant: The role of titin-based stretch sensing complexes in the heart. *Trends Cell Biol.* **2004**, *14*, 119–126. [CrossRef]
79. LeWinter, M.M.; Granzier, H.L. Cardiac titin and heart disease. *J. Cardiovasc. Pharmacol.* **2014**, *63*, 207–212. [CrossRef]
80. Itoh-Satoh, M.; Hayashi, T.; Nishi, H.; Koga, Y.; Arimura, T.; Koyanagi, T.; Takahashi, M.; Hohda, S.; Ueda, K.; Nouchi, T.; et al. Titin mutations as the molecular basis for dilated cardiomyopathy. *Biochem. Biophys. Res. Commun.* **2002**, *291*, 385–393. [CrossRef]
81. Siu, B.L.; Niimura, H.; Osborne, J.A.; Fatkin, D.; MacRae, C.; Solomon, S.; Benson, D.W.; Seidman, J.G.; Seidman, C.E. Familial dilated cardiomyopathy locus maps to chromosome 2q31. *Circulation* **1999**, *99*, 1022–1026. [CrossRef] [PubMed]
82. Guo, W.; Schafer, S.; Greaser, M.L.; Radke, M.H.; Liss, M.; Govindarajan, T.; Maatz, H.; Schulz, H.; Li, S.; Parrish, A.M.; et al. RBM20, a gene for hereditary cardiomyopathy, regulates titin splicing. *Nat. Med.* **2012**, *18*, 766–773. [CrossRef] [PubMed]
83. Guo, W.; Pleitner, J.M.; Saupe, K.W.; Greaser, M.L. Pathophysiological defects and transcriptional profiling in the RBM20-/- rat model. *PLoS ONE* **2013**, *8*, e84281. [CrossRef]
84. Li, S.; Guo, W.; Dewey, C.N.; Greaser, M.L. Rbm20 regulates titin alternative splicing as a splicing repressor. *Nucleic Acids Res.* **2013**, *41*, 2659–2672. [CrossRef]
85. Flashman, E.; Redwood, C.; Moolman-Smook, J.; Watkins, H. Cardiac myosin binding protein C: Its role in physiology and disease. *Circ. Res.* **2004**, *94*, 1279–1289. [CrossRef] [PubMed]
86. Kensler, R.W.; Craig, R.; Moss, R.L. Phosphorylation of cardiac myosin binding protein C releases myosin heads from the surface of cardiac thick filaments. *Proc. Natl. Acad. Sci. USA* **2017**, *114*, E1355–E1364. [CrossRef]
87. Mamidi, R.; Gresham, K.S.; Verma, S.; Stelzer, J.E. Cardiac Myosin Binding Protein-C Phosphorylation Modulates Myofilament Length-Dependent Activation. *Front. Physiol.* **2016**, *7*, 38. [CrossRef]

88. Weber, F.E.; Vaughan, K.T.; Reinach, F.C.; Fischman, D.A. Complete sequence of human fast-type and slow-type muscle myosin-binding-protein C (MyBP-C). Differential expression, conserved domain structure and chromosome assignment. *Eur. J. Biochem.* **1993**, *216*, 661–669. [CrossRef]
89. Gautel, M.; Zuffardi, O.; Freiburg, A.; Labeit, S. Phosphorylation switches specific for the cardiac isoform of myosin binding protein-C: A modulator of cardiac contraction? *EMBO J.* **1995**, *14*, 1952–1960. [CrossRef]
90. Dhoot, G.K.; Hales, M.C.; Grail, B.M.; Perry, S.V. The isoforms of C protein and their distribution in mammalian skeletal muscle. *J. Muscle Res. Cell Motil.* **1985**, *6*, 487–505. [CrossRef]
91. Reinach, F.C.; Masaki, T.; Fischman, D.A. Characterization of the C-protein from posterior latissimus dorsi muscle of the adult chicken: Heterogeneity within a single sarcomere. *J. Cell Biol.* **1983**, *96*, 297–300. [CrossRef] [PubMed]
92. Gautel, M.; Furst, D.O.; Cocco, A.; Schiaffino, S. Isoform transitions of the myosin binding protein C family in developing human and mouse muscles: Lack of isoform transcomplementation in cardiac muscle. *Circ. Res.* **1998**, *82*, 124–129. [CrossRef] [PubMed]
93. James, J.; Robbins, J. Signaling and myosin-binding protein C. *J. Biol. Chem* **2011**, *286*, 9913–9919. [CrossRef] [PubMed]
94. Sadayappan, S.; de Tombe, P.P. Cardiac myosin binding protein-C as a central target of cardiac sarcomere signaling: A special mini review series. *Pflugers Arch.* **2014**, *466*, 195–200. [CrossRef] [PubMed]
95. Seidman, C.E.; Seidman, J.G. Identifying sarcomere gene mutations in hypertrophic cardiomyopathy: A personal history. *Circ. Res.* **2011**, *108*, 743–750. [CrossRef]
96. Sarikas, A.; Carrier, L.; Schenke, C.; Doll, D.; Flavigny, J.; Lindenberg, K.S.; Eschenhagen, T.; Zolk, O. Impairment of the ubiquitin-proteasome system by truncated cardiac myosin binding protein C mutants. *Cardiovasc. Res.* **2005**, *66*, 33–44. [CrossRef]
97. Bulteau, A.L.; Szweda, L.I.; Friguet, B. Age-dependent declines in proteasome activity in the heart. *Arch. Biochem. Biophys.* **2002**, *397*, 298–304. [CrossRef]
98. Okada, K.; Wangpoengtrakul, C.; Osawa, T.; Toyokuni, S.; Tanaka, K.; Uchida, K. 4-Hydroxy-2-nonenal-mediated impairment of intracellular proteolysis during oxidative stress. Identification of proteasomes as target molecules. *J. Biol. Chem.* **1999**, *274*, 23787–23793. [CrossRef]
99. Simonson, T.S.; Zhang, Y.; Huff, C.D.; Xing, J.; Watkins, W.S.; Witherspoon, D.J.; Woodward, S.R.; Jorde, L.B. Limited distribution of a cardiomyopathy-associated variant in India. *Ann. Hum. Genet.* **2010**, *74*, 184–188. [CrossRef]
100. Anand, A.; Chin, C.; Shah, A.S.V.; Kwiecinski, J.; Vesey, A.; Cowell, J.; Weber, E.; Kaier, T.; Newby, D.E.; Dweck, M.; et al. Cardiac myosin-binding protein C is a novel marker of myocardial injury and fibrosis in aortic stenosis. *Heart* **2018**, *104*, 1101–1108. [CrossRef]
101. Mishra, A.; Srivastava, A.; Mittal, T.; Garg, N.; Mittal, B. Impact of renin-angiotensin-aldosterone system gene polymorphisms on left ventricular dysfunction in coronary artery disease patients. *Dis. Markers* **2012**, *32*, 33–41. [CrossRef] [PubMed]
102. Farza, H.; Townsend, P.J.; Carrier, L.; Barton, P.J.; Mesnard, L.; Bahrend, E.; Forissier, J.F.; Fiszman, M.; Yacoub, M.H.; Schwartz, K. Genomic organisation, alternative splicing and polymorphisms of the human cardiac troponin T gene. *J. Mol. Cell Cardiol.* **1998**, *30*, 1247–1253. [CrossRef] [PubMed]
103. Kumar, S.; Mishra, A.; Srivastava, A.; Mittal, T.; Garg, N.; Mittal, B. Significant role of ADRB3 rs4994 towards the development of coronary artery disease. *Coron. Artery Dis.* **2014**, *25*, 29–34. [CrossRef]
104. Mishra, A.; Srivastava, A.; Mittal, T.; Garg, N.; Mittal, B. Genetic predisposition to left ventricular dysfunction: A multigenic and multi-analytical approach. *Gene* **2014**, *546*, 309–317. [CrossRef] [PubMed]
105. Sadayappan, S.; Osinska, H.; Klevitsky, R.; Lorenz, J.N.; Sargent, M.; Molkentin, J.D.; Seidman, C.E.; Seidman, J.G.; Robbins, J. Cardiac myosin binding protein C phosphorylation is cardioprotective. *Proc. Natl. Acad. Sci. USA* **2006**, *103*, 16918–16923. [CrossRef] [PubMed]
106. Mishra, A.; Srivastava, A.; Mittal, T.; Garg, N.; Mittal, B. Association of matrix metalloproteinases (MMP2, MMP7 and MMP9) genetic variants with left ventricular dysfunction in coronary artery disease patients. *Clin. Chim. Acta* **2012**, *413*, 1668–1674. [CrossRef] [PubMed]
107. Mishra, A.; Srivastava, A.; Mittal, T.; Garg, N.; Mittal, B. Role of inflammatory gene polymorphisms in left ventricular dysfunction (LVD) susceptibility in coronary artery disease (CAD) patients. *Cytokine* **2013**, *61*, 856–861. [CrossRef]

108. Akasheva, D.U.; Plokhova, E.V.; Tkacheva, O.N.; Strazhesko, I.D.; Dudinskaya, E.N.; Kruglikova, A.S.; Pykhtina, V.S.; Brailova, N.V.; Pokshubina, I.A.; Sharashkina, N.V.; et al. Age-Related Left Ventricular Changes and Their Association with Leukocyte Telomere Length in Healthy People. *PLoS ONE* **2015**, *10*, e0135883. [CrossRef]
109. Hayward, C.S.; Kalnins, W.V.; Kelly, R.P. Gender-related differences in left ventricular chamber function. *Cardiovasc. Res.* **2001**, *49*, 340–350. [CrossRef]
110. Kishi, S.; Reis, J.P.; Venkatesh, B.A.; Gidding, S.S.; Armstrong, A.C.; Jacobs, D.R., Jr.; Sidney, S.; Wu, C.O.; Cook, N.L.; Lewis, C.E.; et al. Race-ethnic and sex differences in left ventricular structure and function: The Coronary Artery Risk Development in Young Adults (CARDIA) Study. *J. Am. Heart Assoc.* **2015**, *4*, e001264. [CrossRef]
111. Alshehri, A.M.; Azoz, A.M.; Shaheen, H.A.; Farrag, Y.A.; Khalifa, M.A.; Youssef, A. Acute effects of cigarette smoking on the cardiac diastolic functions. *J. Saudi Heart Assoc.* **2013**, *25*, 173–179. [CrossRef] [PubMed]
112. Triposkiadis, F.; Giamouzis, G.; Parissis, J.; Starling, R.C.; Boudoulas, H.; Skoularigis, J.; Butler, J.; Filippatos, G. Reframing the association and significance of co-morbidities in heart failure. *Eur J. Heart Fail.* **2016**, *18*, 744–758. [CrossRef] [PubMed]
113. Mishra, A.; Srivastava, A.; Kumar, S.; Mittal, T.; Garg, N.; Agarwal, S.K.; Pande, S.; Mittal, B. Role of angiotensin II type I (AT1 A1166C) receptor polymorphism in susceptibility of left ventricular dysfunction. *Indian Heart J.* **2015**, *67*, 214–221. [CrossRef] [PubMed]

15

Novel Biomarkers in Patients with Chronic Kidney Disease: An Analysis of Patients Enrolled in the GCKD-Study

Moritz Mirna [1], Albert Topf [1], Bernhard Wernly [1], Richard Rezar [1], Vera Paar [1], Christian Jung [2], Hermann Salmhofer [3], Kristen Kopp [1], Uta C. Hoppe [1], P. Christian Schulze [4], Daniel Kretzschmar [4], Markus P. Schneider [5], Ulla T. Schultheiss [6], Claudia Sommerer [7], Katharina Paul [8], Gunter Wolf [8], Michael Lichtenauer [1,*] and Martin Busch [8]

1 Department of Internal Medicine II, Division of Cardiology, Paracelsus Medical University of Salzburg, 5020 Salzburg, Austria; m.mirna@salk.at (M.M.); a.topf@salk.at (A.T.); b.wernly@salk.at (B.W.); r.rezar@salk.at (R.R.); v.paar@salk.at (V.P.); k.kopp@salk.at (K.K.); u.hoppe@salk.at (U.C.H.)

2 Department of Cardiology, Pulmonology and Vascular Medicine, Medical Faculty, Heinrich Heine University Duesseldorf, 40225 Duesseldorf, Germany; christian.jung@med.uni-duesseldorf.de

3 Department of Internal Medicine I, Division of Nephrology, Paracelsus Medical University of Salzburg, 5020 Salzburg, Austria; h.salmhofer@salk.at

4 Department of Internal Medicine I, Division of Cardiology, Friedrich Schiller University Jena, 07743 Jena, Germany; christian.schulze@med.uni-jena.de (P.C.S.); daniel.kretzschmar@med.uni-jena.de (D.K.)

5 Department of Nephrology and Hypertension, University Hospital Erlangen, Friedrich-Alexander University Erlangen-Nürnberg, 91054 Erlangen, Germany; markus.schneider@klinikum-nuernberg.de

6 Department of Medicine IV – Nephrology and Primary Care, Institute of Genetic Epidemiology, Medical Center–University of Freiburg, Faculty of Medicine, 79106 Freiburg, Germany; ulla.schultheiss@uniklinik-freiburg.de

7 Department of Nephrology, University of Heidelberg, 69117 Heidelberg, Germany; claudia.sommerer@med.uni-heidelberg.de

8 Department of Internal Medicine III, Friedrich Schiller University Jena, 07743 Jena, Germany; katharina.paul@med.uni-jena.de (K.P.); gunter.wolf@med.uni-jena.de (G.W.); martin.busch@med.uni-jena.de (M.B.)

* Correspondence: michael.lichtenauer@chello.at

Abstract: *Background:* Chronic kidney disease (CKD) and cardiovascular diseases (CVD) often occur concomitantly, and CKD is a major risk factor for cardiovascular mortality. Since some of the most commonly used biomarkers in CVD are permanently elevated in patients with CKD, novel biomarkers are warranted for clinical practice. *Methods:* Plasma concentrations of five cardiovascular biomarkers (soluble suppression of tumorigenicity (sST2), growth differentiation factor 15 (GDF-15), heart-type fatty acid-binding protein (H-FABP), insulin-like growth factor-binding protein 2 (IGF-BP2), and soluble urokinase plasminogen activator receptor) were analyzed by means of enzyme-linked immunosorbent assay (ELISA) in 219 patients with CKD enrolled in the German Chronic Kidney Disease (GCKD) study. *Results:* Except for sST2, all of the investigated biomarkers were significantly elevated in patients with CKD (2.0- to 4.4-fold increase in advanced CKD (estimated glomerular filtration rate (eGFR) < 30 mL/min/1.73 m^2 body surface area (BSA)) and showed a significant inverse correlation with eGFR. Moreover, all but H-FABP and sST2 were additionally elevated in patients with micro- and macro-albuminuria. *Conclusions:* Based on our findings, sST2 appears to be the biomarker whose diagnostic performance is least affected by decreased renal function, thus suggesting potential viability in the management of patients with CVD and concomitant CKD. The predictive potential of sST2 remains to be proven in endpoint studies.

Keywords: CKD; CVD; biomarkers; sST2

1. Introduction

Chronic kidney disease (CKD) affects about 11.5% of the overall population with increasing age-dependent prevalence of up to 47% in persons older than 70 years [1]. Apart from old age, CKD is associated with diabetes mellitus and hypertension. Due to an increase of these precipitating and often causative diseases, the prevalence of CKD is expected to rise even further in the future [1]. Because of shared risk factors and the fact that CKD constitutes an independent risk factor itself, CKD and cardiovascular disease (CVD) often occur concomitantly [2–4]. Hence, biomarkers established in the evaluation of patients with CVD are increasingly used in patients with decreased renal function. Unfortunately, some of the most common biomarkers in this field, such as troponin or brain natriuretic peptide (BNP), are chronically elevated in patients with CKD, which may in part be due to impaired renal clearance [5–7]. Therefore, their clinical applicability in patients with CKD is limited and hence, novel biomarkers are warranted to improve diagnosis and risk stratification in these disease entities.

In the following study, plasma concentrations of novel cardiovascular biomarkers (sST2, GDF-15, H-FABP, IGF-BP2 and suPAR) were investigated in patients with various stages of CKD.

Soluble suppression of tumorigenicity (sST2; molecular mass: 36,993 Da [8]; normal reference ranges for male subjects: 4000–31,000 pg/mL; for female subjects: 2000–21,000 pg/mL [9]) is a member of the toll-like/IL-1-receptor family that acts as a scavenger-receptor for IL-33, thus attenuating the effects of this immunomodulatory cytokine [10]. sST2 is secreted in response to mechanical stress, and hence elevated plasma levels are found in patients with acute and chronic heart failure [11]. Increased plasma concentrations of sST2 have been associated with adverse outcomes in patients with coronary artery disease [12] and heart failure [11,13] in previous trials.

Growth differentiation factor 15 (GDF-15; molecular mass: 34,140 Da [14]; normal reference ranges: 310 ± 10 pg/mL [15]) is a member of the transforming growth factor ß (TGF-ß) cytokine family. GDF-15 is secreted in response to tissue injury or by the effect of proinflammatory cytokines and is involved in the regulation of inflammatory and apoptotic processes [16]. Recently, elevated plasma levels of GDF-15 have been associated with an increased risk of mortality in patients with coronary artery disease and chronic heart failure [17–19]. Furthermore, increased plasma concentrations of circulating GDF-15 were associated with a decline of renal function in patients with CKD [20].

Heart-type fatty acid-binding protein (H-FABP; molecular mass: 14,858 Da [21]; normal reference ranges for male subjects: 3.5 ± 0.4; for female subjects: 3.9 ± 0.4 ng/mL [22]) is a small cytoplasmic protein that transports long-chained fatty acids in cardiomyocytes and is considered a biomarker of myocardial ischemia [23]. In case of damage to the cell membrane, H-FABP is rapidly released into circulation and therefore was evaluated for use in diagnosis and risk stratification of coronary artery disease and acute coronary syndrome [24,25]. In fact, increased plasma levels of H-FABP are associated with an elevated risk of adverse outcomes in acute coronary syndrome and heart failure [26,27].

Insulin-like growth factor-binding protein 2 (IGF-BP2; molecular mass: 34,814 Da [28]; normal reference ranges: 321.2 ± 285.0 ng/mL [29]) is an anabolic peptide with extensive structural and functional homology to insulin. IGF-BP2 is a potent effector of growth, proliferation, and metabolism that elicits its effects via autocrine, paracrine, and endocrine mechanisms [30]. Elevated plasma concentrations of IGF-BP2 have been associated with diabetes mellitus [31], metabolic syndrome [32], and progression of CKD [33] in previous studies. Moreover, IGF-BP2 seems to be involved in the pathogenesis of atherosclerosis. In a recent trial, plasma concentrations of IGF-BP2 were inversely correlated with arterial intima-media thickness of the carotid artery in healthy participants [34,35].

Soluble urokinase plasminogen activator receptor (suPAR; molecular mass (depending on the considered isoform): 31,263–36,978 Da [36]; normal reference ranges: 2100 pg/mL, IQR: 1700–2300 pg/mL [37]) is the soluble isoform of the urokinase plasminogen activator receptor (uPAR), a membrane-bound protein in endothelial and immunological cells that plays a role in various inflammatory processes [38]. Recent evidence suggests that suPAR is involved in the formation of atherosclerotic lesions and hence, elevated plasma levels of suPAR have been associated with an increased risk for coronary artery disease and cardiovascular mortality [39]. Furthermore, elevated plasma concentrations of suPAR were recently correlated with the deterioration of renal function in patients with CKD [40,41], and an association between suPAR and primary focal segmental glomerulosclerosis (pFSGS) [42,43] was found.

2. Materials and Methods

Plasma samples from 219 of 245 patients enrolled in the regional center of Jena within the German Chronic Kidney Disease study (GCKD), Germany, were analyzed. The remaining 26 patients were excluded as serum samples were missing. The GCKD study was approved by the local ethics committee, registered in the German national registry for clinical studies (DRKS00003971) and was conducted according to the principles of the Declaration of Helsinki and Good Clinical Practice. Informed consent was obtained from all patients prior to enrollment.

2.1. Study Population

Details of the study design and the enrollment process of the GCKD study have been described previously [44]. Briefly, patients aged 18–74 years with CKD in routine nephrological care were enrolled across nine German study centers between March 2010 and March 2012. Patients were included if they had an estimated glomerular filtration rate (eGFR) of < 60mL/min/1.73m^2 body surface area (BSA) or overt proteinuria in the presence of a higher eGFR (defined as albuminuria of > 300 mg/g creatinine or proteinuria of > 500 g/g creatinine). Exclusion criteria were non-Caucasian race, history of transplantation, active malignancy, New York Heart Association (NYHA) heart failure functional class IV, and/or inability to provide written informed consent [44].

Glomerular filtration rate (GFR) was estimated using the 4-variable modification of diet in renal disease (MDRD) formula, as previously published [45,46]. CKD was categorized according to the clinical practice guidelines from the Kidney Disease: Improving Global Outcomes Initiative (KDIGO) in the following G and A-stages. G-stages: CKD stage G1: eGFR ≥ 90 mL/min/1.73 m^2 BSA, stage G2: eGFR 60–89 mL/min/1.73 m^2 BSA, stage G3a: 45–59 mL/min/1.73 m^2 BSA, stage G3b: eGFR 30–44 mL/min/1.73 m^2 BSA, and stages G4 and G5 (combined): eGFR < 30 mL/min/1.73 m^2 BSA. A-stages: urinary albumin/creatinine ratio (UACR) < 30 mg/g Crea (A1 = normo-albuminuria), 30–300 mg/g Crea (A2 = micro-albuminuria), or > 300 mg/g Crea (A3 = macro-albuminuria) [47,48]. Symptoms of heart failure were estimated by the modified Gothenburg scale, as previously published [47,49].

2.2. Blood Samples and Biomarker Analysis

Blood samples were collected upon study enrollment using a vacuum-containing system. Plasma levels of sST2, GDF-15, H-FABP, IGF-BP2, and suPAR were measured by using commercially available enzyme-linked immunosorbent assay (ELISA) kits (R&D Systems, USA). Preparation of reagents and measurements were performed according to the manufacturer's instructions. In brief, patient samples and standard protein were added to the wells of the ELISA plates (Nunc MaxiSorp flat-bottom 96 well plates, VWR International GmbH, Austria) and incubated for two hours. Plates were then washed using a Tween 20/PBS solution (Sigma Aldrich, USA). Then, a biotin-labelled antibody was added and incubated for another two hours. Plates were washed another time, and streptavidin–horseradish-peroxidase solution was added to the wells. After adding tetramethylbenzidine (TMB; Sigma Aldrich, USA) a color reaction was generated. Values of optical density (OD) were determined at 450 nm on an ELISA plate-reader (iMark Microplate Absorbance Reader, Bio-Rad Laboratories, Austria).

2.3. Statistical Analysis

Statistical analyses were performed using SPSS (Version 24.0, SPSSS Inc., USA) and GraphPad Prism software (GraphPad Software, USA). Normally distributed data was expressed as mean and standard deviation (SD); not normally distributed data was expressed as median and interquartile range (IQR). Medians were compared using a Mann–Whitney U-test or a Kruskal–Wallis test with Dunn's post-hoc test, depending on the number of groups analyzed. Bonferroni–Holm correction was conducted to adjust for multiple comparisons. To assess the association between renal function and biomarker concentrations, correlation analysis was conducted using Spearman's rank correlation test, followed by multiple linear regression analysis to adjust for parameters known for confounding with renal function (age, gender, BMI, diabetes mellitus, and arterial hypertension). Prior to multiple linear regression analysis, normal distribution was assessed by performing a Kolmogorov–Smirnov test, where applicable, and multicollinearity was excluded using the collinearity diagnostics tool by SPSS. A p-value < 0.05 was considered statistically significant.

3. Results

In total, 219 plasma samples of patients enrolled in the GCKD study were analyzed. The mean age was 63 ± 9 years, and the majority of patients were male (60.3%, n = 132). Regarding comorbidities, arterial hypertension was present in 90.4% (n = 198), diabetes mellitus type 2 in 39.3% (n = 86), heart failure in 26.0% (n = 57), and 49.3% had a history of smoking (n = 108) (see Table 1).

3.1. Renal Function and Causes of Renal Disease

Regarding renal function, the majority of patients was in CKD stages G3a (41.6% (n = 91), eGFR 45–59 mL/min/1.73 m^2 BSA) and G3b (32.4% (n = 71), eGFR 30–44 mL/min/1.73 m^2 BSA), followed by CKD stage 2 (13.7% (n = 30), eGFR 60–89 mL/min/1.73 m^2 BSA) and CKD stages 4 and 5 (9.6% (n = 21), eGFR < 30 mL/min/1.73 m^2 BSA); 2.7% (n = 6) of the patients had an eGFR above 90 mL/min/1.73 m^2 BSA while having proteinuria.

Regarding urinary albumin excretion, micro-albuminuria (UACR 30–300 mg/g) was observed in 32% (n = 70) of patients, whereas macro-albuminuria (UACR > 300 mg/g) was evident in 20.5% (n = 45) of the patients at the time of inclusion (see Table 1). Only two patients had an UACR above 3000 mg/g.

The median estimated glomerular filtration rate (eGFR) was 47.7 mL/min/1.73 m^2 (IQR 38.2–55.7), the median level of creatinine was 1.5 mg/dL (IQR 1.2–1.7), and the median level of cystatin-C was 1.4 mg/L (IQR 1.2–1.7). The median plasma level of serum urea was 26.5 mg/dL (IQR 20.6–33.3), the median level of uric acid was 7.1 mg/dL (IQR 6.0–8.3), and the median level of CRP was 2.4 mg/dL (IQR 1.2–4.9).

The leading cause of renal disease was nephrosclerosis (28.8%, n = 63), followed by diabetic nephropathy (diabetes mellitus type 1 and 2 combined: 17.4%, n = 38) and interstitial nephropathy (9.1%, n = 20) (see Table 1).

Table 1. Baseline characteristics, comorbidities, stages of chronic kidney disease (CKD), and causes of renal disease of the overall cohort.

General		
Age, mean (years)	63	±9
BMI, mean (kg/m^2)	30	±5.6
Serum creatinine, median (mg/dl)	1.5	IQR 1.2–1.7
eGFR, median (mL/min/1.73 m^2)	47.7	IQR 38.2–55.7
Urinary albumin/creatinine ratio (UACR), median (mg/g Crea)	44	IQR 7.4–216.7
Comorbidities	**%**	**(n)**
Hypertension	90.4	198
Diabetes mellitus	39.3	86
Heart Failure	26.0	57
CKD stages	**%**	**(n)**
Stage G1 (≥ 90 mL/min/1.73 m^2)	2.7	6
Stage G2 (eGFR 60–89 mL/min/1.73 m^2)	13.7	30
Stage G3a (eGFR 45–59 mL/min/1.73 m^2)	41.6	91
Stage G3b (eGFR 30–44 mL/min/1.73 m^2)	32.4	71
Stages G4 and G5 (eGFR <30 mL/min/1.73 m^2)	9.6	21
Urinary albumin/creatinine ratio (ACR)	**%**	**(n)**
A1 (<30 mg/g)	43.8	96
A2 (30–300 mg/g)	32.0	70
A3 (>300 mg/g)	20.5	45
Missing	4.7	8
Leading cause of renal disease	**%**	**(n)**
Vascular nephrosclerosis	28.8	63
Diabetic nephropathy	17.4	38
Interstitial nephropathy	9.1	20
IgA-nephritis	4.1	9
Autosomal dominant polycystic kidney disease	4.1	9
Membranous glomerulonephritis	2.7	6
Membranoproliferative glomerulonephritis	1.4	3
Other	17.9	40
Missing	14.6	32

BMI = body mass index, DM = diabetes mellitus.

3.2. Biomarker Concentrations

The median plasma levels of sST2, GDF-15, H-FABP, IGF-BP2, and suPAR in our study cohort are depicted in Figure 1 and Supplementary Materials, Table A1 in Appendix A.

Except for sST2, all of the investigated biomarkers showed significantly elevated plasma concentrations in the advanced stages of CKD (GDF-15: 3.6-fold increase, H-FABP: 4.4-fold increase, IGF-BP2: 3.0-fold increase, suPAR 2.0-fold increase when eGFR was <30 mL/min/1.73 m^2 BSA compared to eGFR ≥ 90 mL/min/1.73 m^2 BSA, see Figure 1 and Supplementary Materials, Table A1 in Appendix A). This finding remained statistically significant after applying Bonferroni–Holm correction for multiple comparisons (GDF-15: $p = 0.0005$, H-FABP: $p = 0.0005$, IGF-BP2: $p = 0.002$, suPAR: $p = 0.0005$).

Patients with concomitant symptoms of heart failure had significantly elevated plasma concentrations of sST2 (median 5039 pg/mL vs. 3673 pg/mL, $p = 0.008$).

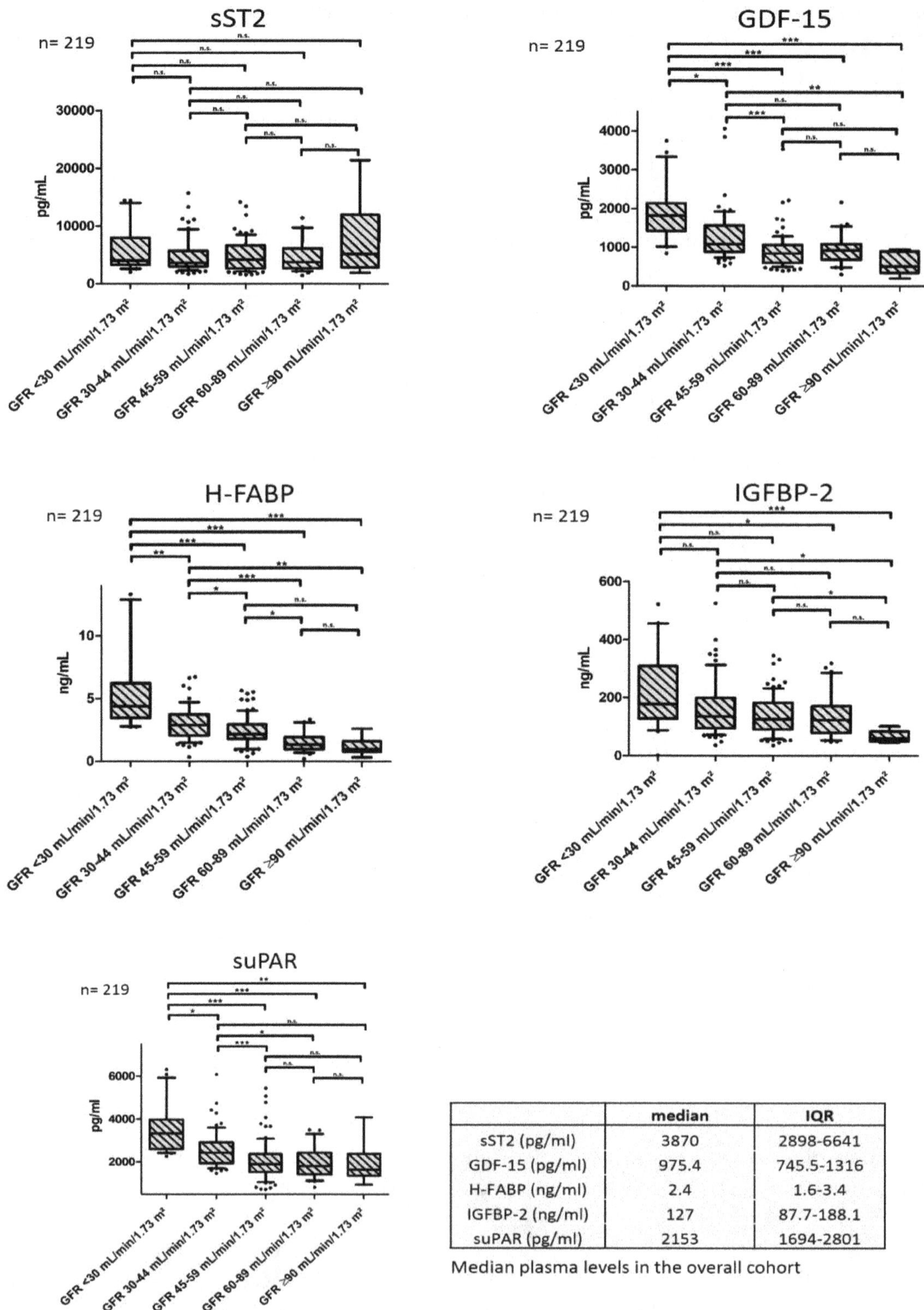

	median	IQR
sST2 (pg/ml)	3870	2898-6641
GDF-15 (pg/ml)	975.4	745.5-1316
H-FABP (ng/ml)	2.4	1.6-3.4
IGFBP-2 (ng/ml)	127	87.7-188.1
suPAR (pg/ml)	2153	1694-2801

Median plasma levels in the overall cohort

Figure 1. Biomarker concentrations throughout the stages of CKD. Median plasma levels and interquartile ranges (IQR) of the overall cohort are depicted in the additional table. * indicates a p of <0.05, ** a p of <0.01 and *** a p of <0.001, n.s.= not significant. Abbreviations: sST2 = soluble suppression of tumorigenicity, GDF-15 = growth differentiation factor 15, H-FABP = heart-type fatty acid binding protein, IGF-BP2= insulin-like growth factor binding protein 2, suPAR = soluble urokinase plasminogen activator receptor, eGFR = estimated glomerular filtration rate, IQR = interquartile range.

3.3. Correlation Analyses and Multiple Linear Regression Analyses

Plasma concentrations of GDF-15, H-FABP, suPAR, and IGF-BP2 showed a significant positive correlation with serum creatinine (GDF-15: rs = 0.566, $p < 0.0001$, H-FABP: rs = 0.584, $p < 0.0001$, suPAR: rs = 0.506, $p < 0.0001$, IGF-BP2: rs = 0.267, $p < 0.0001$; rs = correlation coefficient) and a significant inverse correlation with eGFR (GDF-15: rs = −0.493, $p < 0.0001$, H-FABP: rs = −0.550, $p < 0.0001$, suPAR: rs = −0.485, $p < 0.0001$, IGF-BP2: rs = −0.298, $p < 0.0001$), which remained statistically significant after applying Bonferroni–Holm correction. sST2 showed no correlation with renal function, neither with serum creatinine, nor with eGFR (see Figure 2 and Table 2).

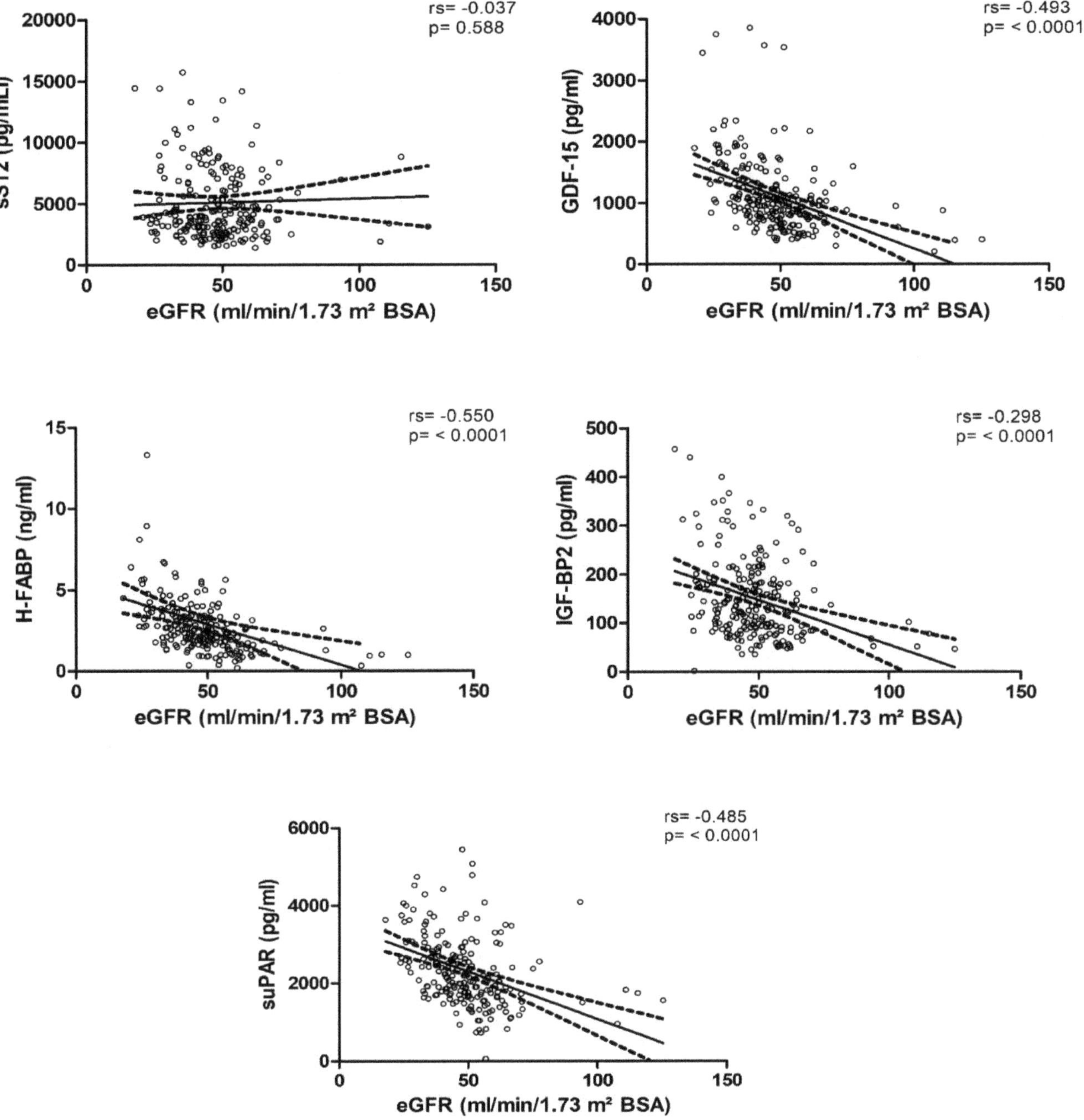

Figure 2. Visual representation of the correlation of biomarker concentrations with estimated glomerular filtration rate (eGFR).

Table 2. Correlation analysis of the investigated biomarkers.

Biomarker		BMI	Creatinine	eGFR	UACR	CRP	sST2	GDF15	H-FABP	IGF-BP2	suPAR
sST2	rs	0.890	0.125	−0.037	0.139	0.087		0.133	0.348	0.151	0.082
	p-value	0.191	0.067	0.588	0.044 *	0.200		0.049	<0.0001	0.025	0.228
GDF-15	rs	0.097	0.566	−0.493	0.251	0.240	0.133		0.491	0.266	0.614
	p-value	0.151	<0.0001	<0.0001	<0.0001	0.0004	0.049		<0.0001	<0.0001	<0.0001
H-FABP	rs	0.314	0.584	−0.550	0.100	0.162	0.348	0.491		0.194	0.516
	p-value	<0.0001	<0.0001	< 0.0001	0.149	0.017	<0.0001	<0.0001		0.004	<0.0001
IGF-BP2	rs	-0.343	0.267	−0.298	0.192	−0.071	0.151	0.266	0.194		0.180
	p-value	<0.0001	<0.0001	<0.0001	0.005	0.296	0.025	<0.0001	0.004		0.007
suPAR	rs	0.243	0.506	−0.485	0.163	0.377	0.082	0.614	0.516	0.180	
	p-value	<0.0001	<0.0001	<0.0001	0.018 *	<0.0001	0.228	<0.0001	<0.0001	0.007	

* Denotes correlations that became statistically insignificant after applying a Bonferroni–Holm correction. Abbreviations: BMI = body mass index, CRP = C-reactive protein, eGFR = estimated glomerular filtration rate, rs = correlation coefficient, UACR = urinary albumin/ creatinine ratio.

The correlation of biomarker concentrations with eGFR remained statistically significant in a multiple linear regression analysis after correction for parameters that are known to confound with renal function (GDF-15: B = −0.10, $p < 0.0001$; H-FABP: B = −1.187, $p < 0.0001$; IGF-BP2: B = −0.064, $p < 0.0001$; suPAR: B = −0.006, $p < 0.0001$; B = regression coefficient, see Supplementary Materials, Table A2 in Appendix A). There was still no significant correlation between plasma concentrations of sST2 and renal function (sST2: B = 0.000, 95% CI 0.000–0.001, $p = 0.643$) after adjusting for the aforementioned confounders.

Except for H-FABP, all of the biomarkers showed a weak, yet statistically significant correlation with the UACR (sST2: rs = 0.139, $p = 0.044$; GDF-15: rs = 0.251, $p < 0.0001$; IGF-BP2 rs = 0.192, $p = 0.005$; suPAR: rs = 0.163, $p = 0.018$, H-FABP: rs = 0.100, $p = 0.149$, see Table 2). Notably, the weak correlations of sST2 and suPAR with the UACR were statistically insignificant after applying the Bonferroni–Holm correction for multiple comparisons (sST2: $p = 0.088$, suPAR: $p = 0.054$).

However, after adjusting for the aforementioned confounders in another multiple linear regression model, all correlations with the UACR, except the ones with suPAR and H-FABP, remained statistically significant (sST2: B = 0.031, $p = 0.007$; GDF-15: B = 0.179, $p = 0.012$; IGF-BP2: B = 2.086, $p < 0.0001$; see Supplementary Materials, Table A2 in Appendix A).

Furthermore, the plasma concentrations of suPAR, H-FABP, and IGF-BP2 showed a significant correlation with BMI and the plasma levels of suPAR, H-FABP, and GDF-15 correlated with CRP. Additionally, the plasma concentrations of H-FABP correlated with the plasma levels of sST2, GDF-15, suPAR, and IGF-BP2, and the concentrations of suPAR correlated with the plasma levels of GDF-15 and IGF-BP2 and vice versa (see Table 2).

3.4. Biomarker Concentrations in Patients with Albuminuria

The plasma levels of GDF-15, IGF-BP2, and suPAR were significantly elevated in patients with micro-and macro-albuminuria, as defined by the UACR (Table 3). In contrast, the plasma concentrations of sST2 and H-FABP were not significantly influenced by the stage of albuminuria (see Table 3). This finding remained statistically significant after applying a Bonferroni–Holm correction for multiple comparisons (GDF-15: $p = 0.01$, IGF-BP2: $p = 0.01$, suPAR: $p = 0.012$).

Table 3. Concentrations in patients with normo-albuminuria, micro-albuminuria (UACR 30–300 mg/g, A2), and macro-albuminuria (UACR > 300 mg/g); the *p*-value represents the statistical differences between the three subgroups of albuminuria.

Biomarker	Total Cohort		Normo-albuminuria (A1)		Micro-albuminuria (A2)		Macro-albuminuria (A3)		
	median	IQR	median	IQR	median	IQR	median	IQR	*p*-Value
sST2 (pg/mL)	3870	2898–6641	3663	2726–6172	3647	2758–5793	4552	8587–3235	0.052
GDF-15 (pg/mL)	975.4	745.5–1316	892.2	675.6–1087	1035	780.9–861.7	1281	861.7–1635	0.002
H-FABP (ng/mL)	2.4	1.6–3.4	2.3	1.6–3.1	2.2	1.7–3.4	2.8	1.6–4.1	0.170
IGF-BP2 (ng/mL)	127	87.7–188.1	112.9	84.2–172.3	126.2	83.6–182.7	172.6	91.5–280.1	0.002
suPAR (pg/mL)	2153	1694–2801	1925	1653–2680	2197	1674–2723	2402	1918–2983	0.044

4. Discussion

In patients with chronic kidney disease (CKD), a high burden of cardiovascular diseases (CVD) is common, and an inverse correlation of renal function with the prevalence of coronary artery disease, congestive heart failure, and cerebrovascular disease is observed [1,50]. Moreover, the incidence of acute kidney injury has been steadily increasing in recent years, leading to higher healthcare costs and mortality and contributing to increasing prevalence rates of CKD [51,52]. With an increasing prevalence of CKD from variable causes, the number of patients with end-stage renal disease is on the rise [1,53]. Furthermore, the presence of CKD markedly increases cardiovascular mortality in a stage-dependent manner [54–56]. According to current evidence, patients with end-stage renal disease (ESRD) undergoing hemodialysis have a 10- to 30-fold higher risk of cardiovascular mortality than the general population [57].

In fact, diagnosis, risk stratification, and treatment of patients with CVD increasingly relies on cardiovascular biomarkers. Since some of the most commonly used biomarkers for these purposes (e.g., troponin or brain natriuretic peptide (BNP)) are chronically elevated in patients with CKD [57,58], novel cardiovascular biomarkers are warranted to facilitate the management of patients with decreased renal function.

In our study cohort, plasma concentrations of GDF-15, H-FABP, IGF-BP2, and suPAR were markedly elevated in patients with decreased renal function, with a 2.0- to 4.4-fold increase in biomarker levels in the advanced stages of CKD (eGFR < 30 mL/min/1.73 m^2 BSA). In contrast, we found no significant elevation of sST2 in patients with CKD. In fact, the plasma levels of sST2 even remained unaltered in advanced CKD (eGFR < 30 mL/min/1.73 m^2 BSA) and showed no correlation with estimated glomerular filtration rate (eGFR). In contrast to sST2, we found significant correlations of the plasma levels of GDF-15, H-FABP, IGF-BP2, and suPAR with serum creatinine and eGFR. Considering potential diagnostic value, it is essential to determine whether a biomarker would accumulate due to impaired renal clearance or increase due to the pathophysiologic process that it is supposed to portray (i.e., troponin in myocardial ischemia). Although the association with renal function does not preclude the predictive ability of a biomarker, its clinical applicability in the evaluation of patients with CVD and concomitant CKD appears to be somewhat limited [59]. Since some of the most commonly used conventional biomarkers in CVD are chronically elevated in patients with CKD, at least partly because of impaired renal clearance, the finding that sST2 acts independently of renal function might be of significant relevance for clinical practice. Nevertheless, this finding needs to be confirmed in large prospective endpoint trials because it to some extent contradicts the findings of a study by Alam et al. In this study, some correlation of sST2 with renal function was observed in a larger, pooled cohort, yet this relationship was very weak [60]. Furthermore, the clinical performance of biomarkers needs to be confirmed in large prospective endpoint trials. In this regard, recent trials investigated the plasma concentrations of NT-proBNP, troponin T, and IGF-BP2 in patients with CKD and reported a higher prognostic value of the investigated biomarkers in these patients [61,62]. However, it is always questionable whether such studies consistently correct their statistical models for kidney function. Hence, the adjustment for renal function may be more valid for biomarkers, which do not primarily correlate with renal function. Interestingly, although the ST2/IL-33 signaling pathway seems to be involved in various inflammatory processes [63–66], the aforementioned study by Alam et al. did not find a statistically significant association of the plasma levels of sST2 with the progression of CKD to end-stage renal disease (ESRD) [60]. Taken together with our results, it seems as if sST2, in contrast to numerous other cytokines or mediators, acts relatively independent from renal function and pathophysiologic processes affecting the kidneys.

Furthermore, all of the investigated biomarkers, except for H-FABP and sST2, were additionally elevated in patients with micro- and macro-albuminuria, as defined by the UACR. This association is of particular interest, since albuminuria is an independent cardiovascular risk factor reflecting endothelial dysfunction [67,68], which might modulate the predictive potential of the biomarkers investigated. Notably, despite no statistical significance, we observed an obvious increase in the plasma concentrations of sST2 between the different stages of albuminuria (see Table 3). This increase was accompanied by a weak, yet statistically significant correlation of sST2 with albuminuria (sST2: rs = 0.139, $p = 0.044$), which became statistically insignificant after applying a Bonferroni–Holm correction for multiple comparisons.

sST2 is a promising new biomarker in risk stratification and therapy guidance [69,70] in patients with acute and chronic heart failure, and was associated with an increased risk of adverse outcomes in previous trials [12,71,72]. According to our present findings, sST2 might be a useful additional biomarker in the management of patients with CVD and concomitant CKD, with or without albuminuria. Although some studies reported similar findings in the plasma levels of sST2 in patients with

CKD [73,74], the innovative value of our manuscript lies in the structured analysis and recording of five novel biomarkers, which portray different pathophysiological pathways, in a well-defined cohort. Furthermore, we investigated and described the respective plasma levels in different stages of CKD as reflected by eGFR and albuminuria.

5. Conclusions

Except for sST2, all of the investigated biomarkers were significantly elevated in patients with CKD, inversely correlating with eGFR. Based on our findings, sST2 appears to be the biomarker whose diagnostic performance is least affected by decreased renal function, hence suggesting potential viability in the management of patients with CVD and concomitant CKD. Whether this may influence its predictive potential in patients with CKD remains to be investigated by endpoint studies.

6. Limitations

A major limitation of this study is the absence of matched healthy controls, which would have further strengthened our findings. Moreover, the Gothenburg scale was found to be not ideal for reliably defining heart failure in patients with CKD in a previous trial due to shared symptoms and medications between the two disease entities [47]. However, a significant proportion of patients had concomitant heart failure, which may have acted as a bias in regard to the median concentrations of sST2. Notably, this trial did not analyze associations of the investigated biomarkers with clinical endpoints. We have to highlight that the conclusions drawn by the findings in this study are primarily of hypothesis-generating character and should be further validated in future trials. A limitation of the study may also be the applicability to populations of patients of non-Caucasian origin, since it is known that the cardiovascular risk also varies depending on ethnicity due to genetic differences. Thus, further investigative and population-specific endpoint trials, i.e., in the total GCKD cohort, seem necessary to confirm our present findings. One minor limitation is the use of estimated GFR instead of direct GFR measurement. Although more accurate, direct GFR measurement is too complex and impractical for everyday clinical use; hence, it appears unsuitable for a large multi-center trial. The use of eGFR by means of the MDRD formula does not represent a large bias regarding our current findings since only a minority of the patients had an eGFR above 60 mL/min/1.73 m^2.

Author Contributions: M.M., A.T. and R.R. were responsible for the study design, writing and correction of the manuscript. V.P. conducted the necessary experiments and B.W. was responsible of the statistical analyses. K.K. provided English language editing, M.L. was involved in the primary design of the study, writing and correction of the manuscript. U.C.H., P.C.S., D.K., M.P.S., U.T.S., C.S., K.P., G.W., M.B., C.J. and H.S. were involved in the design of the study and provided substantial corrections and improvements to the manuscript. All authors have read and agreed to the published version of the manuscript.

Acknowledgments: We are very grateful for the willingness and time of all study participants of the GCKD study. The authors thank all participating patients and the physicians and nurses taking care of them. We also thank the large number of nephrologists for their support of the GCKD study (list of nephrologists currently collaborating with the GCKD study is available at http://www.gckd.org). Current GCKD investigators and collaborators with the GCKD study are: University of Erlangen-Nürnberg: K.-U.E., H.M., M.P.S., M.S., T.D., H.-U.P., B.B., A.B., D.K., A.R., A.B.E., S.A., D.B.-G., U.A.-S., B.H., A.W.; University of Freiburg: Gerd Walz, A. K., U.T.S., F. K., S. M., E. M., U. R.; RWTH Aachen University: J.F., G.S., T.S.; Charité, University Medicine Berlin: E.S., S.B.-A., K.T.; Hannover Medical School: H.H., J.M.; University of Heidelberg: M.Z., C.S., R.W.; University of Jena: G.W., M.B., R.P.; Ludwig-Maximilians University of München: T.S.; University of Würzburg: C.W., V.K., A.B.-K., B.B.; Medical University of Innsbruck, Division of Genetic Epidemiology: F.K., J.R., B.K., L.F., S.S., Hansi Weissensteiner; University of Regensburg, Institute of Functional Genomics: P.O., W.G., H.Z.; Department of Medical Biometry, Informatics and Epidemiology (IMBIE), University Hospital of Bonn: M.S., J.N.

Appendix A

Table A1. Biomarker concentrations by estimated glomerular filtration rate (eGFR).

	eGFR <30 mL/min/1.73 m^2		eGFR 30–44 mL/min/1.73 m^2		eGFR 45–59 mL/min/1.73 m^2		eGFR 60–89 mL/min/1.73 m^2		eGFR ≥ 90 mL/min/1.73 m^2		total cohort		
Biomarker	**median**	**IQR**	**median**	**IQR**	**median**	**IQR**	**median**	**IQR**	**median**	**IQR**	**median**	**IQR**	***p*-value**
sST2 (pg/mL)	3998	3262–7949	3612	2997–5689	4167	2643–6620	3731	2660–6098	5170	2820–11,952	3870	2898–6641	0.788
GDF-15 (pg/mL)	1816	1420–2139	1086	883.4–1567	843.8	602.5–1064	929.7	683.0–1084	506.3	348.3–896.4	975.4	745.5–1316	<0.0001
H-FABP (ng/mL)	4.4	3.5–6.2	2.9	2.1–3.7	2.2	1.8–3.0	1.4	1.0–1.9	1.0	0.8–1.6	2.4	1.6–3.4	<0.0001
IGF-BP2 (ng/mL)	177.8	127.5–309.0	135.4	94.9–198.8	126.0	91.3–182.5	122.6	79.0–171.4	59.9	50.2–83.6	127	87.7–188.1	0.001
suPAR (pg/mL)	3342	2618–3977	2443	1936–2921	1898	1537–2382	1811	1422–2442	1648	1364–2393	2153	1694–2801	<0.0001

Table A2. Multiple linear regression analysis with adjustment for age, gender, BMI, hypertension and diabetes mellitus.

Dependent Variable: eGFR Adjustment for: Age, Gender, BMI, Hypertension, Diabetes					Dependent Variable: UACR Adjustment for: Age, Gender, BMI, Hypertension, Diabetes				
Biomarker	**r**	**Std. Error**	**95% CI**	***p*-Value**	**Biomarker**	**r**	**Std. Error**	**95% CI**	***p*-Value**
sST2 (pg/mL)	0.000	0.000	0.000–0.001	0.643	sST2 (pg/mL)	0.031	0.011	0.008–0.053	0.007
GDF-15 (pg/mL)	−0.010	0.002	−0.013–(−0.007)	<0.0001	GDF-15 (pg/mL)	0.179	0.071	0.040–0.319	0.012
H-FABP (ng/mL)	−1.187	0.321	−1.820–(−0.555)	<0.0001	H-FABP (ng/mL)	17.542	12.923	−7.938–43.02	0.176
IGF-BP2 (ng/mL)	−0.064	0.012	−0.087–(−0.041)	<0.0001	IGF-BP2 (ng/mL)	2.086	0.464	1.170–3.001	<0.0001
suPAR (pg/mL)	−0.006	0.001	−0.008–(−0.004)	<0.0001	suPAR (pg/mL)	0.084	0.045	−0.004–0.171	0.062

Variance inflation factor (VIF): age = 1.037, gender = 1.084, BMI = 1.197, hypertension = 1.122, diabetes mellitus = 1.229. Abbreviations: eGFR = estimated glomerular filtration rate, UACR = urinary albumin/creatinine ratio, B = regression coefficient, BMI = body mass index, eGFR = estimated glomerular filtration rate, 95% CI = 95% confidence interval.

References

1. Levey, A.S.; Coresh, J. Chronic kidney disease. *Lancet* **2012**, *379*, 165–180. [CrossRef]
2. Ardhanari, S.; Alpert, M.A.; Aggarwal, K. Cardiovascular disease in chronic kidney disease: Risk factors, pathogenesis, and prevention. *Adv. Perit. Dial.* **2014**, *30*, 40–53.
3. Di Lullo, L.; House, A.; Gorini, A.; Santoboni, A.; Russo, D.; Ronco, C. Chronic kidney disease and cardiovascular complications. *Heart Fail. Rev.* **2015**, *20*, 259–272. [CrossRef] [PubMed]
4. Suckling, R.; Gallagher, H. Chronic kidney disease, diabetes mellitus and cardiovascular disease: Risks and commonalities. *J. Ren. Care* **2012**, *38*, 4–11. [CrossRef] [PubMed]
5. Kanderian, A.S.; Francis, G.S. Cardiac troponins and chronic kidney disease. *Kidney Int.* **2006**, *69*, 1112–1114. [CrossRef]
6. Stacy, S.R.; Suarez-Cuervo, C.; Berger, Z.; Wilson, L.M.; Yeh, H.-C.; Bass, E.B.; Michos, E.D. Role of Troponin in Patients With Chronic Kidney Disease and Suspected Acute Coronary Syndrome. *Ann. Intern. Med.* **2014**, *161*, 502–512. [CrossRef]
7. Takase, H.; Dohi, Y. Kidney function crucially affects B-type natriuretic peptide (BNP), N-terminal proBNP and their relationship. *Eur. J. Clin. Investig.* **2014**, *44*, 303–308. [CrossRef]
8. Universal Protein Resource (UniProt). Interleukin-1 Receptor-Like 1. Available online: https://www.uniprot.org/uniprot/Q01638#structure (accessed on 6 March 2020).
9. Dieplinger, B.; Januzzi, J.L.; Steinmair, M.; Gabriel, C.; Poelz, W.; Haltmayer, M.; Mueller, T. Analytical and clinical evaluation of a novel high-sensitivity assay for measurement of soluble ST2 in human plasma—The Presage^{TM} ST2 assay. *Clin. Chim. Acta* **2009**, *409*, 33–40. [CrossRef]
10. Mueller, T.; Dieplinger, B. Soluble ST2 and Galectin-3: What We Know and Don't Know Analytically. *EJIFCC* **2016**, *27*, 224–237.
11. Bhardwaj, A.; Januzzi, J.L., Jr. ST2: A novel biomarker for heart failure. *Expert Rev. Mol. Diagn.* **2010**, *10*, 459–464. [CrossRef]
12. Dieplinger, B.; Egger, M.; Haltmayer, M.; Kleber, M.E.; Scharnagl, H.; Silbernagel, G.; de Boer, R.A.; Maerz, W.; Mueller, T. Increased Soluble ST2 Predicts Long-term Mortality in Patients with Stable Coronary Artery Disease: Results from the Ludwigshafen Risk and Cardiovascular Health Study. *Clin. Chem.* **2014**, *60*, 530–540. [CrossRef] [PubMed]
13. Savic-Radojevic, A.; Pljesa-Ercegovac, M.; Matic, M.; Simic, D.; Radovanovic, S.; Simic, T. Novel Biomarkers of Heart Failure. In *Advances in Clinical Chemistry*; Elsevier: Amsterdam, The Netherlands, 2017; Volume 79, pp. 93–152.
14. Universal Protein Resource (UniProt). Growth/Differentiation Factor 15. Available online: https://www.uniprot.org/uniprot/Q99988 (accessed on 6 March 2020).
15. Liu, X.; Chi, X.; Gong, Q.; Gao, L.; Niu, Y.; Chi, X.; Cheng, M.; Si, Y.; Wang, M.; Zhong, J.; et al. Association of serum level of growth differentiation factor 15 with liver cirrhosis and hepatocellular carcinoma. *PLoS ONE* **2015**, *10*, e0127518. [CrossRef] [PubMed]
16. George, M.; Jena, A.; Srivatsan, V.; Muthukumar, R.; Dhandapani, V.E. GDF 15—A Novel Biomarker in the Offing for Heart Failure. *Curr. Cardiol. Rev.* **2016**, *12*, 37–46. [CrossRef] [PubMed]
17. Zeng, X.; Li, L.; Wen, H.; Bi, Q. Growth-differentiation factor 15 as a predictor of mortality in patients with heart failure. *J. Cardiovasc. Med.* **2017**, *18*, 53–59. [CrossRef] [PubMed]
18. Wollert, K.C.; Kempf, T. Growth Differentiation Factor 15 in Heart Failure: An Update. *Curr. Heart Fail. Rep.* **2012**, *9*, 337–345. [CrossRef]
19. Zhang, S.; Dai, D.; Wang, X.; Zhu, H.; Jin, H.; Zhao, R.; Jiang, L.; Lu, Q.; Yi, F.; Wan, X.; et al. Growth differentiation factor—15 predicts the prognoses of patients with acute coronary syndrome: A meta-analysis. *BMC Cardiovasc. Disord.* **2016**, *16*, 82. [CrossRef]
20. Nair, V.; Robinson-Cohen, C.; Smith, M.R.; Bellovich, K.A.; Bhat, Z.Y.; Bobadilla, M.; Brosius, F.; de Boer, I.H.; Essioux, L.; Formentini, I.; et al. Growth Differentiation Factor-15 and Risk of CKD Progression. *J. Am. Soc. Nephrol.* **2017**, *28*, 2233–2240. [CrossRef]
21. Universal Protein Resource (UniProt). Fatty Acid-Binding Protein, Heart. Available online: https://www.uniprot.org/uniprot/P05413 (accessed on 6 March 2020).

22. Ishimura, S.; Furuhashi, M.; Watanabe, Y.; Hoshina, K.; Fuseya, T.; Mita, T.; Okazaki, Y.; Koyama, M.; Tanaka, M.; Akasaka, H.; et al. Circulating levels of fatty acid-binding protein family and metabolic phenotype in the general population. *PLoS ONE* **2013**, *8*, e81318. [CrossRef]
23. Kakoti, A.; Goswami, P. Heart type fatty acid binding protein: Structure, function and biosensing applications for early detection of myocardial infarction. *Biosens. Bioelectron.* **2013**, *43*, 400–411. [CrossRef]
24. Colli, A.; Josa, M.; Pomar, J.L.; Mestres, C.A.; Gherli, T. Heart Fatty Acid Binding Protein in the Diagnosis of Myocardial Infarction: Where Do We Stand Today? *Cardiology* **2007**, *108*, 4–10. [CrossRef]
25. Otaki, Y.; Watanabe, T.; Kubota, I. Heart-type fatty acid-binding protein in cardiovascular disease: A systemic review. *Clin. Chim. Acta* **2017**, *474*, 44–53. [CrossRef] [PubMed]
26. Boscheri, A.; Wunderlich, C.; Langer, M.; Schoen, S.; Wiedemann, B.; Stolte, D.; Elmer, G.; Barthel, P.; Strasser, R.H. Correlation of heart-type fatty acid-binding protein with mortality and echocardiographic data in patients with pulmonary embolism at intermediate risk. *Am. Heart J.* **2010**, *160*, 294–300. [CrossRef]
27. Niizeki, T.; Takeishi, Y.; Arimoto, T.; Nozaki, N. Persistently Increased Serum Concentration of Heart-Type Fatty Acid-Binding Protein Predicts Adverse Clinical Outcomes in Patients with Chronic Heart Failure. *Cric. J.* **2008**, *72*, 109–114. [CrossRef] [PubMed]
28. Universal Protein Resource (UniProt). Insulin-Like Growth Factor-Binding Protein 2. Available online: https://www.uniprot.org/uniprot/P18065 (accessed on 6 March 2020).
29. Kendrick, Z.W.; Firpo, M.A.; Repko, R.C.; Scaife, C.L.; Adler, D.G.; Boucher, K.M.; Mulvihill, S.J. Serum IGFBP2 and MSLN as diagnostic and prognostic biomarkers for pancreatic cancer. *HPB* **2014**, *16*, 670–676. [CrossRef]
30. Hoeflich, A.; Russo, V.C. Physiology and pathophysiology of IGFBP-1 and IGFBP-2—Consensus and dissent on metabolic control and malignant potential. *Best Pract. Res. Clin. Endocrinol. Metab.* **2015**, *29*, 685–700. [CrossRef] [PubMed]
31. Rajpathak, S.N.; He, M.; Sun, Q.; Kaplan, R.C.; Muzumdar, R.; Rohan, T.E.; Gunter, M.J.; Pollak, M.; Kim, M.; Pessin, J.E.; et al. Insulin-like growth factor axis and risk of type 2 diabetes in women. *Diabetes* **2012**, *61*, 2248–2254. [CrossRef]
32. Heald, A.; Kaushal, K.; Siddals, K.; Rudenski, A.; Anderson, S.; Gibson, J. Insulin-like Growth Factor Binding Protein-2 (IGFBP-2) is a Marker for the Metabolic Syndrome. *Exp. Clin. Endocrinol. Diabetes* **2006**, *114*, 371–376. [CrossRef]
33. Vasylyeva, T.L.; Ferry, R.J. Novel roles of the IGF–IGFBP axis in etiopathophysiology of diabetic nephropathy. *Diabetes Res. Clin. Pract.* **2007**, *76*, 177–186. [CrossRef]
34. Hoeflich, A.; David, R.; Hjortebjerg, R. Current IGFBP-Related Biomarker Research in Cardiovascular Disease-We Need More Structural and Functional Information in Clinical Studies. *Front. Endocrinol.* **2018**, *9*, 388. [CrossRef]
35. Martin, R.M.; Gunnell, D.; Whitley, E.; Nicolaides, A.; Griffin, M.; Georgiou, N.; Davey Smith, G.; Ebrahim, S.; Holly, J.M.P. Associations of Insulin-Like Growth Factor (IGF)-I, IGF-II, IGF Binding Protein (IGFBP)-2 and IGFBP-3 with Ultrasound Measures of Atherosclerosis and Plaque Stability in an Older Adult Population. *J. Clin. Endocrinol. Metab.* **2008**, *93*, 1331–1338. [CrossRef]
36. Universal Protein Resource (UniProt). Urokinase Plasminogen Activator Surface Receptor. Available online: https://www.uniprot.org/uniprot/Q03405 (accessed on 6 March 2020).
37. Chew-Harris, J.; Appleby, S.; Richards, A.M.; Troughton, R.W.; Pemberton, C.J. Analytical, biochemical and clearance considerations of soluble urokinase plasminogen activator receptor (suPAR) in healthy individuals. *Clin. Biochem.* **2019**, *69*, 36–44. [CrossRef] [PubMed]
38. Huai, Q.; Mazar, A.P.; Kuo, A.; Parry, G.C.; Shaw, D.E.; Callahan, J.; Li, Y.; Yuan, C.; Bian, C.; Chen, L.; et al. Structure of human urokinase plasminogen activator in complex with its receptor. *Science* **2006**, *311*, 656–659. [CrossRef] [PubMed]
39. Eapen, D.J.; Manocha, P.; Ghasemzadeh, N.; Patel, R.S.; Al Kassem, H.; Hammadah, M.; Hammadah, M.; Veledar, E.; Le, N.-A.; Pielak, T.; et al. Soluble Urokinase Plasminogen Activator Receptor Level Is an Independent Predictor of the Presence and Severity of Coronary Artery Disease and of Future Adverse Events. *J. Am. Heart Assoc.* **2014**, *3*, e001118. [CrossRef] [PubMed]
40. Hayek, S.S.; Sever, S.; Ko, Y.A.; Trachtman, H.; Awad, M.; Wadhwani, S.; Altintas, M.M.; Wei, C.; Hotton, A.L.; French, A.L.; et al. Soluble Urokinase Receptor and Chronic Kidney Disease. *N. Engl. J. Med.* **2015**, *373*, 1916–1925. [CrossRef]

41. Skorecki, K.L.; Freedman, B.I. A suPAR Biomarker for Chronic Kidney Disease. *N. Engl. J. Med.* **2015**, *373*, 1971–1972. [CrossRef]
42. Wei, C.; Trachtman, H.; Li, J.; Dong, C.; Friedman, A.L.; Gassman, J.J.; McMahan, J.L.; Radeva, M.; Heil, K.M.; Trautmann, A.; et al. Circulating suPAR in Two Cohorts of Primary FSGS. *J. Am. Soc. Nephrol.* **2012**, *23*, 2051–2059. [CrossRef]
43. Lee, J.M.; Yang, J.W.; Kronbichler, A.; Eisenhut, M.; Kim, G.; Lee, K.H.; Shin, J.I. Increased Serum Soluble Urokinase-Type Plasminogen Activator Receptor (suPAR) Levels in FSGS: A Meta-Analysis. *J. Immunol. Res.* **2019**, *2019*, 1–11. [CrossRef]
44. Eckardt, K.U.; Bärthlein, B.; Baid-Agrawal, S.; Beck, A.; Busch, M.; Eitner, F.; Ekici, A.B.; Floege, J.; Gefeller, O.; Haller, H.; et al. The German Chronic Kidney Disease (GCKD) study: Design and methods. *Nephrol. Dial. Transplant.* **2012**, *27*, 1454–1460. [CrossRef]
45. Titze, S.; Schmid, M.; Köttgen, A.; Busch, M.; Floege, J.; Wanner, C.; Kronenberg, F.; Eckardt, K.U.; Titze, S.; Prokosch, H.U.; et al. Disease burden and risk profile in referred patients with moderate chronic kidney disease: Composition of the German Chronic Kidney Disease (GCKD) cohort. *Nephrol. Dial. Transplant.* **2015**, *30*, 441–451. [CrossRef]
46. Levey, A.S.; Greene, T.; Beck, G.J.; Caggiula, A.W.; Kusek, J.W.; Hunsicker, L.G.; Klahr, S. Dietary protein restriction and the progression of chronic renal disease: What have all of the results of the MDRD study shown? Modification of Diet in Renal Disease Study group. *J. Am. Soc. Nephrol.* **1999**, *10*, 2426–2439.
47. Beck, H.; Titze, S.I.; Hübner, S.; Busch, M.; Schlieper, G.; Schultheiss, U.T.; Wanner, C.; Kronenberg, F.; Krane, V.; Eckardt, K.-U.; et al. Heart Failure in a Cohort of Patients with Chronic Kidney Disease: The GCKD Study. *PLoS ONE* **2015**, *10*, e0122552.
48. Wheeler, D.C.; Winkelmayer, W.C.; Kidney Disease: Improving Global Outcomes (KDIGO) CKD-MBD Update Work Group. KDIGO 2017 Clinical Practice Guideline Update for the Diagnosis, Evaluation, Prevention, and Treatment of Chronic Kidney Disease–Mineral and Bone Disorder (CKD-MBD). *Kidney Int. Suppl.* **2017**, *7*, 1–59.
49. Eriksson, H.; Caidahl, K.; Larsson, B.; Ohlson, L.O.; Welin, L.; Wilhelmsen, L.; Svärdsudd, K. Cardiac and pulmonary causes of dyspnea—Validation of a scoring test for clinical-epidemiological use: The Study of Men Born in 1913. *Eur. Heart J.* **1987**, *8*, 1007–1014. [CrossRef]
50. Herzog, C.A.; Asinger, R.W.; Berger, A.K.; Charytan, D.M.; Díez, J.; Hart, R.G.; Eckardt, K.-U.; Kasiske, B.L.; McCullough, P.A.; Passman, R.S.; et al. Cardiovascular disease in chronic kidney disease. A clinical update from Kidney Disease: Improving Global Outcomes (KDIGO). *Kidney Int.* **2011**, *80*, 572–586. [CrossRef]
51. Thongprayoon, C.; Kaewput, W.; Thamcharoen, N.; Bathini, T.; Watthanasuntorn, K.; Salim, S.A.; Ungprasert, P.; Lertjitbanjong, P.; Aeddula, N.R.; Torres-Ortiz, A.; et al. Acute Kidney Injury in Patients Undergoing Total Hip Arthroplasty: A Systematic Review and Meta-Analysis. *J. Clin. Med.* **2019**, *8*, 66. [CrossRef]
52. Thongprayoon, C.; Kaewput, W.; Thamcharoen, N.; Bathini, T.; Watthanasuntorn, K.; Lertjitbanjong, P.; Sharma, K.; Salim, S.A.; Ungprasert, P.; Wijarnpreecha, K.; et al. Incidence and Impact of Acute Kidney Injury after Liver Transplantation: A Meta-Analysis. *J. Clin. Med.* **2019**, *8*, 372. [CrossRef] [PubMed]
53. Salim, S.A.; Zsom, L.; Cheungpasitporn, W.; Fülöp, T. Benefits, challenges, and opportunities using home hemodialysis with a focus on Mississippi, a rural southern state. *Semin. Dial.* **2019**, *32*, 80–84. [CrossRef] [PubMed]
54. Shulman, N.B.; Ford, C.E.; Hall, W.D.; Blaufox, M.D.; Simon, D.; Langford, H.G.; Schneider, K.A. Prognostic value of serum creatinine and effect of treatment of hypertension on renal function. Results from the hypertension detection and follow-up program. The Hypertension Detection and Follow-up Program Cooperative Group. *Hypertension* **1989**, *13*, I80–I93. [CrossRef] [PubMed]
55. Foley, R.N.; Parfrey, P.S.; Sarnak, M.J. Epidemiology of cardiovascular disease in chronic renal disease. *J. Am. Soc. Nephrol.* **1998**, *9*, S16–S23. [CrossRef]
56. Go, A.S.; Chertow, G.M.; Fan, D.; McCulloch, C.E.; Hsu, C. Chronic Kidney Disease and the Risks of Death, Cardiovascular Events, and Hospitalization. *N. Engl. J. Med.* **2004**, *351*, 1296–1305. [CrossRef]
57. Sarnak, M.J.; Levey, A.S.; Schoolwerth, A.C.; Coresh, J.; Culleton, B.; Hamm, L.L.; McCullough, P.A.; Kasiske, B.L.; Kelepouris, E.; Klag, M.J.; et al. Kidney Disease as a Risk Factor for Development of Cardiovascular Disease. *Circulation* **2003**, *108*, 2154–2169. [CrossRef] [PubMed]

58. Srisawasdi, P.; Vanavanan, S.; Charoenpanichkit, C.; Kroll, M.H. The Effect of Renal Dysfunction on BNP, NT-proBNP, and Their Ratio. *Am. J. Clin. Pathol.* **2010**, *133*, 14–23. [CrossRef] [PubMed]
59. Colbert, G.; Jain, N.; de Lemos, J.A.; Hedayati, S.S. Utility of Traditional Circulating and Imaging-Based Cardiac Biomarkers in Patients with Predialysis CKD. *Clin. J. Am. Soc. Nephrol.* **2015**, *10*, 515. [CrossRef]
60. Alam, M.L.; Katz, R.; Bellovich, K.A.; Bhat, Z.Y.; Brosius, F.C.; de Boer, I.H.; Gadegbeku, C.A.; Gipson, D.S.; Hawkins, J.J.; Himmelfarb, J.; et al. Soluble ST2 and Galectin-3 and Progression of CKD. *Kidney Int. Rep.* **2019**, *4*, 103–111. [CrossRef] [PubMed]
61. Gregg, L.P.; Adams-Huet, B.; Li, X.; Colbert, G.; Jain, N.; de Lemos, A.J.; Hedayati, S.S. Effect modification of chronic kidney disease on the association of circulating and imaging cardiac biomarkers with outcomes. *J. Am. Heart Assoc.* **2017**, *6*, 7. [CrossRef] [PubMed]
62. Ravassa, S.; Beaumont, J.; Cediel, G.; Lupón, J.; López, B.; Querejeta, R.; Díez, J.; Bayés-Genís, A.; González, A. Cardiorenal interaction and heart failure outcomes. A role for insulin-like growth factor binding protein 2? *Rev. Esp. Cardiol. (Engl. Ed.)* **2020**. [CrossRef]
63. Griesenauer, B.; Paczesny, S. The ST2/IL-33 Axis in Immune Cells during Inflammatory Diseases. *Front. Immunol.* **2017**, *8*, 475. [CrossRef]
64. Stankovic, M.S.; Janjetovic, K.; Velimirovic, M.; Milenkovic, M.; Stojkovic, T.; Puskas, N.; Zaletel, I.; De Luka, S.R.; Jankovic, S.; Stefanovic, S.; et al. Effects of IL-33/ST2 pathway in acute inflammation on tissue damage, antioxidative parameters, magnesium concentration and cytokines profile. *Exp. Mol. Pathol.* **2016**, *101*, 31–37. [CrossRef]
65. Chen, W.-Y.; Tsai, T.-H.; Yang, J.-L.; Li, L.-C. Therapeutic Strategies for Targeting IL-33/ST2 Signalling for the Treatment of Inflammatory Diseases. *Cell. Physiol. Biochem.* **2018**, *49*, 349–358. [CrossRef]
66. Xu, H.; Turnquist, H.R.; Hoffman, R.; Billiar, T.R. Role of the IL-33-ST2 axis in sepsis. *Mil. Med. Res.* **2017**, *4*, 3. [CrossRef]
67. Kunimura, A.; Ishii, H.; Uetani, T.; Harada, K.; Kataoka, T.; Takeshita, M.; Harada, K.; Okumura, S.; Shinoda, N.; Kato, B.; et al. Prognostic Value of Albuminuria on Cardiovascular Outcomes after Elective Percutaneous Coronary Intervention. *Am. J. Cardiol.* **2016**, *117*, 714–719. [CrossRef] [PubMed]
68. Stephen, R.; Jolly, S.E.; Nally, J.V.; Navaneethan, S.D. Albuminuria: When urine predicts kidney and cardiovascular disease. *Cleve. Clin. J. Med.* **2014**, *81*, 41–50. [CrossRef]
69. Januzzi, J.L.; Pascual-Figal, D.; Daniels, L.B. ST2 Testing for Chronic Heart Failure Therapy Monitoring: The International ST2 Consensus Panel. *Am. J. Cardiol.* **2015**, *115*, 70B–75B. [CrossRef] [PubMed]
70. Gaggin, H.K.; Januzzi, J.L. Biomarkers and diagnostics in heart failure. *Biochim. Biophys. Acta Mol. Basis Dis.* **2013**, *1832*, 2442–2450. [CrossRef] [PubMed]
71. Aimo, A.; Vergaro, G.; Ripoli, A.; Bayes-Genis, A.; Figal, D.A.P.; de Boer, R.A.; Lassus, J.; Mebazaa, A.; Gayat, E.; Breidthardt, T.; et al. Meta-Analysis of Soluble Suppression of Tumorigenicity-2 and Prognosis in Acute Heart Failure. *JACC Heart Fail.* **2017**, *5*, 287–296. [CrossRef] [PubMed]
72. Dalal, J.J.; Digrajkar, A.; Das, B.; Bansal, M.; Toomu, A.; Maisel, A.S. ST2 elevation in heart failure, predictive of a high early mortality. *Indian Heart J.* **2018**, *70*, 822–827. [CrossRef]
73. Mueller, T.; Leitner, I.; Egger, M.; Haltmayer, M.; Dieplinger, B. Association of the biomarkers soluble ST2, galectin-3 and growth-differentiation factor-15 with heart failure and other non-cardiac diseases. *Clin. Chim. Acta* **2015**, *445*, 155–160. [CrossRef]
74. Bayes-Genis, A.; Zamora, E.; De Antonio, M.; Galán, A.; Vila, J.; Urrutia, A.; Díez, C.; Coll, R.; Altimir, S.; Lupón, J. Soluble ST2 serum concentration and renal function in heart failure. *J. Card. Fail.* **2013**, *19*, 768–775. [CrossRef]

The c.*52 *A/G* and c.*773 *A/G* Genetic Variants in the UTR'3 of the *LDLR* Gene are Associated with the Risk of Acute Coronary Syndrome and Lower Plasma HDL-Cholesterol Concentration

Gilberto Vargas-Alarcon [1], Oscar Perez-Mendez [1,2], Julian Ramirez-Bello [3], Rosalinda Posadas-Sanchez [4], Hector Gonzalez-Pacheco [5], Galileo Escobedo [6], Betzabe Nieto-Lima [1], Elizabeth Carreon-Torres [1] and Jose Manuel Fragoso [1,*]

1 Department of Molecular Biology, Instituto Nacional de Cardiología Ignacio Chavez, Mexico City 14080, Mexico; gvargas63@yahoo.com (G.V.-A.); opmendez@yahoo.com (O.P.-M.); betsy@ciencias.unam.mx (B.N.-L.); qfbelizabethcm@yahoo.es (E.C.-T.)
2 School of Engineering and Sciences, Tecnologico de Monterrey, Campus Ciudad de Mexico, Mexico City 14380, Mexico
3 Research Unit on Endocrine and Metabolic Diseases, Hospital Juarez de México, Mexico City 01460, Mexico; dr.julian.ramirez.hjm@gmail.com
4 Department of Endocrinology, Instituto Nacional de Cardiología Ignacio Chavez, Mexico City 14080, Mexico; rossy_posadas_s@yahoo.it
5 Unit Coronary, Instituto Nacional de Cardiología Ignacio Chavez, Mexico City 14080, Mexico; hectorglezp@hotmail.com
6 Unit of the Experimental Medicine, Hospital General de Mexico, Dr. Eduardo Liceaga, Mexico City 06726, Mexico; gescobedog@msn.com
* Correspondence: mfragoso1275@yahoo.com.mx

Abstract: Dyslipidemia has a substantial role in the development of acute coronary syndrome (ACS). Low-density lipoprotein receptor (LDLR) plays a critical role in plasma lipoprotein hemostasis, which is involved in the formation of atherosclerotic plaque. This study aimed to evaluate whether *LDLR* gene polymorphisms are significantly associated with ACS and the plasma lipids profile. Three *LDLR* gene polymorphisms located in the *UTR'3* region (c.*52 *A/G*, c.*504 *A/G*, and c.* 773 *A/G*) were determined using TaqMan genotyping assays in a group of 618 ACS patients and 666 healthy controls. Plasma lipids profile concentrations were determined by enzymatic/colorimetric assays. Under co-dominant and recessive models, the *c.*52 A* allele of the *c.*52 A/G* polymorphism was associated with a higher risk of ACS (OR = 2.02, $pC_{\text{Co-dom}} = 0.033$, and OR = 2.00, $pC_{\text{Res}} = 0.009$, respectively). In the same way, under co-dominant and recessive models, the *c.*773 G* allele of the *c.*773 A/G* polymorphism was associated with a high risk of ACS (OR = 2.04, $pC_{\text{Co-dom}} = 0.027$, and OR = 2.01, $pC_{\text{Res}} = 0.007$, respectively). The *"AAG"* haplotype was associated with a high risk of ACS (OR = 1.22, $pC = 0.016$). The *c.*52 AA* genotype showed a lower HDL-C concentration than individuals with the *GG* genotype. In addition, carriers of *c.*773 GG* genotype carriers had a lower concentration of the high-density lipoprotein-cholesterol (HDL-C) than subjects with the *AA* genotype. Our data suggest the association of the *LDLR c.*773 A/G* and *LDLR c.*52 A/G* polymorphisms with both the risk of developing ACS and with a lower concentration of HDL-C in the study population.

Keywords: genetics; single nucleotide polymorphism; acute coronary syndrome

1. Introduction

Acute coronary syndrome (ACS) constitutes a worldwide public health problem. It is a complex disease resulting from the interaction of genetic and environmental factors, as well as traditional cardiovascular risk factors [1,2]. This syndrome is a consequence of atherosclerosis by the excessive accumulation of cholesterol, which results in the formation of the atherosclerotic plaque associated with a strong inflammatory component [1–3]. The low-density lipoprotein receptor (LDLR) is a cell membrane glycoprotein that functions in the binding and internalization of circulating cholesterol-containing lipoprotein particles. The LDL receptor is ubiquitously expressed and is a key receptor for maintaining cholesterol homeostasis in humans [3–5]. This receptor mediates endocytosis of plasma lipoproteins containing apolipoprotein B, as well as remnants of triglyceride-rich lipoprotein metabolism, which are the precursors of plasma low-density lipoprotein cholesterol (LDL-C), which plays an important role in the atherosclerotic plaque [4–6].

Previous reports have shown a large number of the genetic variants in the *LDLR* gene that play an important role in the development of hypercholesterolemia and cardiovascular diseases in different populations; however, less than 15% have functional evidence [7,8]. Nonetheless, in recent years, three novel single nucleotide polymorphisms [*LDLR* UTR'3 c.*52 *A/G* (rs14158), *LDLR* UTR'3 c.*504 *A/G* (rs2738465), and *LDLR* UTR'3 c.* 773 *A/G* (rs2738466)] in the 3′ untranslated region (UTR'3) of the *LDLR* gene (located in p13.1-13.3 of the chromosome 19) have been associated with higher levels of LDL-C and a greater risk of the developing hypercholesterolemia, the principal cardiovascular risk factor in atherosclerosis [9–11].

In this context, considering the important role of the LDL receptor in the uptake of low-density lipoprotein cholesterol (LDL-C) associated with the atherosclerotic plaque formation, the present study aimed to establish the role of the *LDLR* c.*52 *A/G*, *LDLR* c.*504 *A/G*, and *LDLR* c.* 773 *A/G* polymorphisms in the susceptibility to develop ACS. Furthermore, we evaluated whether these polymorphisms are associated with lipid profile plasma concentrations in a Mexican population sample.

2. Materials and Methods

2.1. Characteristics of the Study Population

We used the sample size calculation for unmatched cases and controls study with a power of 80% and an alpha error of 0.05 [12]. The study included 618 patients with ACS and 666 healthy controls unmatched by age or gender. From July 2010 to July 2015, 618 patients with ACS (82% men and 18% women, with a mean age of 58 ± 10.5 years) were referred to the Instituto Nacional de Cardiologia Ignacio Chavez. The patient inclusion criterion was the diagnosis of ACS; this disease was identified and classified by either an ST-elevation myocardial infarction (STEMI) or a non-ST-elevation ACS (NSTE-ACS) based on clinical characteristics, electrocardiographic changes, and biochemical markers of cardiac necrosis (creatinine kinase isoenzymes, creatinine phosphokinase, or troponin I above the upper limit of normal). The European Society of Cardiology (ESC) and American College of Cardiology (ACC) definitions were followed [13,14]. The diagnosis of NSTE-ACS included non-STEMI and unstable angina. The diagnosis of non-STEMI was angina or discomfort at rest with ST-segment changes on ECG indicating ischemia [ST-segment depression or transient elevation (≥1 mm) in at least two contiguous leads and/or prominent T-wave inversion] with a positive biomarker indicating myocardial necrosis. Patients with clinical features and/or electrocardiographic expression of non-STEMI (albeit with normal cardiac biomarker levels) were diagnosed with unstable angina [13,14]. Moreover, 666 healthy controls were included (68% men and 32% women with a mean age of 54 ± 7.65 years) from the cohort of the Genetics of Atherosclerotic Disease (GEA) Mexican study. The GEA study investigates the genetic factors associated with premature coronary artery disease (CAD), atherosclerosis, and other coronary risk factors in the Mexican population [15]. All subjects were asymptomatic and healthy individuals without a family history of premature CAD or atherosclerosis; they were recruited from June 2009 to June 2013 from blood bank donors and with the assistance of brochures posted in social service centers.

The exclusion criteria included the use of anti-dyslipidemic and anti-hypertensive drugs at the time of the study, congestive heart failure, and liver, renal, thyroid, or oncological disease. Additionally, the control subjects had a zero coronary calcium score determined by computed tomography, indicating the absence of subclinical atherosclerosis [15]. To assess the contributions of the *LDLR* UTR'3 c.*52 *A/G*, *LDLR* UTR'3 c.*504 *A/G*, and *LDLR* UTR'3 c.* 773 *A/G* SNPs genotypes on the plasma lipids levels, we selected only the healthy controls group. All the included subjects were ethnically matched and considered Mexican mestizos only if they and their ancestors (at last three generations) had been born in the country. The study complies with the Declaration of Helsinki and was approved by the Ethics and Research commission of Instituto Nacional de Cardiologia Ignacio Chavez. Written informed consent was obtained from all individuals enrolled in the study.

2.2. *Laboratory Analyses*

Cholesterol and triglycerides plasma concentrations were determined by enzymatic/colorimetric assays (Randox Laboratories, Crumlin, Country Antrim, UK). HDL-cholesterol (C) concentrations were determined after precipitation of the apo B-containing lipoproteins by the method of the phosphotungstic acid-Mg^{2+}. The LDL-C concentration was determined in samples with a triglyceride level lower than 400 mg/dL with the Friedewald formula [16]. Dyslipidemia was defined as the presence of one or more of the following conditions: cholesterol > 200 mg/dL, LDL-C > 130 mg/dL, HDL-C < 40 mg/dL, or triglycerides > 150 mg/dL, according to the guidelines of the National Cholesterol Education Project (NCEP) Adult Treatment Panel (ATP III) [17]. Type 2 diabetes mellitus (T2DM) was defined with a fasting glucose ≥ 126 mg/dL; it was also considered when participants reported glucose-lowering treatment or a physician diagnosis of T2DM. Hypertension was defined by a systolic blood pressure ≥ 140 mmHg, diastolic blood pressure ≥ 90 mmHg, or the use of oral antihypertensive therapy [15].

2.3. *Genetic Analysis*

DNA extraction was performed from peripheral blood in agreement with the method described by Lahiri and Nurnberger [18]. The *LDLR* UTR'3 c.*52 *A/G* (rs14158), *LDLR* UTR'3 c.*504 *A/G* (rs2738465), and *LDLR* UTR'3 c.* 773 *A/G* (rs2738466) SNPs were genotyped using 5' exonuclease TaqMan genotyping assays on a 7900HT Fast Real-Time PCR System according to manufacturer's instructions (Applied Biosystems, Foster City, CA, USA). To avoid genotyping errors, 10% of the samples were assayed in duplicate; the results were concordant for all cases.

2.4. *Inheritance Models Analysis*

The association of the c.*52 *A/G*, c.*504 *A/G*, and c.* 773 *A/G* SNPs with ACS patients was perform under the following inheritance model: additive (major allele homozygotes versus heterozygotes versus minor allele homozygotes), codominant (major allele homozygotes versus minor allele homozygotes), dominant (major allele homozygotes versus heterozygotes + minor allele homozygotes), over-dominant (heterozygotes versus major allele homozygotes + minor allele homozygotes), and recessive (major allele homozygotes + heterozygotes versus minor allele homozygotes) using logistic regression, adjusting for cardiovascular risk factors.

2.5. *Analysis of the Haplotypes*

The linkage disequilibrium analysis (LD, D") and haplotypes construction were performed using Haploview version 4.1 (Broad Institute of Massachusetts Institute of Technology and Harvard University, Cambridge, MA, USA).

2.6. Functional Prediction Analysis

Two in silico programs, the ESEfinder 3.0 and SNP Function Prediction, were used to predict the possible functional effect of the LDLR SNPs. Both web-based tools (ESEfinder2.0 and SNPinfo) analyze the localization of the SNPs (e.g., 5′-upstream, 3′-untranslated regions, intronic) and their possible functional effects, such as amino acid changes in protein structure, transcription factor binding sites in the promoter or intronic enhancer regions, and alternative splicing regulation by disrupting exonic splicing enhancers (ESE) or silencers [19,20].

2.7. Statistical Analysis

All statistical analyses in this study were performed using SPSS version 18.0 (SPSS, Chicago, IL, USA). The Mann-Whitney *U* test was used to compare the continuous variables (e.g., age, body mass index (BMI), blood pressure, glucose, total cholesterol, HDL-C, LDL-C, and triglycerides) between control and ACS groups. For the categorical variables (e.g., gender, hypertension, T2DM, dyslipidemia, and smoking habit), chi-squared or Fisher's exact tests were performed. All *p*-values were corrected (pC) by the Bonferroni test. The values of $pC < 0.05$ were considered statistically significant, and all odds ratios (OR) were presented with 95% confidence intervals. The occurrence of the ACS in our study was based in the OR values: (a) OR = 1 does not affect the odds of developing ACS, (b) OR > 1 is associated with higher odds of developing ACS, and (c) OR < 1 is associated with lower odds of developing ACS. To evaluate Hardy-Weinberg equilibrium (HWE), we used the chi-squared test. The Mann-Whitney U test was used for establishing the contributions of the genotypes on the lipid plasma levels. Values were expressed as means ± SD, and statistical significance was set at $p < 0.05$. The statistical power to detect an association with ACS was 0.80 according to the QUANTO software [21].

3. Results

3.1. Characteristics of the Study Population

Anthropometrics and biochemical parameters of the ACS patients and healthy controls are presented in Table 1. Patients with ACS have higher levels of blood pressure, glucose, and higher prevalence of hypertension, diabetes, and dyslipidemias than control subjects. On the other hand, ACS patients presented lower levels of total cholesterol, LDL-C, and triglycerides than healthy controls. This phenomenon could be due to the treatment with statins received by the group of patients.

3.2. Allele and Genotype Frequencies

Genotype frequencies in the polymorphic sites were in HWE. The allele and genotype frequencies of the *LDLR* SNPs in ACS patients and healthy controls are shown in Table 2. The frequencies allelic of the *c.**52 *A/G*, c.*504 A/G, and *c.**773 *A/G* SNPs located in the *LDLR* gene showed that the *c.**52 *A*, c.*504 A, and *c.**773 *G* alleles were associated with the risk of developing ACS (OR = 1.20, $pC = 0.02$, OR = 1.18, $pC = 0.02$, and OR = 1.22, $pC = 0.01$ respectively) (Table 2). In addition, we corroborated the association according to the inheritance models. In this context, the association of the c.*504 A/G polymorphism loses significance statistically ($pC > 0.05$). Nonetheless, the *c.**52 *A/G* and *c.**773 *A/G* polymorphisms were associated with the presence of ACS (Table 2). Under co-dominant and recessive models, the c.*52 *AA* genotype of the *c.**52 *A/G* polymorphism was associated with a greater risk of ACS (OR = 2.02, $pC_{\text{Co-dom}} = 0.033$, and OR = 2.00, $pC_{\text{Res}} = 0.009$, respectively). In the same way, under co-dominant and recessive models, the *c.**773 *G* genotype of the *c.**773 *A/G* polymorphism was associated with a high risk of ACS (OR = 2.04, $pC_{\text{Co-dom}} = 0.027$, and OR = 2.01, $pC_{\text{Res}} = 0.007$, respectively). All models were adjusted for gender, age, blood pressure, BMI, glucose, total cholesterol, HDL-C, LDL-C, triglycerides, and smoking habits.

Table 1. Anthropometrics and biochemical parameters of the study individuals.

Characteristic		ACS Patients (n = 618)	Healthy Controls (n = 666)	*p*-Value
		Median (percentile 25–75)	Median (percentile 25–75)	
Age (years)		58 (51–65)	54 (49–59)	0.001
Gender n (%)	Male	505 (82)	453 (68)	<0.001
	Female	113 (18)	213 (32)	
BMI (kg/m2)		27 (25–29)	28 (26–31)	0.521
Blood pressure (mmHg)	Systolic	132 (114–144)	117 (106–126)	<0.001
	Diastolic	80 (70–90)	73 (67–78)	<0.001
Glucose (mg/dL)		159 (102–188)	98 (84–99)	<0.001
Total cholesterol (mg/dL)		164(128–199)	191 (165–210)	<0.001
HDL-C (mg/dL)		39 (34–45)	44 (35–53)	0.017
LDL-C (mg/dL)		106 (75–132)	116 (94–134)	<0.001
Triglycerides (mg/dL)		169 (109–201)	176 (113–208)	0.301
Hypertension n (%)	Yes	350 (57)	201 (30)	<0.001
Type II diabetes mellitus n (%)	Yes	216 (35)	63 (9)	<0.001
Dyslipidemia n (%)	Yes	528 (85)	479 (72)	<0.001
Smoking n (%)	Yes	222 (36)	147 (22)	<0.001

Data are expressed as median and percentiles (25th–75th). *p* values were estimated using the Mann-Whitney *U* test for continuous variables and the chi-squared test for categorical values. ACS: Acute coronary syndrome.

Table 2. Distribution of *LDLR* polymorphisms in ACS patients and healthy controls.

Polymorphic Site		n (Genotype Frequency)		Model	OR (95%CI)	*pC*	n (Allele Frequency)		*OR*	*95%CI*	*pC*
LDLR UTR'3	*c.*52 A/G* (rs14158)							**Risk allele*			
Control	*GG*	*AG*	*AA*				*G*	**A*	*A vs. G*		
(n = 666)	385 (0.578)	252 (0.378)	29 (0.043)	Co-dominant	2.02 (1.18–3.46)	0.033	1022 (0.766)	310 (0.232)			
				Dominant	1.13 (0.88–1.45)	0.35			1.20	1.00–1.44	0.02
ACS	337 (0.545)	231 (0.374)	50 (0.081)	Recessive	2.00 (1.18–3.39)	0.009	905 (0.732)	331 (0.267)			
(n = 618)				Over-dominant	0.96 (0.74–1.24)	0.73					
				Additive	1.20 (0.98–1.45)	0.075					
LDLR UTR'3	*c.*504 A/G* (rs2738465)										
Control	*GG*	*AG*	*AA*				*G*	**A*	*A vs. G*		
(n = 666)	323 (0.485)	283 (0.425)	60 (0.090)	Co-dominant	1.50 (0.99–2.26)	0.16	929 (0.696)	403 (0.302)			
				Dominant	1.15 (0.90–1.47)	0.27			1.18	1.00–1.40	0.02
ACS	280 (0.453)	256 (0.414)	82 (0.133)	Recessive	1.45 (0.98–2.16)	0.06	816 (0.660)	420 (0.339)			
(n = 618)				Over-dominant	0.99 (0.77–1.27)	0.94					
				Additive	1.17 (0.97–1.41)	0.09					
LDLR UTR'3	*c.*773 A/G* (rs2738466)										
Control	*AA*	*AG*	*GG*				*A*	**G*	*G vs. A*		
(n = 666)	386 (0.580)	250 (0.375)	30 (0.045)	Co-dominant	2.04 (1.35–3.45)	0.027	1022 (0.766)	310 (0.232)			
				Dominant	1.14 (0.88–1.46)	0.32			1.22	1.02–1.146	0.01
ACS	335 (0.542)	231 (0.374)	52 (0.084)	Recessive	2.01 (1.20–3.38)	0.007	901 (0.728)	335 (0.271)			
(n = 618)				Over-dominant	0.96 (0.74–1.24)	0.73					
				Additive	1.21 (0.99–1.48)	0.062					

ACS, Acute coronary syndrome; OR, odds ratio; CI, confidence interval; *pC*, *p*-value. The *p*-values were calculated with the logistic regression analysis, and ORs were adjusted for gender, age, blood pressure, BMI, glucose, total cholesterol, HDL-C, LDL-C, triglycerides, and smoking habit.

3.3. Linkage Disequilibrium Analysis

The linkage disequilibrium analysis between the c.*52 *A/G*, c.*504 *A/G*, and c.* 773 *A/G* SNPs located in the *LDLR* gene showed three common haplotypes (Table 3). Two of them showed significant differences between patients with ACS and healthy controls. The "*GGA*" haplotype was associated with a low risk of developing ACS (OR = 0.84, 95% CI: 0.71–0.99, *pC* = 0.023), whereas the "*AAG*" haplotype was associated with high risk of developing the same syndrome (OR = 1.22, 95% CI: 1.02–1.46, *pC* = 0.016). In this study, we did not find any other haplotype because these SNPs are in almost complete linkage disequilibrium (D′ ≈ 1), which results in the joint co-segregation of these polymorphisms in the cases and controls (data not shown).

Table 3. Frequencies of *LDLR* haplotypes in patients with ACS and healthy controls.

c.*52 A/G	c.*504 A/G	c.*773 A/G	ACS (n = 618)	Controls (n = 666)	OR	95%CI	*pC*
Haplotype			Hf	Hf			
G	*G*	*A*	0.658	0.695	0.84	0.71–0.99	0.023
A	*A*	*G*	0.267	0.230	1.22	1.02–1.46	0.016
A	*G*	*A*	0.070	0.069	1.03	0.76–1.39	0.446

Abbreviations: ACS: acute coronary syndrome; Hf = Haplotype frequency, *pC* = *p* corrected. The order of the polymorphisms in the haplotypes is according to the positions in the chromosome (rs14158, rs2738465, rs2738466).

3.4. Functional Prediction

According, with the in silico programs ESEfinder 3.0 and SNP Function Prediction [19,20], the functional prediction analysis showed that the presence of the *A* allele of the c.*504 *A/G* polymorphism potentially produced a binding motif for the miR-200a microRNA. Moreover, a binding motif for miR-638 is predicted for the *G* allele of the c.* 773 *A/G* SNP. This analysis suggest that these polymorphisms located in the UTR′3 of the LDLR gene could be influence splicing or mRNA stability altering expression levels.

3.5. Association of Polymorphisms and Haplotypes with Plasma Lipids Levels

To define the possible functional effect of c.*52 *A/G*, c.*504 *A/G*, and c.* 773 *A/G* SNPs, we determined the plasma lipids levels (total cholesterol, LDL-C, HDL-C, and triglycerides), as well as the risk cardiovascular factors (BMI, blood pressure, glucose) in individuals with different genotypes of these three polymorphisms. For this analysis, we selected only the healthy controls group. We did not include the plasma-lipid level analysis in patients with ACS because, in the setting of the coronary syndrome, these levels may be altered using anti-dyslipidemic or anti-hypertensive drugs [8–10]. The analysis showed that the c.*52 *A/G*, c.*504 *A/G*, and c.* 773 *A/G* SNPs were not associated with the following parameters: total cholesterol, LDL-C, triglycerides, BMI, blood pressure, and glucose (Supplementary Table S1). However, we observed significant differences in HDL-C plasma levels when subjects were grouped by these SNPs. As for the c.*52 *A/G* SNP, individuals with the *AA* genotype showed a lower concentration of HDL-C in plasma (38 ± 10.4 mg/dL) than individuals with either *AG* (45.5 ± 13.7 mg/dL, *p* = 0.002) or *GG* genotypes (44.3 ± 13.2 mg/dL, *p* = 0.007) (Figure 1A). Alternatively, subjects carrying c.*773 *GG* genotype had a lower HDL-C plasma concentration (38 ± 10.3 mg/dL) than carriers of either the *AA* (44.4 ± 13.1 mg/dL, *p* = 0.007) or *AG* genotype (45.4 ± 14.9 mg/dL, *p* = 0.003) (Figure 1C). Although the c.*504 *A/G* polymorphism was not associated with ACS development, individuals with the c.*504 *AA* genotype had a lower HDL-C plasma concentration than individuals with the *AG* genotype (41.7 ± 13.8 mg/dL, *p* = 0.039) (Figure 1B). In addition, the analysis of the haplotypes (*GGA* and *AAG*) showed significant differences when compared with HDL-C plasma concentrations. The "*AAG*" haplotype risk showed a lower concentration of HDL-C in plasma (39.9 ± 12.3 mg/dL) when compared to "*GGA*" haplotype of low risk (44.5 ± 13.24, *p* = 0.004) (Figure 2).

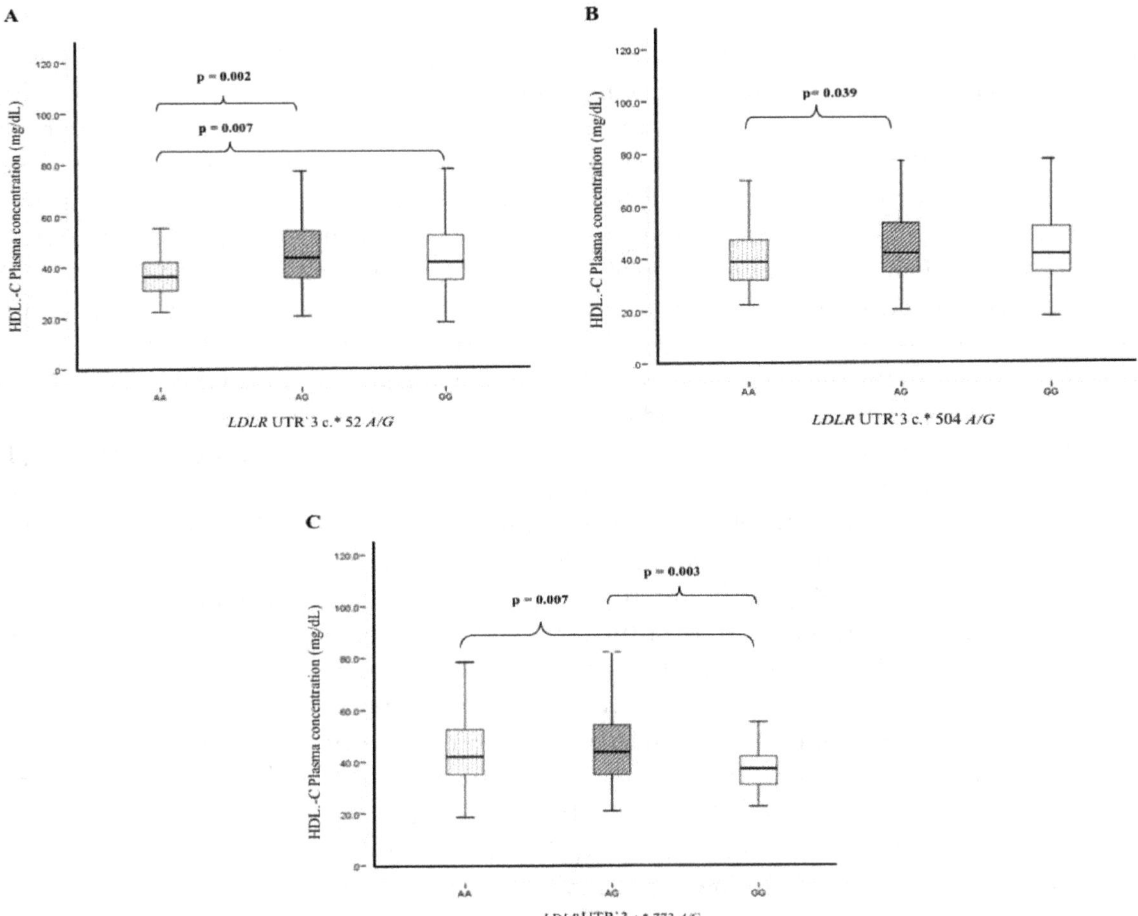

Figure 1. Genetic contribution of the *LDLR* UTR'3 c.*52 A/G, *LDLR* UTR'3 c.*504 *A/G*, and *LDLR* UTR'3 c.* 773 *A/G* polymorphisms on HDL-C levels. (**A**) The *AA* genotype of the *LDLR* UTR'3 c.*52 *A/G* SNP showed low HDL-C levels in plasma when compared to *AG/GG* genotypes. (**B**) The *AA* genotype of the *LDLR* UTR'3 c.*504 *A/G* polymorphism showed lower HDL-C levels in plasma than the *AG* genotype. (**C**) The *GG* genotype of the *LDLR* UTR'3 c.* 773 *A/G* showed low HDL-C levels in plasma when compared to *AA/AG* genotypes.

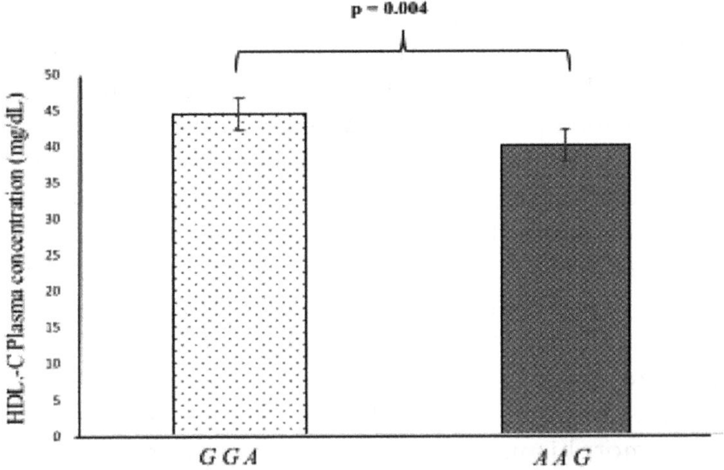

Figure 2. Contribution of the "*GGA*" and "*AAG*" on HDL-C levels. The "*AAG*" haplotype risk showed a lower concentration of HDL-C in plasma when compared to "*GGA*" haplotype of low risk ($p = 0.004$).

4. Discussion

ACS is a multifactorial and polygenic disorder consequence of atherosclerosis, in which the excessive accumulation of cholesterol plays an important role. In the present study, we focused on the LDL receptor, which is a cell membrane glycoprotein that functions in the binding and internalization of circulating cholesterol-containing lipoprotein particles. The LDL receptor is ubiquitously expressed and is a key receptor for maintaining cholesterol homeostasis in humans [3–5]. We studied three polymorphisms (c.*52 *A/G*, c.*504 *A/G*, and c.*773 *A/G)* located in the 3′ untranslated region of the *LDLR* gene in ACS patients and healthy controls. According to our analysis, the c.*52 *A/G* and c.*773 *A/G* SNPs were associated with the risk of developing ACS, as well as with lower plasma HDL-C concentrations. To the best of our knowledge, this study is the first to describe the association between these polymorphisms and the presence of ACS. In this context, the association of these SNPs with several diseases in different populations is scarce and controversial. For example, in agreement with our data, van Zyl et al. reported that the *A* allele of the c.*52 *A/G* SNP increased the risk of developing familial hypercholesterolemia in the African population [11]. In the same way, De Castro-Oros et al. reported that the hypercholesterolemic subjects with the c.*52 *A*, c.*504 *A*, and c.*773 *G* alleles have a lower response to the anti-dyslipidemic drug Armolipid Plus; in their study, the authors suggested that these SNPs increased the risk of developing hypercholesterolemia in a Spanish population [10]. In contrast, Zambrano et al. reported that the *A* allele of the c.*52 *A/G* SNP decreased the risk of the developing hypercholesterolemia in a Brazilian population [9]. By the same token, Chen et al. reported that c.*52 *A/G*, c.*504 *A/G*, and c.*773 *A/G* polymorphisms were not associated with the risk of developing coronary heart diseases in a Chinese population [22]. Although in our study the c.*504 A/G polymorphism showed a moderate association with the risk of developing ACS ($pC = 0.06$), van Zyl et al. reported that this polymorphism increased the risk of developing familial hypercholesterolemia in an African population ($p = 0.051$) [11]. In addition, we found that the "AAG" haplotype was associated with a high risk of developing ACS and with lower plasma HDL-C levels, whereas the "GGA" haplotype was associated with a low risk and higher plasma HDL-C levels.

According to data in the literature, the impact of the *LDLR* gene polymorphisms on lipid plasma concentration has been proposed as the mechanism that explains the relationship between these SNPs and the higher risk of developing familial hypercholesterolemia [7,8]. In this context, recent studies have associated the *LDLR* polymorphisms (c.*52 *A/G*, c.*504 *A/G*, and c.*773 *A/G*) with low levels of plasma lipids and the risk of developing familial hypercholesterolemia [9–11,23]. For example, Li et al. reported that c.*773 *G/G* genotype is associated with decreased plasma levels of HDL-C in healthy individuals of China [23]. In the same way, van Zyl et al. documented that c.*52 *A/A* and c.*504 *A/A* genotypes are associated with increased levels of LDL-C in the healthy black South African population [11]. Our results showed that c.*52 *A/A*, c.*504 *A/A*, and c.*773 *G/G* genotypes were associated with low HDL-C levels. In contrast, Chen et al., studying a Chinese population, reported that these polymorphisms were not associated with altered plasma lipid levels in patients with coronary heart diseases and healthy controls [22]. As far as we know, the precise mechanism by which low HDL-C levels are associated with hypercholesterolemia and adverse events, such as ACS, remains to be elucidated. Nonetheless, data in the literature provide evidence that the reduction of plasma HDL-C is due to the defective assembly of nascent HDL by hepatocyte Abca1 (ATP binding cassette transport A1) and increased plasma clearance of HDL protein and cholesteryl ester [24,25]. Moreover, experimental studies in mice have shown that (i) the hepatic LDL receptor stimulated plasma HDL selective cholesteryl ester uptake, and (ii) sterol trafficking into reverse cholesterol transport decreased HDL-C levels, when hepatocyte Abca1 was deficient [24–26]. Additionally, using bioinformatics tools, we determined the potential effect of the *LDLR* gene polymorphisms; no evidence of a functional motif was found for the c.*52 *A/G* polymorphism. Nonetheless, the analysis of the c.*504 *A/G* polymorphism showed that *A* allele produced a binding motif for miR-200a; this microRNA regulates the kelch-like EHC-associated protein 1 (Keap1)/nuclear factor erythroid 2-related factor (Nrf2) signaling axis, which plays an important role in regulating ischemic myocardial oxidative stress. Furthermore, the overexpression of miR-200a was found to protect cardiomyocytes from hypoxia-induced cell damage and the excessive production of reactive oxygen species [27]. On the other hand, the *G* allele of the *c.*773 A/G* polymorphism produced a binding site for miR-638; this microRNA plays an important role in the vascular smooth muscle cell (VSMC) proliferation and migration in atherosclerotic plaque vulnerability through the regulation of the cyclin D and NOR1. Alternatively, miR-638 is a regulator of the platelet-derived growth factor-BB (PDGF-BB), which is released primarily by vascular endothelial cells and platelets at the sites of vascular injury. Of note, this miRNA has been identified as one of the most potent stimulants for the VSMC proliferation and migration, through the modulation of several transcription factors and key molecular signaling pathways [28,29]. However, the effects of miR-200a or miR-638 on plasma lipid levels has not been previously reported. Mechanistically, using bioinformatics tools, miRNAs predicted to recognize the polymorphic site were expected to decrease the LDL-R-mRNA half-life in the cytoplasm [19,20]. Consequently, LDL-cholesterol should have been higher in the risk allele carriers, but such difference was not observed. Speculative explanations to these observations include a mRNA stabilizing role of the micro RNAs or a limited or null association of the miRNA to the 3'UTR region. Based in the LDL-cholesterol plasma levels it is likely that the second result is more acceptable; the miR-200a and miR-638 seem to have a little impact on regulating LDL-R gene expression. Nevertheless, it cannot be discarded a contribution of these miRNAS to increasing LDL-cholesterol plasma levels. To our knowledge, there are no data describing the possible pathways altered specifically in ACS and/or other cardiovascular events by the miR-200a and miR-638, and binding sites harboring to the alleles c. * 52 A and c. * 773 G. Nonetheless, recent data have identified several SNPs that generates binding sites with microRNAs such as miR-33, miR-148a, and miR.128-1 that play an important role in the LDLR expression [30]. Future investigations are needed to understand the effect of these polymorphisms on LDL-R and HDL-C plasma levels and its potential relationship with miRNAs.

Finally, in our study, the c.*52 *A/G* and c.*773 *A/G* polymorphisms were associated with the presence of ACS; however, the participation of these polymorphisms is controversial in other populations. We think that the association of the *LDLR* polymorphisms with ACS could be due to the role of this receptor in the regulation of the circulating cholesterol-containing lipoprotein particles, which is, in turn, an important cardiovascular risk factor [11,23]. It is important to notice that the allele distribution of these polymorphisms varies according to the ethnic origin of the study populations. In this context, data obtained from the National Center for Biotechnology Information revealed that the individuals from Los Angeles with Mexican ancestry, Mexican mestizos, Caucasian, and Africans had a lower frequency of the c.*52 A allele (26, 23, 23, and 15%, respectively) than Asians (41%). Moreover, Mexican mestizos, Europeans, Africans, as well as individuals from Los Angeles with Mexican ancestry, have a lower frequency of the c.*773 G allele (23, 22, 16, and 26%, respectively) than the Asian population (41%) [31]. Of note, the Mexican population has a characteristic genetic background with important ethnic differences compared to other populations [32–34]. Therefore, we consider that studies with a greater sample in populations with different ethnic origins may explain the true role of *LDLR* SNPs in the risk of developing ACS.

In summary, this study demonstrated that the *c.*52 A/G* and *c.*773 A/G* polymorphisms of the *LDLR* gene are associated with the risk of developing ACS in a Mexican population. In addition, it was possible to distinguish one haplotype (*AAG*) associated with a higher risk of developing ACS. There was a statistically significant association of both c.*52 A/G and c.*773 A/G polymorphisms with lower HDL-C levels in plasma. Lastly, because of the specific genetic characteristics of the Mexican population, we consider that additional studies need to be undertaken in a larger number of individuals and in populations with different ethnic origins. This future research could help define the true role of these polymorphisms as markers of risk or protection from developing ACS and other cardiovascular events.

Author Contributions: Conceptualization, G.V.-A., O.P.-M., and J.M.F.; Data curation, O.P.-M., J.R.-B., H.G.-P., and E.C.-T.; Formal analysis, R.P.-S., G.E., B.N.-L., E.C.-T., and J.M.F.; Investigation, G.V.-A., O.P.-M., and J.M.F.; Methodology, O.P.-M., R.P.-S., G.E., and B.N.-L.; Resources, O.P.-M., J.R.-B., R.P.-S., H.G.-P., B.N.-L., and J.M.F.; Software, J.R.-B., R.P.-S., and G.E.; Supervision, J.M.F.; Validation, G.V.-A., O.P.-M., and J.M.F.; Writing—original draft, J.M.F.; Writing—review and editing, G.V.-A. and J.M.F. All authors have read and agreed to the published version of the manuscript.

Acknowledgments: The authors are grateful to the study participants. Institutional Review Board approval was obtained for all sample collections. The authors are grateful to the technicians Silvestre Ramirez-Fuentes and Marva Arellano-Gonzalez for their participation in the collection of samples and extraction of DNA.

Abbreviations

LDLR	Low-density lipoprotein receptor
UTR'3	Untranslated region-'3
HDL-C	High-density lipoprotein-cholesterol
LDL-C	Low-density lipoprotein-cholesterol
T2DM	Type 2 diabetes mellitus
SNP	Single nucleotide polymorphism
ACS	Acute coronary syndrome

References

1. Libby, P.; Ridker, P.M.; Maseri, A. Inflammation and Atherosclerosis. *Circulation* **2002**, *105*, 1135–1143. [CrossRef] [PubMed]
2. Virmani, R.; Kolodgie, F.D.; Burke, A.; Finn, A.V.; Gold, H.K.; Tulenko, T.N.; Wrenn, S.P.; Narula, J. Atherosclerotic Plaque Progression and Vulnerability to Rupture. *Arter. Thromb. Vasc. Biol.* **2005**, *25*, 2054–2061. [CrossRef] [PubMed]
3. Zhang, Y.; Ma, K.; Ruan, X.Z.; Liu, B.C. Dysregulation of the Low-Density Lipoprotein Receptor Pathway Is Involved in Lipid Disorder-Mediated Organ Injury. *Int. J. Biol. Sci.* **2016**, *12*, 569–579. [CrossRef]
4. Litvinov, D.Y.; Savushkin, E.V.; Dergunov, A.D. Intracellular and Plasma Membrane Events in Cholesterol Transport and Homeostasis. *J. Lipids* **2018**, *2018*, 1–22. [CrossRef]
5. Abisambra, J.F.; Fiorelli, T.; Padmanabhan, J.; Neame, P.; Wefes, I.; Potter, H. LDLR Expression and Localization Are Altered in Mouse and Human Cell Culture Models of Alzheimer's Disease. *PLoS ONE* **2010**, *5*, e8556. [CrossRef] [PubMed]
6. Nikolic, J.; Belot, L.; Raux, H.; Legrand, P.; Gaudin, Y.; Albertini, A.A. Structural basis for the recognition of LDL-receptor family members by VSV glycoprotein. *Nat. Commun.* **2018**, *9*, 1029. [CrossRef] [PubMed]
7. Bourbon, M.; Alves, A.C.; Sijbrands, E.J.G. Low-density lipoprotein receptor mutational analysis in diagnosis of familial hypercholesterolemia. *Curr. Opin. Lipidol.* **2017**, *28*, 120–129. [CrossRef]
8. Defesche, J.C.; Gidding, S.S.; Harada-Shiba, M.; Hegele, R.A.; Santos, R.D.; Wierzbicki, A.S. Familial hypercholesterolaemia. *Nat. Rev. Dis. Primers* **2017**, *3*, 17093. [CrossRef]
9. Zambrano, T.; Hirata, M.H.; Cerda, Á.; Dorea, E.L.; Pinto, G.A.; Gusukuma, M.C.; Bertolami, M.C.; Salazar, L.A.; Hirata, R.D.C. Impact of 3'UTR genetic variants in PCSK9 and LDLR genes on plasma lipid traits and response to atorvastatin in Brazilian subjects: A pilot study. *Int. J. Clin. Exp. Med.* **2015**, *8*, 5978–5988.
10. De Castro-Orós, I.; Solà, R.; Valls, R.-M.; Brea, Á.; Mozas, P.; Puzo, J.; Pocovi, M. Genetic Variants of LDLR and PCSK9 Associated with Variations in Response to Antihypercholesterolemic Effects of Armolipid Plus with Berberine. *PLoS ONE* **2016**, *11*, e0150785. [CrossRef]

11. Van Zyl, T.; Jerling, J.C.; Conradie, K.R.; Feskens, E.J. Common and rare single nucleotide polymorphisms in the LDLR gene are present in a black South African population and associate with low-density lipoprotein cholesterol levels. *J. Hum. Genet.* **2013**, *59*, 88–94. [CrossRef] [PubMed]
12. Openepi.com. Available online: http://www.openepi.com/SampleSize/SSCC.html (accessed on 1 April 2020).
13. Cannon, C.P.; Battler, A.; Brindis, R.G.; Cox, J.L.; Ellis, S.G.; Every, N.R.; Flaherty, J.T.; Harrington, R.A.; Krumholz, H.M.; Simoons, M.L.; et al. American College of Cardiology key data elements and definitions for measuring the clinical management and outcomes of patients with acute coronary syndromes: A report of the American College of Cardiology Task Force on Clinical Data Standards (Acute Coronary Syndromes Writing Committee) Endorsed by the American Association of Cardiovascular and Pulmonary Rehabilitation, American College of Emergency Physicians, American Heart Association, Cardiac Society of Australia & New Zealand, National Heart Foundation of Australia, Society for Cardiac Angiography and Interventions, and the Taiwan Society of Cardiology. *J. Am. Coll. Cardiol.* **2001**, *38*, 2114–2130. [CrossRef]
14. Hamm, C.W.; Bassand, J.-P.; Agewall, S.; Bax, J.; Boersma, E.; Bueno, H.; Caso, P.; Dudek, D.; Gielen, S.; Huber, K.; et al. ESC Guidelines for the management of acute coronary syndromes in patients presenting without persistent ST-segment elevation: The Task Force for the management of acute coronary syndromes (ACS) in patients presenting without persistent ST-segment elevation of the European Society of Cardiology (ESC). *Eur. Heart J.* **2011**, *32*, 2999–3054. [CrossRef]
15. Posadas-Sánchez, R.; Pérez-Hernández, N.; Angeles-Martinez, J.; López-Bautista, F.; Villarreal-Molina, T.; Rodriguez-Perez, J.M.; Fragoso, J.M.; Posadas-Romero, C.; Vargas-Alarcón, G. Interleukin 35 Polymorphisms Are Associated with Decreased Risk of Premature Coronary Artery Disease, Metabolic Parameters, and IL-35 Levels: The Genetics of Atherosclerotic Disease (GEA) Study. *Mediat. Inflamm.* **2017**, *2017*, 1–10. [CrossRef] [PubMed]
16. Delong, D.M.; Delong, E.R.; Wood, P.D.; Lippel, K.; Rifkind, B.M. A Comparison of Methods for the Estimation of Plasma Low- and Very Low-Density Lipoprotein Cholesterol. *JAMA* **1986**, *256*, 2372–2377. [CrossRef] [PubMed]
17. ATP III Guidelines At-A-Glance Quick Desk Reference. Available online: https://www.nhlbi.nih.gov/files/docs/guidelines/atglance.pdf (accessed on 29 April 2020).
18. Lahiri, D.K.; Numberger, J.I. A rapid non-enzymatic method for the preparation of HMW DNA from blood for RFLP studies. *Nucleic Acids Res.* **1991**, *19*, 5444. [CrossRef]
19. Smith, P.J.; Zhang, C.; Wang, J.; Chew, S.L.; Zhang, M.Q.; Krainer, A. An increased specificity score matrix for the prediction of SF2/ASF-specific exonic splicing enhancers. *Hum. Mol. Genet.* **2006**, *15*, 2490–2508. [CrossRef]
20. Xu, Z.; Taylor, J.A. SNPinfo: Integrating GWAS and candidate gene information into functional SNP selection for genetic association studies. *Nucleic Acids Res.* **2009**, *37*, W600–W605. [CrossRef]
21. QUANTO. Available online: https://preventivemedicine.usc.edu/download-quanto/ (accessed on 3 April 2020).
22. Chen, W.; Wang, S.; Ma, Y.; Zhou, Y.; Liu, H.; Strnad, P.; Kraemer, F.B.; Krauss, R.M.; Liu, J. Analysis of polymorphisms in the 3′ untranslated region of the LDL receptor gene and their effect on plasma cholesterol levels and drug response. *Int. J. Mol. Med.* **2008**, *21*, 345–353. [CrossRef]
23. Li, Z.; Zhao, T.-Y.; Tan, X.-H.; Lei, S.; Huang, L.; Yang, L. Polymorphisms in PCSK9, LDLR, BCMO1, SLC12A3, and KCNJ1 are Associated with Serum Lipid Profile in Chinese Han Population. *Int. J. Environ. Res. Public Health* **2019**, *16*, 3207. [CrossRef]
24. Bashore, A.C.; Liu, M.; Key, C.-C.C.; Boudyguina, E.; Wang, X.; Carroll, C.M.; Sawyer, J.K.; Mullick, A.E.; Lee, R.G.; Macauley, S.L.; et al. Targeted Deletion of Hepatocyte Abca1 Increases Plasma HDL (High-Density Lipoprotein) Reverse Cholesterol Transport via the LDL (Low-Density Lipoprotein) Receptor. *Arter. Thromb. Vasc. Biol.* **2019**, *39*, 1747–1761. [CrossRef]
25. Joyce, C.; Wagner, E.M.; Basso, F.; Amar, M.J.; Freeman, L.A.; Shamburek, R.D.; Knapper, C.L.; Syed, J.; Wu, J.; Vaisman, B.L.; et al. ABCA1 Overexpression in the Liver of LDLr-KO Mice Leads to Accumulation of Pro-atherogenic Lipoproteins and Enhanced Atherosclerosis. *J. Biol. Chem.* **2006**, *281*, 33053–33065. [CrossRef] [PubMed]
26. Rinninger, F.; Heine, M.; Singaraja, R.; Hayden, M.; Brundert, M.; Ramakrishnan, R.; Heeren, J. High density lipoprotein metabolism in low density lipoprotein receptor-deficient mice. *J. Lipid Res.* **2014**, *55*, 1914–1924. [CrossRef] [PubMed]

27. Sun, X.; Zuo, H.; Liu, C.; Yang, Y. Overexpression of miR-200a protects cardiomyocytes against hypoxia-induced apoptosis by modulating the kelch-like ECH-associated protein 1-nuclear factor erythroid 2-related factor 2 signaling axis. *Int. J. Mol. Med.* **2016**, *38*, 1303–1311. [CrossRef]
28. Li, P.; Liu, Y.; Yi, B.; Wang, G.; You, X.; Zhao, X.; Summer, R.; Qin, Y.; Sun, J. MicroRNA-638 is highly expressed in human vascular smooth muscle cells and inhibits PDGF-BB-induced cell proliferation and migration through targeting orphan nuclear receptor NOR1. *Cardiovasc. Res.* **2013**, *99*, 185–193. [CrossRef]
29. Luque, A.; Farwati, A.; Krupinski, J.; Aran, J.M. Association between low levels of serum miR-638 and atherosclerotic plaque vulnerability in patients with high-grade carotid stenosis. *J. Neurosurg.* **2019**, *131*, 72–79. [CrossRef]
30. Aryal, B.; Singh, A.K.; Rotllan, N.; Price, N.D.; Fernández-Hernando, C. MicroRNAs and lipid metabolism. *Curr. Opin. Lipidol.* **2017**, *28*, 273–280. [CrossRef]
31. Ensembl.org. Available online: https://www.ensembl.org/Multi/Search/Results (accessed on 3 April 2020).
32. Lisker, R.; Granados, J.; Babinsky, V.; De Rubens, J.; Armendares, S.; Buentello, L.; Perez-Briceño, R. Gene frequencies and admixture estimates in a Mexico City population. *Am. J. Phys. Anthr.* **1986**, *71*, 203–207. [CrossRef]
33. Lisker, R.; Ramirez, E.; Briceño, R.P.; Granados, J.; Babinsky, V. Gene frequencies and admixture estimates in four Mexican urban centers. *Hum. Biol.* **1990**, *62*, 791–801. [PubMed]
34. Juárez-Cedillo, T.; Zúñiga, J.; Acuña-Alonzo, V.; Pérez-Hernández, N.; Rodriguez-Perez, J.M.; Barquera, R.; Gallardo, G.J.; Arenas, R.S.; García-Peña, M.D.C.; Granados, J.; et al. Genetic admixture and diversity estimations in the Mexican Mestizo population from Mexico City using 15 STR polymorphic markers. *Forensic Sci. Int. Genet.* **2008**, *2*, e37–e39. [CrossRef] [PubMed]

Permissions

All chapters in this book were first published by MDPI; hereby published with permission under the Creative Commons Attribution License or equivalent. Every chapter published in this book has been scrutinized by our experts. Their significance has been extensively debated. The topics covered herein carry significant findings which will fuel the growth of the discipline. They may even be implemented as practical applications or may be referred to as a beginning point for another development.

The contributors of this book come from diverse backgrounds, making this book a truly international effort. This book will bring forth new frontiers with its revolutionizing research information and detailed analysis of the nascent developments around the world.

We would like to thank all the contributing authors for lending their expertise to make the book truly unique. They have played a crucial role in the development of this book. Without their invaluable contributions this book wouldn't have been possible. They have made vital efforts to compile up to date information on the varied aspects of this subject to make this book a valuable addition to the collection of many professionals and students.

This book was conceptualized with the vision of imparting up-to-date information and advanced data in this field. To ensure the same, a matchless editorial board was set up. Every individual on the board went through rigorous rounds of assessment to prove their worth. After which they invested a large part of their time researching and compiling the most relevant data for our readers.

The editorial board has been involved in producing this book since its inception. They have spent rigorous hours researching and exploring the diverse topics which have resulted in the successful publishing of this book. They have passed on their knowledge of decades through this book. To expedite this challenging task, the publisher supported the team at every step. A small team of assistant editors was also appointed to further simplify the editing procedure and attain best results for the readers.

Apart from the editorial board, the designing team has also invested a significant amount of their time in understanding the subject and creating the most relevant covers. They scrutinized every image to scout for the most suitable representation of the subject and create an appropriate cover for the book.

The publishing team has been an ardent support to the editorial, designing and production team. Their endless efforts to recruit the best for this project, has resulted in the accomplishment of this book. They are a veteran in the field of academics and their pool of knowledge is as vast as their experience in printing. Their expertise and guidance has proved useful at every step. Their uncompromising quality standards have made this book an exceptional effort. Their encouragement from time to time has been an inspiration for everyone.

The publisher and the editorial board hope that this book will prove to be a valuable piece of knowledge for researchers, students, practitioners and scholars across the globe.

List of Contributors

Kobchai Santisukwongchote, Yutti Amornlertwatana and Churdsak Jaikang
Department of Forensic Medicine, Faculty of Medicine, Chiang Mai University, Chiang Mai 50200, Thailand

Thanapat Sastraruji
Center of Excellence in Oral and Maxillofacial Biology, Faculty of Dentistry, Chiang Mai University, Chiang Mai 50200, Thailand

Raquel Figuinha Videira and Paula A. da Costa Martins
CARIM School for Cardiovascular Diseases, Faculty of Health, Medicine and Life Sciences, Maastricht University, 6229 ER Maastricht, The Netherlands
Department of Molecular Genetics, Faculty of Science and Engineering, Maastricht University, 6229 ER Maastricht, The Netherlands
Cardiovascular Research and Development Center, Faculty of Medicine, University of Porto, 4200-319 Porto, Portugal

Inês Falcão-Pires
Cardiovascular Research and Development Center, Faculty of Medicine, University of Porto, 4200-319 Porto, Portugal

Toshiaki Nakajima, Tatsuya Sawaguchi, Akiko Haruyama, Hiroyuki Kaneda, Takafumi Nakajima, Takaaki Hasegawa, Takuo Arikawa, Syotaro Obi, Masashi Sakuma, Shigeru Toyoda, Shichiro Abe and Teruo Inoue
Department of Cardiovascular Medicine, School of Medicine, Dokkyo Medical University, Shimotsuga-gun, Tochigi 321-0293, Japan

Ikuko Shibasaki, Hironaga Ogawa and Hirotsugu Fukuda
Department of Cardiovascular Surgery, School of Medicine, Dokkyo Medical University, Shimotsuga-gun, Tochigi 321-0293, Japan

Fumitaka Nakamura
Third Department of Internal Medicine, Teikyo University, Chiba Medical Center, Ichihara, Chiba 299-0111, Japan

Yu-Ching Lin and Koon-Kwan Ng
Department of Radiology, Chang Gung Memorial Hospital, Keelung and Chang Gung University, Keelung 20401, Taiwan

Kuang-Fu Chang
Department of Radiology, Chang Gung Memorial Hospital, Keelung and Chang Gung University, Keelung 20401, Taiwan
Department of Medical Imaging and Intervention, Chang Gung Memorial Hospital, Linkou and Chang Gung University, Taoyuan 33305, Taiwan

Pei-Ching Huang, Yu-Hsiang Juan, Pen-An Liao and Shu-Hang Ng
Department of Medical Imaging and Intervention, Chang Gung Memorial Hospital, Linkou and Chang Gung University, Taoyuan 33305, Taiwan

Yu-Chun Lin and Jiun-Jie Wang
Department of Medical Imaging and Intervention, Chang Gung Memorial Hospital, Linkou and Chang Gung University, Taoyuan 33305, Taiwan
Imaging Core Lab, Institute for Radiological Research, Chang Gung University, Taoyuan 333, Taiwan

Gigin Lin
Department of Medical Imaging and Intervention, Chang Gung Memorial Hospital, Linkou and Chang Gung University, Taoyuan 33305, Taiwan
Imaging Core Lab, Institute for Radiological Research, Chang Gung University, Taoyuan 333, Taiwan
Clinical Metabolomics Core Lab, Chang Gung Memorial Hospital, Taoyuan 333, Taiwan

Chao-Hung Wang and Min-Hui Liu
Department of Cardiology and Heart Failure Center, Chang Gung Memorial Hospital, Keelung 20401, Taiwan

Shang-Yueh Tsai
Graduate Institute of Applied Physics, National Chengchi University, Taipei 11605, Taiwan

Ming-Ting Wu
Department of Radiology, Kaohsiung Veterans General Hospital, Kaohsiung 81362, Taiwan

Lan-Yan Yang
Clinical Trial Center, Chang Gung Memorial Hospital at Linkou, Taoyuan 333, Taiwan

Valerie Samouillan and Jany Dandurand
CIRIMAT, Université de Toulouse, Université Paul Sabatier, Equipe PHYPOL, 31062 Toulouse, France

Ignacio Miguel Martinez de Lejarza Samper, David Vilades, Esther Jorge, Jose Maria Guerra, Francesc Carreras and Ruben Leta
Department of Cardiology, Hospital de la Santa Creu i Sant Pau, Biomedical Research Institute Sant Pau (IIB Sant Pau), Universitat Autonoma de Barcelona, 08193 Barcelona, Spain
CIBERCV, Institute of Health Carlos III, 28029 Madrid, Spain

Aleyda Benitez Amaro and David de Gonzalo Calvo
Institute of Biomedical Research of Barcelona (IIBB), Spanish National Research Council (CSIC), 08036 Barcelona, Spain
Group of Lipids and Cardiovascular Pathology, Biomedical Research Institute Sant Pau (IIB Sant Pau), Hospital de la Santa Creu i Sant Pau, 08041 Barcelona, Spain

Vicenta Llorente Cortes
CIBERCV, Institute of Health Carlos III, 28029 Madrid, Spain
Institute of Biomedical Research of Barcelona (IIBB), Spanish National Research Council (CSIC), 08036 Barcelona, Spain
Group of Lipids and Cardiovascular Pathology, Biomedical Research Institute Sant Pau (IIB Sant Pau), Hospital de la Santa Creu i Sant Pau, 08041 Barcelona, Spain

Josefina Casas
Research Unit on BioActive Molecules (RUBAM), Department of Biological Chemistry, Institute for Advanced Chemistry of Catalonia (IQAC-CSIC), 08034 Barcelona, Spain
CIBEREHD Institute of Health Carlos III, 28029 Madrid, Spain

Alberto Gallardo and Enrique Lerma
Department of Pathology, Hospital de la Santa Creu i Sant Pau, 08041 Barcelona, Spain

Stasė Gasiulė, Vaidotas Stankevičius, Raimundas Ražanskas and Giedrius Vilkaitis
Institute of Biotechnology, Vilnius University, LT-10257 Vilnius, Lithuania

Vaiva Patamsytė, Rimantas Benetis and Vaiva Lesauskaitė
Institute of Cardiology, Lithuanian University of Health Sciences, LT-50103 Kaunas, Lithuania

Giedrius Žukovas
Department of Cardiac, Thoracic and Vascular Surgery, Lithuanian University of Health Sciences, LT-50103 Kaunas, Lithuania

Žana Kapustina
Thermo Fisher Scientific Baltics, LT-02241 Vilnius, Lithuania

Diana Žaliaduonytė
Department of Cardiology, Lithuanian University of Health Sciences, LT-50161 Kaunas, Lithuania

Erik Nilsson
Department of Medical Epidemiology and Biostatistics, Karolinska Institutet, 17177 Stockholm, Sweden
School of Medical Sciences, Örebro University, 70182 Örebro, Sweden

Jens Kastrup
Department of Cardiology, Rigshospitalet University of Copenhagen, 2100 Copenhagen, Denmark

Ahmad Sajadieh
Department of Cardiology, Copenhagen University Hospital of Bispebjerg and Frederiksberg, 2000 Frederiksberg, Denmark

Gorm Boje Jensen
Department of Cardiology, Hvidovre Hospital University of Copenhagen, 2650 Hvidovre, Denmark

Kasper K Iversen
Department of Cardiology S, Herlev Hospital University of Copenhagen, 2730 Herlev, Denmark

Hans Jørn Kolmos
Department of Clinical Microbiology, Odense University Hospital, 5000 Odense, Denmark

Jonas Wuopio
Department of Medicine, Mora County Hospital, 79251 Mora, Sweden

Christoph Nowak and Axel C. Carlsson
Division for Family Medicine and Primary Care, Department of Neurobiology, Care Sciences and Society, Karolinska Institutet, 14183 Huddinge, Sweden

Anders Larsson
Department of Medical Sciences, Uppsala University, 75185 Uppsala, Sweden

Per Winkel and Christian Gluud
Copenhagen Trial Unit, Centre for Clinical Intervention Research, Rigshospitalet, Copenhagen University Hospital, 2100 Copenhagen, Denmark

Laura Tribouillard
Department of Cardiology, University Hospital of Dijon, 21000 Dijon, France

Erik Kjøller
Department of Cardiology S, Herlev Hospital University of Copenhagen, 2730 Herlev, Denmark
Copenhagen Trial Unit, Centre for Clinical Intervention Research, Rigshospitalet, Copenhagen University Hospital, 2100 Copenhagen, Denmark

Janus Christian Jakobsen
Copenhagen Trial Unit, Centre for Clinical Intervention Research, Rigshospitalet, Copenhagen University Hospital, 2100 Copenhagen, Denmark
Department of Cardiology, Holbæk Hospital, 4300 Holbæk, Denmark

Johan Ärnlöv
Division for Family Medicine and Primary Care, Department of Neurobiology, Care Sciences and Society, Karolinska Institutet, 14183 Huddinge, Sweden
School of Health and Social Studies, Dalarna University, 79131 Falun, Sweden

Georgiana-Aura Giurgea
Department of Angiology, Internal Medicine II, Medical University of Vienna, 1090 Vienna, Austria

Katrin Zlabinger, Alfred Gugerell, Dominika Lukovic, Bonni Syeda, Ljubica Mandic, Noemi Pavo, Julia Mester-Tonczar, Denise Traxler-Weidenauer, Andreas Spannbauer, Nina Kastner, Claudia Müller, Anahit Anvari, Jutta Bergler-Klein and Mariann Gyöngyösi
Department of Cardiology, Internal Medicine II, Medical University of Vienna, 1090 Vienna, Austria

Luc Rochette, Marianne Zeller and Catherine Vergely
Laboratoire Physiopathologie et Epidémiologie Cérébro-Cardiovasculaires (PEC2, EA 7460), Université de Bourgogne-Franche-Comté, UFR des Sciences de Santé; 7 Bd Jeanne d'Arc, 21000 Dijon, France

Alexandre Meloux, Maud Maza, Florence Bichat and Yves Cottin
Laboratoire Physiopathologie et Epidémiologie Cérébro-Cardiovasculaires (PEC2, EA 7460), Université de Bourgogne-Franche-Comté, UFR des Sciences de Santé; 7 Bd Jeanne d'Arc, 21000 Dijon, France
Department of Cardiology, University Hospital of Dijon, 21000 Dijon, France

Peter Jirak, Michael Lichtenauer, Bernhard Wernly, Vera Paar, Lukas J. Motloch, Richard Rezar and Uta C. Hoppe
Clinic of Internal Medicine II, Department of Cardiology, Paracelsus Medical University of Salzburg, 5020 Salzburg, Austria

Rudin Pistulli
Division of Vascular Medicine, Department of Cardiology and Angiology, University Hospital Muenster, Albert-Schweitzer-Campus 1, Munster, North Rhine-Westphalia, 48149 Münster, Germany

Christian Jung
Division of Cardiology, Pulmonology, and Vascular Medicine, Medical Faculty, University Duesseldorf, 40225 Duesseldorf, Germany

P. Christian Schulze and Daniel Kretzschmar
Department of Internal Medicine I, Division of Cardiology, Angiology, Pneumology and Intensive Medical Care, University Hospital Jena, Friedrich Schiller University Jena, 07740 Jena, Germany

Rüdiger C. Braun-Dullaeus and Tarek Bekfani
Department of Internal Medicine I, Division of Cardiology, Angiology and Intensive Medical Care, University Hospital Magdeburg, Otto von Gericke University, Magdeburg, 39120 Magdeburg, Germany

Gabriel Herrera-Maya, Gilberto Vargas-Alarcón, Oscar Pérez-Méndez, Andros Vázquez-Montero and José Manuel Fragoso
Department of Molecular Biology, Instituto Nacional de Cardiología Ignacio Chávez, Mexico City 14080, Mexico

Rosalinda Posadas-Sánchez
Department of Endocrinology, Instituto Nacional de Cardiología Ignacio Chávez, Mexico City 14080, Mexico

Felipe Masso
Laboratory of Translational Medicine, UNAM-INC Research Unit, Instituto Nacional de Cardiología, Ignacio Chávez, Mexico City 14080, Mexico

Teresa Juárez-Cedillo
Commissioned of the Research Unit in Clinical Epidemiology, Hospital Regional No. 1, Dr. Carlos McGregor Sánchez Navarro, Instituto Mexicano del Seguro Social, Mexico City 14080, Mexico

Ewa Romuk
Department of Biochemistry, Faculty of Medical Sciences in Zabrze, Medical University of Silesia, 40-055 Katowice, Poland

Wojciech Jacheć and Celina Wojciechowska
Second Department of Cardiology, Faculty of Medical Sciences in Zabrze, Medical University of Silesia, 40-055 Katowice, Poland

Ewa Zbrojkiewicz and Alina Mroczek
Department of Toxicology and Health Protection, Faculty of Health Sciences in Bytom, Medical University of Silesia, 40-055 Katowice, Poland

Jacek Niedziela and Mariusz Gąsior
3rd Department of Cardiology, Faculty of Medical Sciences in Zabrze, Medical University of Silesia, Silesian Centre for Heart Disease, 41-800 Zabrze, Poland

Piotr Rozentryt
Department of Toxicology and Health Protection, Faculty of Health Sciences in Bytom, Medical University of Silesia, 40-055 Katowice, Poland
3rd Department of Cardiology, Faculty of Medical Sciences in Zabrze, Medical University of Silesia, Silesian Centre for Heart Disease, 41-800 Zabrze, Poland

David Niederseer, Adam Bakula and Christian Schmied
Department of Cardiology, University Heart Center Zurich, University of Zurich, University Hospital Zurich, 8091 Zurich, Switzerland

Sarah Wernly, Sebastian Bachmayer, Ursula Huber-Schönauer, Georg Semmler and Christian Datz
Department of Internal Medicine, General Hospital Oberndorf, Teaching Hospital of the Paracelsus Medical University Salzburg, 5110 Oberndorf, Austria

Elmar Aigner
Department of Internal Medicine I, Paracelsus Medical University Salzburg, 5020 Salzburg, Austria

Surendra Kumar
Department of Anatomy, All India Institute of Medical Sciences, New Delhi 110029, India

Christian Jung
Department of Cardiology, Pulmonology and Vascular Medicine, Medical Faculty, Heinrich Heine University Duesseldorf, 40225 Duesseldorf, Germany

Moritz Mirna, Albert Topf, Bernhard Wernly, Richard Rezar, Vera Paar, Kristen Kopp, Uta C. Hoppe and Michael Lichtenauer
Department of Internal Medicine II, Division of Cardiology, Paracelsus Medical University of Salzburg, 5020 Salzburg, Austria

Gilberto Vargas-Alarcon, Betzabe Nieto-Lima, Elizabeth Carreon-Torres and Jose Manuel Fragoso
Department of Molecular Biology, Instituto Nacional de Cardiología Ignacio Chavez, Mexico City 14080, Mexico

Vijay Kumar and Jong-Joo Kim
Department of Biotechnology, Yeungnam University, Gyeongsan, Gyeongbuk 38541, Korea

Hermann Salmhofer
Department of Internal Medicine I, Division of Nephrology, Paracelsus Medical University of Salzburg, 5020 Salzburg, Austria

Markus P. Schneider
Department of Nephrology and Hypertension, University Hospital Erlangen, Friedrich-Alexander University Erlangen-Nürnberg, 91054 Erlangen, Germany

Ulla T. Schultheiss
Department of Medicine IV - Nephrology and Primary Care, Institute of Genetic Epidemiology, Medical Center–University of Freiburg, Faculty of Medicine, 79106 Freiburg, Germany

Katharina Paul, Gunter Wolf and Martin Busch
Department of Internal Medicine III, Friedrich Schiller University Jena, 07743 Jena, Germany

Claudia Sommerer
Department of Nephrology, University of Heidelberg, 69117 Heidelberg, Germany

Oscar Perez-Mendez
Department of Molecular Biology, Instituto Nacional de Cardiología Ignacio Chavez, Mexico City 14080, Mexico
School of Engineering and Sciênses, Tecnologico de Monterrey, Campus Ciudad de Mexico, Mexico City 14380, Mexico

Julian Ramirez-Bello
Research Unit on Endocrine and Metabolic Diseases, Hospital Juarez de México, Mexico City 01460, Mexico

Rosalinda Posadas-Sanchez
Department of Endocrinology, Instituto Nacional de Cardiología Ignacio Chavez, Mexico City 14080, Mexico

Hector Gonzalez-Pacheco
Unit Coronary, Instituto Nacional de Cardiología Ignacio Chavez, Mexico City 14080, Mexico

Galileo Escobedo
Unit of the Experimental Medicine, Hospital General de Mexico, Dr. Eduardo Liceaga, Mexico City 06726, Mexico
Unit of the Experimental Medicine, Hospital General de Mexico, Dr. Eduardo Liceaga, Mexico City 14080, Mexico

Index

Printed in the USA
CPSIA information can be obtained
at www.ICGtesting.com
JSHW051359091023
49903JS00006B/201